AF782594

GERIATRICS, GERONTOLOGY AND ELDERLY ISSUES

# FIFTY-FIVE CASE HISTORIES IN ACUTE GERIATRIC CARE

## BEDSIDE SKILLS AND BEYOND

# Geriatrics, Gerontology and Elderly Issues

Additional books in this series can be found on Nova's website under the Series tab.

Additional e-books in this series can be found on Nova's website under the e-book tab.

GERIATRICS, GERONTOLOGY AND ELDERLY ISSUES

# FIFTY-FIVE CASE HISTORIES IN ACUTE GERIATRIC CARE

## BEDSIDE SKILLS AND BEYOND

JOCHANAN E. NASCHITZ
AND
YITSHAL N. BERNER

NOVA BIOMEDICAL
*New York*

Copyright © 2012 by Nova Science Publishers, Inc.

**All rights reserved.** No part of this book may be reproduced, stored in a retrieval system or transmitted in any form or by any means: electronic, electrostatic, magnetic, tape, mechanical photocopying, recording or otherwise without the written permission of the Publisher.

For permission to use material from this book please contact us:
Telephone 631-231-7269; Fax 631-231-8175
Web Site: http://www.novapublishers.com

**NOTICE TO THE READER**

The Publisher has taken reasonable care in the preparation of this book, but makes no expressed or implied warranty of any kind and assumes no responsibility for any errors or omissions. No liability is assumed for incidental or consequential damages in connection with or arising out of information contained in this book. The Publisher shall not be liable for any special, consequential, or exemplary damages resulting, in whole or in part, from the readers' use of, or reliance upon, this material. Any parts of this book based on government reports are so indicated and copyright is claimed for those parts to the extent applicable to compilations of such works.

Independent verification should be sought for any data, advice or recommendations contained in this book. In addition, no responsibility is assumed by the publisher for any injury and/or damage to persons or property arising from any methods, products, instructions, ideas or otherwise contained in this publication.

This publication is designed to provide accurate and authoritative information with regard to the subject matter covered herein. It is sold with the clear understanding that the Publisher is not engaged in rendering legal or any other professional services. If legal or any other expert assistance is required, the services of a competent person should be sought. FROM A DECLARATION OF PARTICIPANTS JOINTLY ADOPTED BY A COMMITTEE OF THE AMERICAN BAR ASSOCIATION AND A COMMITTEE OF PUBLISHERS.

Additional color graphics may be available in the e-book version of this book.

**Library of Congress Cataloging-in-Publication Data**

ISBN 978-1-62257-141-3

Library of Congress Control Number: 2012943799

*Published by Nova Science Publishers, Inc. † New York*

# Contents

# Preface

During the last decades, as the population grew older, gerontologically adjusted services became the norm for the highest standard of care. The Acute Care for Elderly Unit has been specifically devised to provide trained acute hospital care for elderly patients with geriatric syndromes, disabilities and frailty. Teamwork here is a routine based on collaboration between hospitalists, geriatricians, nurses, social workers, pharmacist, physical therapist, occupational therapists, speech therapists and dietician, who cooperate to improve the patients' hospital course, to minimize functional decline and to advance discharge planning.

Internists and geriatricians dedicated to acute geriatric care have cultivated, along with classical bedside aptitudes, a variety of novel skills. Such are the skills to make pertinent choices among imaging modalities, laboratory tests, endoscopic procedures, tissue sampling, and than to critically appraise the data obtained. Integral to the clinician's skills are the abilities to consult electronic sources of information, select cost-effective options, discern between different levels of evidence and act according to the best evidence, or in special situations to proceed judiciously unlike guideline recommendations. Yet, the physician's clinical practice, necessarily being selective and unbalanced, produces personal bias and sets hidden traps.

Hospitalists and geriatricians find only limited guidance in the literature referring specifically to the management of acute disorders in elderly persons, having multiple comorbidities, geriatric syndromes, disabilities and frailty. For such conditions we have attempted to update the most recent evidence and define the frontiers of knowledge in the volumes 'Challenges in Acute Geriatric Care' in 2009 and 'Acute Geriatric Care' published in 2012. Fifty five case histories in this tome provide an insight into acute geriatric care: the patients, the problems and the physicians' skills concerned. With the present tome the trilogy on acute geriatric care is completed. In submitting this work we hope to have bridged a number of gaps in the literature and to have answered problems and needs encountered in practice. We believe that this text will be helpful for hospitalists, geriatricians, physicians, residents-in-training, and medical students.

# Abbreviations

| | |
|---|---|
| ACE | angiotensin converting enzyme |
| ADL | activities of daily living |
| ALT | alanine transaminase |
| ARB | angiotensin II receptor blocker |
| AST | aspartate transaminase |
| BP | blood pressure |
| BUN | blood urea nitrogen |
| CBC | complete blood count |
| CNS | central nervous system |
| CRP | C reactive protein |
| CT | computerized tomography |
| ECG | electrocardiogram |
| ESR | erythrocyte sedimentation rate |
| GGT | gamma glutamyl transpeptidase |
| MIC | minimum inhibitory concentration |
| PT-INR | prothrombin time international normalized ratio |
| WBC | white blood cells |

# Introduction to Acute Geriatric Care

The profile of aging has changed dramatically over the last century. The average life expectancy in the United States has increased from 47 years in 1900 to over 78 years in 2008. By 2030, the percentage of the population over 65 years of age will exceed 20 percent [1]. Elderly persons suffer from high rates of chronic illness; 80 percent have at least one and 50 percent have at least two chronic conditions [1]. Elderly people need increasing numbers of emergency visits, hospital admissions and re-admissions in the older age groups. Compared with the younger, elderly persons have more severe illness and more severe functional impairments and often necessitate a transitional stay either in a subacute skilled-care facility or in long-term care facility. The rising healthcare costs associated with an aging population have become an urgent fiscal difficulty.

In an attempt to outmaneuver the problem, politicians have raised the claim that many acute admissions are 'social', that geriatric care is simple and can be managed effectively and cheaper in the community, that many acute admissions are avoidable, and unpleasant investigations and demanding treatments for old people are inappropriate [2]. The geriatrician's beliefs are different, in recognizing that acutely ill old people present complex medical problems which require accurate diagnosis; delayed admission compromises recovery; that rehabilitation should begin on the first day of acute illness in order to preserve functioning; to the end, good care turns out to be cheaper than bad care. Therefore, acute medical care of elderly people should allow access to investigations and specialist advice on fully equipped wards, and should be conducted by doctors and nurses trained in geriatrics [2].

Two approaches are currently in use to provide specialized care for elderly patients with geriatric problems, when hospitalization is required for acute illness: specialized wards for acute care for elderly [3] and geriatrics multidisciplinary consultation teams [4].

## The Acute Care for Elderly Unit

The Acute Care for Elderly Unit (ward for acute geriatric care) is designed to provide skilled acute hospital care for elderly patients, who are likely to have multiple comorbidities, geriatric syndromes, disabilities or frailty. A multidisciplinary team comprising hospitalists, geriatricians, nurses, social worker, pharmacist, physical therapist, occupational and speech therapist, and dietician cooperate to improve the patients' hospital course, minimize functional decline, and advance discharge planning. In addition to customary hospital care, acute geriatric care focuses on the management of geriatric problems, promotes early ambulation, and supports interventions to limit hospitalization-associated disability. Among the latter, four components are particularly important: provision of a prepared environment to promote mobility and orientation, such as carpeting, raised toilet seats, low beds, clocks, calendars, pictures to promote orientation; nursing initiated protocols for patients self-care, nutrition, sleep hygiene, skin care and cognition; discharge planning with early social worker intervention; review of medications to promote optimal prescribing.

The Acute Care for Elderly Unit may function either as an integral section of the department of medicine in a general hospital, as an outside unit of a general hospital, or within the framework of a long-term care facility. Consequently, there may be variation in the standards of care and disparity in the length of hospital stay between so greatly different institutions. There is no uniform policy as to which patients should be referred to Acute Care for Elderly Units.

The main indications for patient admission to the Acute Care for Elderly Unit are: acute infections, exacerbation of heart failure, exacerbation of chronic obstructive pulmonary disease, uncontrolled diabetes mellitus, falls, syncope, hyponatremia, hypernatremia, and prerenal azotemia. Patients are referred for acute care or subacute care by physicians working on the wards of general hospitals (departments of emergency medicine, internal medicine, surgery, orthopedics, urology, neurology and psychiatry), or from nursing homes or family practices. The indication for the patient's admission is settled between the referring physician and a senior staff member from the Acute Care for Elderly Unit.

*Not suitable* to admission to the Acute Care for Elderly Unit are considered patients with unstable cardiac conditions (candidates for cardiac catheterization, cardioversion, pacing, ablation therapy), severe respiratory distress (in anticipation of assisted ventilation), impending stroke or stroke in evolution, shock, acute gastrointestinal bleeding, decompensated liver cirrhosis, patients who are in need of invasive procedures, and patients who necessitate comprehensive diagnostic work-up (protracted fever, suspected neoplasia or hematological malignancies, vasculitides, glomerulonephritis, certain endocrine disorders, etc).

A French study [5] examined factors that contributed on emergency to the referral of elderly patients to Acute Care for Elderly Units or to other acute hospital units. The study population comprised 1283 patients aged >75 years. Admissions to Acute Care for Elderly Units represented 40.3% of cases. Four factors correlated with admission to the Acute Care for Elderly Units: cognitive disorders (OR =1.79), 'failure to thrive' syndrome (OR=1.54), depression (OR=1.42), and loss of activities of daily living (OR=1.35).

Several trials have demonstrated improved outcomes when elderly patients were treated in Acute Care for Elderly Units as compare to similar patients who were treated in the general medicine ward [5, 6]. Baztan's recent meta-analysis [7] including 11 studies (5 randomized trials, 4 non-randomized trials, 2 case-control studies) showed that people aged 65 or older with acute medical disorders being treated in acute geriatric units had better functional outcome and increased likelihood of living at home after discharge, as compared with similar patients who received conventional acute hospital care. Randomized trials showed that elderly people admitted to acute geriatric units had lower risk of functional decline at discharge as compared to general internal medicine wards (combined odds ratio 0.82, 95% confidence interval 0.68 to 0.99) and were more likely to live at home after discharge (OR 1.30, 95%

confidence interval 1.11 to 1.52), with no differences in case fatality (OR 0.83, 95% confidence interval 0.60 to 1.14).

There are no widely accepted guidelines for the referral of patients. Patient referral is driven primarily by physician practice patterns. Are we referring out patients presenting issues that are not in our core practice? Are our patients demanding more referrals? Are we referring more because of concerns of malpractice? Improved communication between physicians is expected to improve our referral patterns, change the nature of treatment and cost of care that patients receive [8].

*The 'virtual' acute care for elderly team* is an alternative model of acute care for elderly. This is a multidisciplinary geriatrics consult team involving physician, nurse, social worker, pharmacist and physical therapist. The multidisciplinary geriatrics consult team provides the expertise and systems approach to elderly patients admitted to hospitals that are not specialized in geriatric care, particularly for patients thought to be vulnerable [9]. In a multicenter randomized trial, activities of daily living (ADL) and physical performance improved by involvement of a 'virtual' acute care for elderly team as compared with usual hospital care. The field of acute hospital care is undergoing reorganization in Europe as well as in the USA. It is now recognized that in the discipline of acute care, physicians with broader general experience utilize hospital resources in a more efficient and cost-effective manner than sub-specialists. Three positive features contribute to the better performance of hospitalists in acute care: availability, comprehensive skills and continuity in care [10]. The role of acute geriatric care in the context of the contemporary crisis in acute hospital medicine needs to be clarified.

## Clinical Examination of the Geriatric Patient - In What Does It Differ?

*Obtaining the patient history* in the old may be more demanding than usually in adults, because of barriers to communication, the often atypical presentation of illness, and multiple comorbidities. Elderly patients often present with a combination of nonspecific complaints. Sometimes they have no complaint at all. The reliability of the patient's account history should be tactfully assessed early during history taking. This should be done even with the most credible patients. Families and care givers can provide corroboration of the medical history.

Physicians should be aware of atypical manifestations of diseases in the elderly, such as presentation of sepsis with delirium, dyspnea or falls in the absence of fever; ischemic heart disease presenting with apathetic delirium and without chest pain; hypoglycemia presenting with sleepiness in the absence of signs of autonomic arousal; fecal impaction presenting with diarrhea or with delirium; orthostatic hypotension masked by supine hypertension; unrecognized postprandial hypotension mistaken for a habitual postprandial nap; adverse effects of medications confused with organic or functional disorders. Pitfalls in history taking should be anticipated, such as the patient confusing illness with normal aging, denying illness, accepting illness as inevitable, fear of tests and medicines, or financial problems causing the patient avoiding to see the physician.

The circumstances of a symptom's appearance, their association with specific triggers, and the time elapsed between the eliciting factor and the onset of the symptom may provide important clues for the diagnosis. These attributes may be relevant to the assessment of symptoms which return stereotypically, for example postprandial symptoms associated with peptic ulcer disease, postcholecystectomy, dumping syndrome, gastroparesis, chronic intestinal angina, partial small bowel obstruction, reactive hypoglycemia, and postprandial hypotension. Specific triggers of syncope (upright posture, effort, deglutition, pain, compression of the neck) and specific triggers of chest pain (walking, emotion, deep respiration) may hint to the underlying disorder.

An inventory of the medications taken by the patient deserves special emphasis. Patients and care givers should be encouraged to bring the medications for the physician's appraisal. This allows the physician to review the therapy. Specific inquiry about use of over-the-counter medicine and nutrient additives is mandatory, such as glucosamine, ginseng, ginkgo balboa, garlic, saw palmetto, kava, valerian root. Herbal medicines may interact with prescribed drugs. Examples are interactions of ginkgo balboa with warfarin causing an increased risk of bleeding, and St. John's wart taken with serotonin-reuptake inhibitors increasing the risk of serotonin syndrome. Data on pharmacology and interactions of herbal remedies can be found free of charge on internet: http:/nccam.nih.gow.

*Social assessment* is particularly important in the elderly. The occupational history can uncover the patient's exposure to health hazards. Living arrangements and dependence for assistance on family or others should be identified. Issues of abuse or neglect, caregiver stress, and advance directives should be reviewed.

*Functional assessment* is part of the evaluation in acute geriatric care, including the anamnestic and recent functional status, which should be compared to the functional status prior to hospital discharge. At a minimum, the activities of daily living (ADLs) should be assessed, usually by a trained nurse, according to the indices of Katz or Barthel. The ADLs include personal self-care activities (feeding oneself, bathing, dressing, toileting, control of bladder and bowel function) and activities involving moving around independently (from bed to a walker or wheelchair, locomotion). The lack of ability to perform any of these activities does mean that some external assistance must be provided. The instrumental activities of daily living (IADL) involve the ability of a person to manage his or her living environment; the IADLs comprise cooking, housecleaning, laundry, management of medications, management of personal accounts, shopping and use of transportations. In addressing these issues it is essential to corroborate the patient's account with reports by a reliable observer and by direct observation.

*Obtaining clues of cognitive decline* is an issue of major importance, but may be problematic in practice. One study from a general medical ward found that the diagnosis of cognitive decline was missed in 21 percent of demented or delirious patients, while 20 percent of nondemented patients were misjudged as demented [11]. The initial step in the evaluation of a patient with suspected dementia should focus on interrogating persons who know the patient and can provide an adequate history of cognitive and behavioral changes. Any one or several of the following may be initial manifestations of dementia: impaired recent memory (the patient forgets what was heard or read, repeats himself, misplaces things), poor decision-making and poor problem-solving, difficulty in performing routine tasks or new tasks, problems with managing money or household, difficulties in word finding or in participating in conversation, getting lost in familiar areas, forgetting known routes while driving, change in behavior, personality, or mood. The Folstein Mini-Mental State Examination (MMSE) is the most widely used cognitive test for dementia in clinical practice. The examination takes approximately seven minutes to complete. The MMSE is a 30-point standardized screening tool for assessing orientation, attention, short-term recall, naming, repetition, simple verbal and written commands, writing, and construction. Interpretation of the MMSE is subordinate to the patient's state of arousal, attention and motivation, all of them being possibly affected by acute illness and delirium.

The diagnosis of delirium takes advantage of the Confusion Assessment Method (CAM) which is based on four cardinal features of delirium: feature 1- acute onset and fluctuating course; feature 2 inattention, the patient being easily distractible, or having difficulty keeping track of what was being said; feature 3 - disorganized thinking, the patient's thinking appearing disorganized, unclear or illogical; feature 4 - altered level of consciousness, the patient appearing either hyperalert or lethargic. The diagnosis of delirium requires the presence of features 1 and 2 and either 3 or 4.

The MMSE is accurate for distinguishing moderate or severe dementia from normal cognitive states, but the MMSE lacks sensitivity for mild dementia. A MMSE score less than 24 points is suggestive of dementia or delirium. The addition of a clock drawing test (very useful for assessment of the patient's executive functions) and a test of verbal fluency (categorical naming) can improve the sensitivity of the MMSE as a screening test. Specific defects on MMSE are more important than is the total score. A normal MMSE score does not necessarily mean competence, as patients who score well may have deficits in completing common tasks of daily living. In a population with a probable diagnosis of Alzheimer's disease, 50% of patients scoring between 26 and 30 on MMSE had difficulty with tasks such as coping with small sums of money or finding their way around familiar streets. Also, an abnormal MMSE does not necessarily mean incompetence. Many patients with cognitive limitations develop alternative means of coping with their deficits, which allows them to live fairly independent lives. Hence, the MMSE is only one piece of evidence in the assessment of competence.

In recent years, the Montreal Cognitive Assessment (MOCA) has gained priority over the MMSE, in being more sensitive and specific. It evaluates the following domains: delayed recall, verbal fluency, visuospatial skills, clock drawing, executive functions, calculation, abstraction, language, orientation, attention and concentration. In a validation study involving 277 participants recruited from a memory clinic, the test achieved a sensitivity of 90% and specificity of 87% to detect mild cognitive impairment in patients and distinguish them from normal controls. The positive predictive value was 89%, and the negative predictive value was 91%.

Collateral history helps to determine whether the patient is able to provide for his basic needs. Comprehensive evaluation of acquired intellectual impairment and associated behavioral and mood disturbances should be postponed after remission of the acute illness.

*The geriatric systems-review* gives emphasize on cognitive impairment, falls, gait abnormalities, foot problems, nutrition, dental status, osteoporosis, pressure sores, psychiatric illness, sleep disorders, and hearing loss. Depressive symptoms are common in hospitalized elderly patients and it is important to consider depression in all hospitalized elderly persons.

*The physical examination* should strive to be complete, even in patients who are uncooperative. Interpretation of vital signs varies by age. First, a lower threshold of the febrile state has been proposed for older persons by The Clinical Practice Guideline for the

Evaluation of Fever and Infection in Older Adult Residents of Long-Term Care Facilities, 2008 [12]. In elderly persons, typically institutionalized, with multiple chronic comorbidities and functional disabilities, fever is defined as: (1) a single oral temperature 37.8$^0$C; or (2) repeated oral temperatures 37.2$^0$C or rectal temperatures 37.5$^0$C); or (3) increase in temperature by 1.1$^0$C over the baseline temperature. Second, measurement of the BP should be routinely supplemented with determination of postural BP changes. Third, pulse oximetry which is largely used as an estimate of the arterial oxygen saturation ($SaO_2$), may be subject to errors. While in general, a $SaO_2$ 90% corresponds to a $PaO_2$ 60 mmHg, the relationship depends on body temperature, pH, $PaCO_2$, and 2,3-diphosphoglycerate. The accuracy of pulse oxymetry is adversely affected by low perfusion states, peripheral vasoconstriction, dark skin pigmentation, nail polish, dyshemoglobins (carboxyhemoglobin, methemoglobin), intravascular dyes, motion, and ambient light. Patient non-compliance with physical examination can interfere with quality and completeness. In particular, palpation of the abdomen in assessing for tenderness and organomegaly might be affected by non-compliance and cause delay in diagnosis.

*Comprehensive geriatric assessment* is the diagnostic process devised to quantify an elderly individual's medical, psychosocial, and functional capabilities and problems, with the intention of arriving at a wide-ranging plan for therapy and follow-up. The comprehensive geriatric assessment is put into action when a patient's physical, mental, or social condition is deteriorating. The comprehensive geriatric assessment helps to define the patient's goals within the context of the family and social support system, as well as the pinpoint the patient's preferences for care. A family member or close friend should accompany and support the patient through the process of the assessment. The most important components of comprehensive geriatric assessment are:

1. Appraisal of the need for chronic medical treatment, e.g. oxygen, intravenous fluids or medications, treatments by a respiratory therapist, physical therapist, occupational therapist, speech therapist, specialized nursing, management of a tracheostomy, management of other stomas.
2. Appraisal the level of physical functioning with the aid of ADLs and IADLs.
3. Appraisal the level of mental functioning.
4. Mood.
5. Vision/hearing: it should be routine to ask if the patient has difficulty in seeing and hearing and to perform a whisper test of hearing.
6. Nutrition/weight change. The simplest screen for nutritional adequacy is obtained by serial measurements of body weight. The Simplified Nutrition Assessment Questionnaire (SNAQ) is a four item screener which has a sensitivity and specificity of 88.2 and 83.5 percent, respectively, for identification of older persons at risk for 10 percent weight loss. A food diary is very useful. The plasma albumin concentration correlates reasonably well with body protein stores. However, hypoalbuminemia is a relatively late manifestation of malnutrition, since hepatic synthetic reserve is very large. An unfavourable 'calorie distribution shift' occurs during hypercatabolic states, because approximately 25% of the caloric demands are delivered on expense of tissue proteins as compared to 15% under normal metabolic conditions. Well-nourished individuals have a 7- to 10-day reserve of energy and protein to resist a moderate systemic inflammatory response without adverse nutritional conse-

quences. Greater degrees of systemic inflammatory response and preexisting protein-energy malnutrition considerably shorten the period that semistarvation can be tolerated.
7. Dentition.
8. Polypharmacy.
9. Availability of family and social supports.
10. Environmental/home features.
11. Advance care directives.

*In planning the diagnostic work-up and patient management,* the benefits and risks of intervention should be carefully considered. The clinician should not deny effective treatment when it can benefit a patient, and should not initiate an evaluation or treatment when it will not result in a significantly improved outcome for the patient. Geriatric patients are often more prone to complications resulting from invasive diagnostic procedures. Pharmacotherapy also is more problematic. Adverse drug reactions are more likely to occur as the number of drugs taken by a patient increases. The risks of surgery are increased in the old. It is widely accepted that patients with end-stage dementia should receive mainly palliative care; feeding tubes and ventilatory support should not be considered.

*Geriatric prescribing guidelines of medications* include the following:

1. Taking a thorough history of medications, vitamins and herbal products before prescribing a new medication.
2. Before adding new medications to a patient's drug regimen, the diagnosis should be confirmed.
3. Medications considered inappropriate for older patients (Beers criteria) should be avoided or administered with caution. The list of inappropriate medications can be divided into three groups: those that should always be avoided (e.g. barbiturates, chlorpropamide); medications that are rarely appropriate (e.g. diazepam); and medications with some indications but that are often misused (e.g. oxybutirin, methyldopa, reserpine, indomethacin). However, some of the inappropriate drug therapies identified on the Beers list are available as over-the-counter products. Beer's criteria are increasingly being used to monitor quality of care for the elderly.
4. Screening for possible interactions should be performed (drug-drug, drug-disease, and drug-food interactions). Softwares can help clinicians to detect drug interactions, but many programs have not been updated with the evolving knowledge of these interactions, and do not take into consideration important factors needed to optimize drug treatment in elderly patients. Methods such as computerized physician order entry (CPOE), computerized drug interaction software, and computerized decision support systems (CDSS) that detect and alert the physician and pharmacist to potentially serious outcomes can decrease the risk of drug errors. Softwares for personal digital assistants and websites are available for clinicians (Lexi-Comp, Drug interactions handbook: drug interactions software http://www.lexi.com/web/index.jsp; Drug interactions: defining genetic influences on pharmacologic responses http://www.drug-interactions.com). None of the commercial systems is designed specifically for use in elderly patients.

5. Estimate CCT should be computed and guide dosing of drugs excreted by the kidneys. The pharmacists' involvement in patient care can improve the appropriateness of prescribing in elderly patients.
6. If possible, only one medication should be changed at a time, in order to assess the response to that medication.
7. 'Start low and go slow' rule should be followed, i.e. allowing for longer than usual time between dose adjustments to compensate for unpredictable pharmacodynamic and pharmacokinetic inter-patient variability.
8. When a patient does not respond to a medication, it is important to ascertain that the patient was taking that medication an adequate time and dose.
9. Dosing once a day is recommended whenever possible in order to increase patient adherence to treatment; fixed drug combinations when available may help to lower pill burden and increase adherence.
10. Use of a pill box/medication organizer is recommended.
11. The patient or caregiver should be encouraged to always carry a current list of medications including the name, dose and frequency of administration.
12. Pharmacogenetics plays a limited role at present in individualizing drug therapy. The Food and Drug Administration recommends genotyping to guide warfarin dosing (in considering the roles of CYP2C9 and VKORC1) as well as dosing of azathioprine and 6-mercaptopurine (genotyping or phenotyping thiopurine *S*-methyltransferase to reduce myelosuppression).
13. Transitions in care between hospital - nursing home - home are a common source of medication errors and confusions. Adverse drug events attributed to medication changes occurred in 20 percent of patients on transfer from hospital to a nursing home [13]. During acute illness it may be necessary to change the patient's basic medications. Indeed, elderly patients presenting one or several chronic diseases, when admitted to hospital because an acute infection are often dehydrated, hypotensive, oliguric; in such situation it is appropriate to taper down antihypertensive medications, diuretics and withhold digoxin. In the following, when the infection subsides and the patient becomes euvolemic, the BP increases and renal function is improving, it might be indicated to return to the prior treatment schedule. Down tapering of certain medications is often done in the hospital, while medication up-titration is often left to the family physician. On transition from hospital care to ambulatory care, close monitoring of clinical and laboratory parameters is necessary in order to optimize treatment and avoid adverse drug effects.

*Information for patients* should be provided with respect to the ethical principle of autonomy, which entails truth telling and active involvement; so patients are informed, can make the best possible decisions, and cope with illness. Withholding information, however, may be preferable or necessary if a patient lacks the cognitive capacity to understand the information. Then, full information should be provided to a surrogate. Withholding information should be reconsidered if a patient asks directly for information or if the perception of the patient and his or her family about the clinical situation appear to be discordant. Further, if there is a need to intervene urgently, the potential benefits of early intervention often outweigh the potential harms of incomplete or delayed disclosure [14]. If there is no evidence of an advance care planning then the patient should be treated in accordance with their best interests at the outset, until such information becomes available.

Advance care planning is a way of documenting the individuals' preferences about health care while they still retain decision-making capacity. In order to be legally binding, advance decisions to refuse treatment must be 'valid' and 'applicable'. The MCA 2005 gives specific criteria for this, also summarized in GMC guidance on end of life care. On these grounds, it may sometimes be decided that an advance decision need not be followed [15].

## References

[1] Centers for Disease Control and Prevention and The Merck Company Foundation. The State of Aging and Health in America 2007. The Merck Company Foundation, Whitehouse Station, NJ 2007.

[2] Donald I, Hamilton S, for BGS Policy Committee. Assessment of older people for continuing care. BGS Best Practice Guide 4.6, 2009.

[3] Palmer RM, Counsell S, Landefeld CS. Clinical intervention trials: The ACE unit. *Clin. Geriatr. Med. Acute Hosp. Care* 1998, 14:831-849.

[4] Sinoff G, Clarfield AM, Bergman H, Beaudet M. A two-year follow-up of geriatric consults in the emergency department. *J. Amer. Geriatr. Assoc.* 1998;46:716-720.

[5] Somme D, Lazarovici C, Dramé M, Blanc P, Lang PO, Gauvain JB, Voisin T, Gonthier R, De Wazières B, Jeandel C, Couturier P, Blanchard F, Saint-Jean O. The geriatric patient: Use of acute geriatrics units in the emergency care of elderly patients in France. *Arch. Gerontol. Geriat.* 2011;52:40-45.

[6] Counsell SR, Holder CM, Liebenauer LL, Palmer RM, Fortinsky RH, Kresevic DM, Quinn LM, Allen KR, Covinsky KE, Landefeld CS. Effects of a multicomponent intervention on functional outcomes and process of care in hospitalized older patients: a randomized controlled trial of Acute Care for Elders (ACE) in a community hospital. *J. Amer. Geriatr. Assoc.* 2000;48:1572-1581.

[7] Baztán JJ, Suárez-García FM, López-Arrieta J, Rodríguez-Mañas L, Rodríguez-Artalejo F. Effectiveness of acute geriatric units on functional decline, living at home, and case fatality among older patients admitted to hospital for acute medical disorders: meta-analysis. *BMJ* 2009;338:b50.

[8] Katz MH. How Can We Know So Little About Physician Referrals? *Arch. Intern. Med.* 2012;172:100.

[9] Rubenstein LZ, Josephson KR, Wieland GD, English PA, Sayre JA, Kane RL. Effectiveness of the geriatric evaluation unit. A randomized clinical trial. *N. Engl. J. Med.* 1984;311:1664-1670.

[10] Kellett J. Acute hospital medicine - A new sub-speciality of internal medicine re-born? *Eur. J. Intern. Med.* 2011;22: 334-338.

[11] Barrett JJ, Haley WE, Harrell LE, Powers RE. Knowledge about Alzheimer disease among primary care physicians, psychologists, nurses, and social workers. *Alzheimer Dis. Assoc. Disord.* 1997;11:99-106.

[12] High KP, Bradley SF, Gravenstein S, Mehr DR, Quagliarello VJ, Richards C,Yoshikawa TT. Clinical Practice Guideline for the Evaluation of Fever and Infection

in Older Adult Residents of Long-Term Care Facilities: 2008 Update by the Infectious Diseases Society of America. *Clinical Infectious Diseases* 2009; 48:149–171.

[13] Boockvar K, Fishman E, Kyriacou CK, Monias A, Gavi S, Cortes T. Adverse events due to discontinuations in drug use and dose changes in patients transferred between acute and long-term care facilities. *Arch. Intern. Med.* 2004;164:545-550.

[14] Epstein RM, Korones DN, Quill TE. Withholding information from patients - when less is more. *N. Engl. J. Med.* 2010; 362:380-381.

[15] Hayhoe DA, Smajdor A, Boqker LK, Conroy SP, Myint PK. Advance care planning and the older patient. *QJM* 2011, November.

*Chapter I*

# Diagnosis on First Glance

A focused physical examination plays an essential role in all medical fields. A skilled physician may be able to recognize typical disease patterns at once and thus expedite the diagnostic work-up. Findings through laboratory testing or imaging may provide an enlightening hint to the diagnosis, sometimes perceived only by the experienced. Thus, a physician's long-time accumulated clinical skills help to advance the diagnostic work-up. Also, in facing more difficult conundrums the impression of 'deja vue' might provide the physician with useful hints to the solution. Yet, the physician's past clinical experience, necessarily being selective and unbalanced, produces bias and sets hidden traps. Therefore, a quick first impression needs often to be supplemented by a second examination, a second impression, and a second thought, as illustrated in the followings.

## Case 1. Diffuse Melanic Hyperpigmentation-Addison's Disease?

An 84-year-old black woman of Ethiopian origin was admitted for evaluation of fatigue, abdominal discomfort, and delirium. Relevant in her medical history were diabetes mellitus type 2, cryptogenic cirrhosis, and upper gastrointestinal bleeding.

On physical examination, the patient appeared thin and tired.

There was melanic pigmentation of the skin folds on the palms and brownish spots on the soles, bucal mucosa and gingiva (Figure 1). The liver edge was palpable at the costal margin. A search for pigmented nevi and melanoma was unrewarding. Two daughters of the patient had similar dark skin tone, but in distinction from the patient, there was no pigmentation of their palms, soles and bucal mucosa. Ancillary laboratory tests showed hemoglobin 10 g/dL, WBC 4000, serum glucose 140-180 mg/dL, albumin 3.1 g/L, PT-INR 1.8. Results of liver function tests (AST, ALT, GGT and alkaline phosphatase), thyrotropin, vitamin B12, folate, and ferritin were within the normal range. Tests for HBsAg, anti hepatitis B and C antibodies, and HIV were negative. The possibility of adrenal insufficiency was considered, as it might explain the patient's symptoms; but could be excluded based on values of basic serum cortisol 15 μg/dL and ACTH stimulated serum cortisol 25 μg/dL. On chest and abdominal CT there was no evidence of tumor, and the appearance of the liver was consistent with fatty transformation. Cerebral CT showed cortical atrophy and periventricular lucency.

*The differential diagnosis of diffuse melanic hyperpigmentation,* as observed in this patient, includes drug reactions (cyclophosphamide, zidovudine), Addison's disease, ectopic adrenocorticotropic hormone production (e.g. small cell lung cancer), hemochromatosis, primary biliary cirrhosis, hyperthyroidism, vitamin B12 or folate deficiency, diabetic dermopathy, porphyria cutanea tarda, melanosis secondary to metastatic melanoma, and argyria [1]. The differential diagnosis of circumscribed melanic hyperpigmentation, not relevant to this patient, entails postinflammatory pigmentation (e.g. acne vulgaris, arthropod bites, dermatitis, lichen planus), melasma, pityriasis versicolor, mastocytosis, fixed drug reactions, and deposits of drugs and their metabolites.

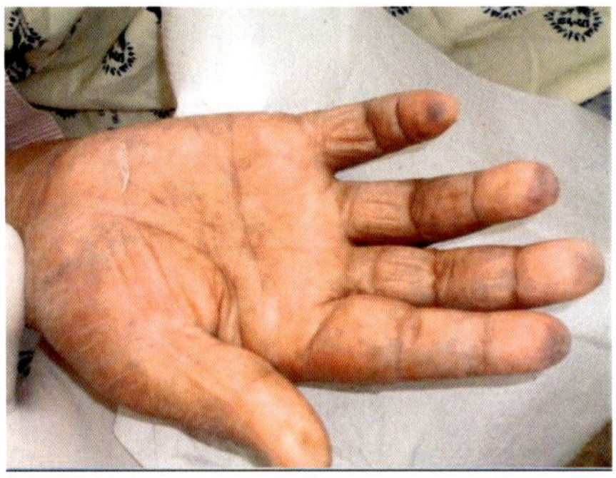

A.

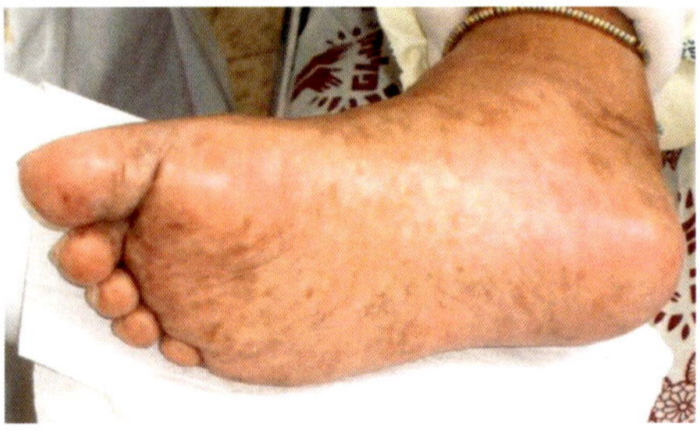

B.

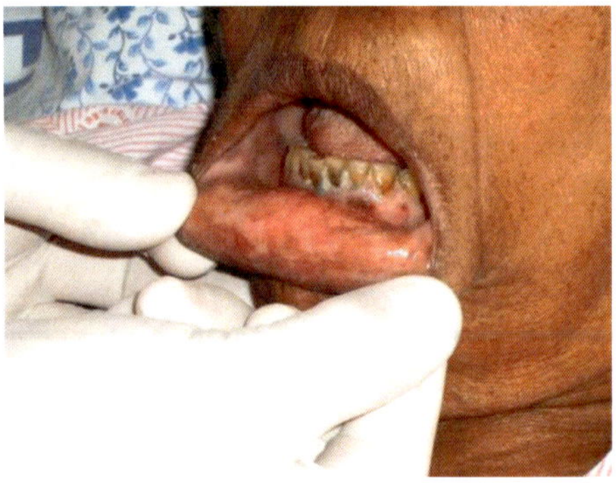

C.

Figure 1 (A, B, C). Melanic pigmentation is seen in palmar creases, pressure points, labial mucosa and gums, not involving the marginal gingiva.

*Diabetic dermopathy* is present in 40% of diabetic patients. Lesions are asymptomatic, round, atrophic hyperpigmented areas on the shins, lower thighs, the sides of the feet, and forearms. They may be initiated by trauma. At onset the lesions are round or oval, red, flat, scaly papules that may become eroded. The lesions heal with epidermal atrophy or hyperpigmentation.

*Porphyria cutanea tarda* presents with hyperpigmentation and blistering in sun-exposed areas, increased skin fragility, facial hypertrichosis, sclerodermoid changes, and dystrophic calcification with ulceration. Healing results in scars and hyperpigmented and hypopigmented atrophic patches. The patient's urine may have a red-brown discoloration from high levels of porphyrin pigments ('port-wine urine'). Assays of fecal, plasma, urinary, and red blood cell porphyrins should be ordered.

*Pellagra* is characterized by the "three D" dynfrome: dermatitis, diarrhea, and dementia. Dermatitis is bilateral, symmetric, confined to sun exposed areas. The changes at first consist of erythema, thickening, and roughening of the skin, which may be followed by extensive scaling, desquamation, and chronic inflammation. Similar lesions may occur in the mouth and vagina.

*Peutz Jager's syndrome* is characterized by mucocutaneous pigmented macules and gastrointestinal hamartomatous polyposis. It is inherited as an autosomal dominant trait with a high degree of penetrance. Pigmented macules, often confluent, varying in size and shades of brown, appear periorally and on the lips and bucal mucosa. The degree of pigmentation and oral involvement varies among affected individuals. Pigmented oral fibromas may also be present. Pigmented macules on the extremities and face are less frequently seen.

*Physiologic (racial) pigmentation* is characterized by pigmented macules of various sizes and is commonly found in African-Americans, Indians, and other dark-skinned persons such as Greeks and Italians. The gingiva is the most commonly affected site (there is no pigmentation of the marginal gingiva in distinction from addisonian pigmentation), followed by the bucal mucosa, lips and palate. Indeed, the color of the normal oral mucosa varies considerably. In healthy dark-skinned individuals, a light brown to dark pigmentation may be considered constitutional, while the same oral pigmentation in Caucasians is viewed as abnormal.

*Primary adrenal insufficiency* is a condition in which the adrenal glands produce inadequate amounts of cortisol and also may include impaired mineralcorticoid production. Craving for salt is common due to the urinary loss of sodium. Addison's disease (chronic primary adrenal insufficiency) is characterized by generalized hyperpigmentation, especially prominent in the palmar skin creases, nails and gums [2, 3]. The pigmentation in Addison's disease involves the marginal gingiva, while physiological pigmentation usually does not – a feature useful in the preliminary differential diagnosis. In developed countries, the most frequent cause of primary adrenal insufficiency is autoimmune adrenalitis. In the developing world, tuberculosis remains the more common cause of primary adrenal insufficiency.

Secondary adrenal insufficiency is caused by lack of production of ACTH by the pituitary or lack of corticotropin-releasing hormone in the hypothalamus. The most common cause of secondary adrenal insufficiency is the abrupt discontinuation of long-term glucocorticoid treatment. Patients with primary adrenal failure usually have both glucocorticoid and mineralocorticoid deficiency. In contrast, those with secondary adrenal insufficiency have an intact renin-angiotensin-aldosterone system. This accounts for differences in salt and water balance in the two groups of patients, which in turn result in different clinical presentations. The most obvious feature that differentiates primary from secondary hypoadrenalism is skin pigmentation which is almost always present in cases of primary adrenal insufficiency and absent in secondary insufficiency.

There is a great individual variability in susceptibility to suppression of the hypothalamic-pituitary axis by exogenous glucocorticoids. Therefore, the presence of adrenal insufficiency cannot be predicted by the dose and duration of glucocorticoid use. Intramuscular, intra-articular, inhaled or topical glucocorticoids can cause significant suppression of the hypothalamic-pituitary axis. Several weeks of exogenous glucocorticoid administration are required for the development of adrenal insufficiency. Patients with secondary adrenocortical insufficiency are often able to function well during unstressed periods, but they may develop cardiovascular instability or hypoglycemia when they undergo physical stress.

The symptoms of adrenal insufficiency are nonspecific and the disease may go undiagnosed for long periods of time, with the risk of potential serious consequences. The diagnosis should be considered when one or several of the following symptoms are present: unexplained malaise, tiredness, anorexia, nausea and vomiting, abdominal pain, melanic pigmentation, weight loss, postural dizziness, craving for salt and hypoglycemic episodes. Pigmentation, when present, is an important clue to the diagnosis. Hyponatremia is often found, although it may be attributed to other causes as it is a common finding in hospitalized patients. Subclinical hypothyroidism may coexist with Addison disease. As thyroid disease is much more common than Addison disease, the patient's symptoms of hyponatremia may be attributed to hypothyroidism. Initiation of thyroxine therapy in such cases can precipitate an adrenal crisis, and physicians should think about Addison disease in patients whose symptoms deteriorate after thyroxin administration.

Adrenal crisis is a life-threatening complication in patients suffering from chronic adrenal insufficiency; it develops when endogenous glucocorticoids or exogenously supply does not cover the increased demands during stressful situations. Precipitating causes were mainly gastrointestinal infection and fever (45%) but also other stressful events such as major pain, surgery, psychic distress. In many cases the cause of adrenal crisis remained unknown [4].

The diagnosis of adrenal insufficiency, in nonacute situations, is based on obtaining cortisol levels early in the morning (because of the known diurnal variation). Normal morning total cortisol levels are between 10 and 20 μg/dL. Values less than 3 μg/dL are highly suggestive of adrenal insufficiency and values less than 10 μg/dL require further adrenal evaluation. Stimulation of adrenal function is recommended in case of suspicion of primary adrenal insufficiency: 1μg or 250μg corticotrophin (according to two different protocols) is injected intravenously, followed by cortisol measurements after 30 and 60 minutes. A serum cortisol level more than 18 μg/dL at either time point constitutes a normal response, independent of the baseline level and time of the day. In acutely stressed persons due to severe illness, cortisol levels should be high. Levels greater than 20 μg/dL in a nonacutely stressed person exclude adrenal insufficiency.

Acute adrenocortical insufficiency is dominated by hypotension or shock, mainly caused by sodium and plasma volume depletion. Acute adrenocortical insufficiency is potentially lethal. The physician must consider adrenocortical insufficiency as a possible cause of unexplained deterioration of the cardiovascular status. When suspecting acute adrenal insufficiency, blood should be sampled for plasma concentration of sodium, potassium, and cortisol, followed immediately by high volume infusion of sodium chloride 0.9% and glucose 5%, and subsequent short corticotropin stimulation. Then, hydrocortisol 100 mg should be administered intravenously or intramuscularly every 8 hours or until results of diagnostic screening are available. If diagnostic screening shows basal or stimulated cortisol greater than 20 μg/dL, hydrocortisone therapy can be discontinued unless the patient is still critically ill. If low basal and stimulated cortisol levels indicate a likelihood of Addison's disease, hydrocortisone treatment should be continued, followed by oral substitution. Final confirmation of Addison disease and evaluation of its etiology may be postponed after resolution of the acute crisis.

Hyperpigmentation in the patient presented in this report had all the attributes of physiological pigmentation. While the clinical context of chronic fatigue, lack of appetite, unintentional weight loss, abdominal discomfort, and delirium suggested chronic adrenal insufficiency, the latter diagnosis could be discarded based on normal results of the corticotropin stimulation test.

### Learning Points

- Physiologic (racial pigmentation) is common in dark-skinned persons. The palmar skin creases, gingiva, bucal mucosa, and lips are most often affected. The same oral pigmentation in Caucasians is abnormal.
- Pigmentation in Addison's disease resembles physiologic pigmentation, but when present in persons of Caucasian extraction should suggest the possible diagnosis of adrenal insufficiency.
- Other causes of diffuse hyperpigmentation include drug reactions, ectopic adrenocorticotropic hormone production by small cell lung carcinoma or other neoplasia, hemochromatosis, hyperthyroidism, vitamin B12 or folate deficiency, porphyria cutanea tarda, pellagra, melanosis secondary to metastatic melanoma, and argyria.
- The possibility of chronic adrenal insufficiency should be considered in patients with unexplained malaise, tiredness, anorexia, nausea and vomiting, abdominal pain, melanic pigmentation, weight loss, postural dizziness, craving for salt and hypoglycemic episodes.
- The symptoms of chronic adrenal insufficiency are nonspecific and the disease may go undiagnosed for long periods of time, with the risk of serious consequences.
- Acute adrenocortical insufficiency is dominated by hypotension; it is potentially lethal and requires immediate treatment.

## References

[1] Eisen D. Disorders of pigmentation in the oral cavity. *Clin. Dermatol.* 2000;18: 579-587.

[2] Salvatori R. Adrenal insufficiency. *JAMA* 2005;294:2481-2488.

[3] Chakera AJ, Vaidya B. Addison disease in adults: diagnosis and management. *Amer. J. Med.* 2010;123:409-413.

[4] Hahner S, Loeffler M, Bleicken B, Drechsler C, Milovanovic D, Fassnacht M, Ventz M, Quinkler M, Allolio B. Epidemiology of adrenal crisis in chronic adrenal insufficiency: the need for new prevention strategies. *Eur. J. Endocrinol.* 2010; 162:597-602.

## Case 2. Hereditary Hemorrhagic Telangiectasia

A 72-year-old woman was admitted to our department for evaluation of dizziness and fatigue. Since young adulthood she had repeated nosebleed and black stools. She had received iron replacement therapy and red blood cell transfusions as required, during the last year two units of blood every second month. The patient's family history was scarce: she had lost her parents and sister in extermination camps in 1944; she had not married. On previous examinations a clinical diagnosis of Osler-Weber-Rendu syndrome was posited. She was currently receiving a ferum sulfate and folic acid oral preparation. The patient was pale but in good nutritional state. A few bright red telangiectasias were dispersed on her fingers, lips and face, presenting as eccentrically placed spots with radiating legs. The upper surface of the tongue was scattered with numerous bright red vascular ectasias (Figure 2).

There was neither sclerodactily nor organomegaly. Laboratory examinations showed hematocrit was 23% and the mean corpuscular volume was 72 fL; no antimitochondrial and anticentromere antibodies were found. The patient received two units of blood, oral folate, i.v. iron and started treatment with topical estrogen applications t.i.d. to the oral mucosa. On six month follow-up examination the hematocrit was 32% without the patient receiving further transfusions.

Hereditary hemorrhagic telangiectasia (Osler-Weber-Rendu syndrome) is often diagnosed on first glance, by right or by mistake. It is an autosomal dominant disorder, characterized by telangiectasia and arteriovenous malformations involving the skin, mucous membranes, and solid organs. Large arteriovenous malformations can involve the lung, liver, and brain. The vascular lesions usually become apparent during the second or third decades of life. The lesions look as red spots that blanch on pressure, and are scattered on the face, lips, nares, fingers, tongue, and oral mucosa. Epistaxis occurs in 90% of patients, upper or lower gastointestinal bleeding in 50%, and hematuria in 15%. Arteriovenous fistulas in the lung may result in right-to-left shunting, hypoxemia, pulmonary hypertension, and clubbing. Arteriovenous fistulas in the liver can cause high-output heart failure. Neurological symptoms may occur, most often due to paradoxical emboli. Telangiectasias are seen easily on endoscopy, although in the presence of severe anemia, blood loss, or hypotension, they transiently may become less obvious or even invisible.

The clinical diagnosis of hereditary hemorrhagic telangiectasia requires the presence of at least three of four clinical criteria: epistaxis (spontaneous and recurrent nosebleeds), multiple telangiectasias at characteristic sites (lips, oral cavity, fingers or nose), visceral lesions (pulmonary, hepatic, cerebral, spinal, or gastrointestinal vascular malformations), and one or several first-degree relative with hereditary hemorrhagic telangiectasia [1]. The clinical differential diagnosis involves mainly telangiectasia of systemic sclerosis and primary biliary cirrhosis. An eccentrically placed red punctum with radiating legs is the characteristic feature of Rendu-Osler-Weber disease; this pattern may be better visualized by stretching the lip.

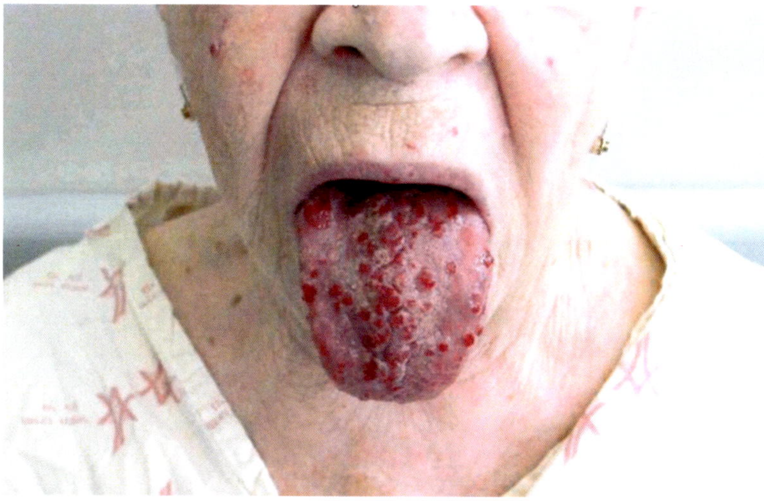

Figure 2. A few telangiectasias are seen on the face and lips, while the upper surface of the tongue is scattered with numerous, prominent cherry red vascular ectasias.

Telangiectasia in scleroderma (CREST syndrome) has a unique morphology: the lesion is a polyangular mat without punctum and radiating legs. The distinction from trivial lesions is clear: such are cherry angiomas, venous lakes presenting as dark blue vascular marks, and caviar spots arising on the undersurface of the tongue as spherical varicose enlargements. The clinical diagnosis of hereditary hemorrhagic telangiectasia can be confirmed by molecular genetic analysis.

The treatment is supportive. Patients with bleeding should receive supplemental iron and folate. Treatment with desmopressin, danazol, and aminocaproic acid has been used with varied success. Endoscopic ablation is promising when the lesions are within reach of the endoscope and not too diffuse. Endoscopic therapy may be performed during active bleeding or between bleeding episodes. Embolization of arteriovenous fistulas may be required. Estrogen or progesterone treatment has been used, but no benefit was demonstrated in a placebo-controlled trial, while other studies were promising [2, 3].

The attempted diagnosis in the propositus was hereditary hemorrhagic telangiectasia, although only two criteria out of four were met: spontaneous and recurrent nosebleeds and telangiectasias at characteristic sites. This diagnosis was also supported by the lengthy benign course of the disease over more than four decades, and by exclusion of other disorders that may be associated with telangiectasias.

## Learning Points

- Spontaneous and recurrent epistaxis, telangiectasias on lips, oral cavity, fingers or nose, visceral vascular malformations, and a first-degree relative with hereditary hemorrhagic telangiectasia constitute the clinical syndrome of hereditary hemorrhagic telangiectasia.
- Typical consequences of this disorder may be anemia, hypoxemia, transient ischemic attacks, or liver disease.
- The treatment is supportive.

## References


[1] Shovlin CL, Guttmacher AE, Buscarini E, Faughnan ME, Hyland RH, Westermann CJ, Kjeldsen AD, Plauchu H. Diagnostic criteria for hereditary hemorrhagic telangiectasia (Rendu-Osler-Weber syndrome). *Am. J. Med. Genet.* 2000; 91:66-67.

[2] Van Cutsam E, Rutgeerts P, Geboes K, Van Gompel F, Vantrappen G. Estrogen-progesterone treatment of Osler-Weber-Rendu disease. *J. Clin. Gastroenterol.* 1988; 10:676-679.

[3] Bergler W, Sadick H, Gotte K, Riedel F, Hörmann K. Topical estrogens combined with argon plasma coagulation in the management of epistaxis in hereditary hemorrhagic telangiectasia. *Ann. Otol. Rhinol. Laryngo*l. 2002;111(3 Pt 1):222-228.


## Case 3. Contact Dermatitis

A 70-year old man was working on a hot summer day in a fig orchard, the bare chest coming in contact with the leaves of the tree. Four hours later he developed a burning and itching erythematous eruptions on his chest (Figure 3). On examination, the patient's temperature and BP were normal and his general state was fairly good. Obviously, the diagnosis was contact dermatitis. The symptoms resolved over a week.

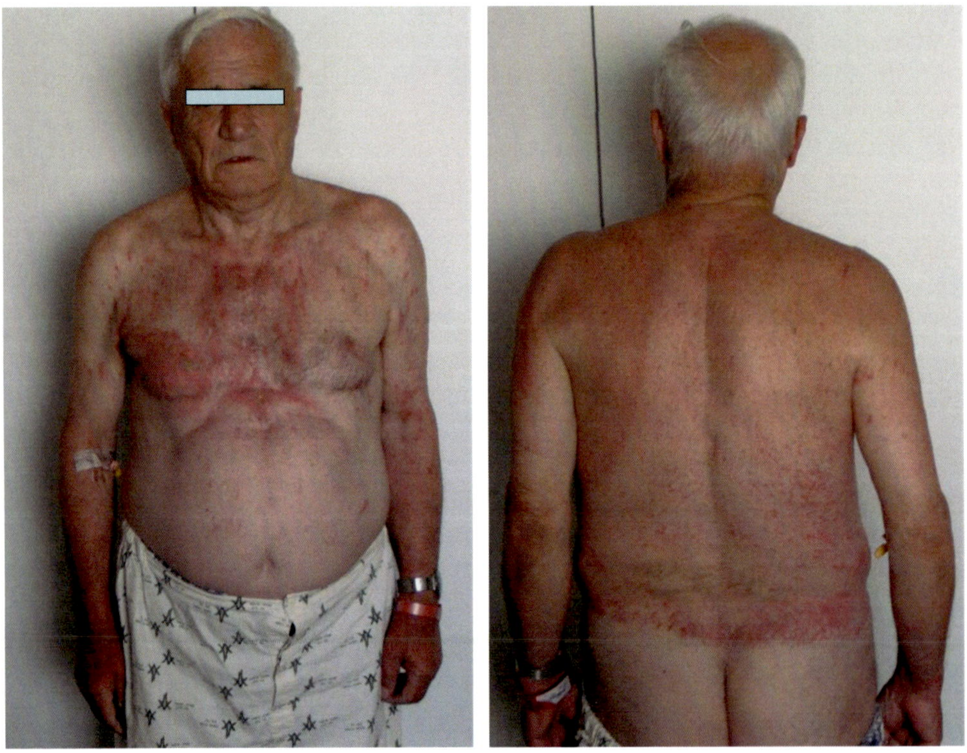

Figure 3. Contact dermatitis.

Irritant dermatitis has been reported from contact with fig (Ficus carica) leaves. The latex contains ficin, a proteolytic enzyme that acts as an irritant. Also, contact with plant-derived phototoxic substances (furocoumarins or psoralens) followed by sunlight exposure produce lesions of phototoxic dermatitis [1, 2]. These reactions occur in persons who cultivate, gather, pack, or consume figs. Therefore, it is prudent to use gloves and protective clothing while working with plants containing furocoumarins and to avoid simultaneous exposure to sunlight.

Contact dermatitis is not uncommon. It is easily recognizable, but unfortunately the diagnosis is often missed. In the present case the diagnosis was straightforward.

### Learning Points

- Contact dermatitis is an inflammation of the skin induced by contact with a specific allergen and resulting in edema and erythema, usually with superimposed vesicles or bullae. Contact dermatitis may be further categorized as allergic or irritant.
- Common causes of allergic contact dermatitis are latex, cosmetics, perfumes, propylene glycol (found in many topical medications), neomycin, bacitracin, poison ivy, and oak.

## References

[1] Goitre M, Bedello PG, Cane D, Alovisi V. Phytophotodermatitis caused by fig tree. *G. Ital. Dermatol. Venereol.* 1984;119:435-436.

[2] Polat M, Oztas P, Dikilitas MC, Alli N. Phytophotodermatitis due to *Ficus carica. Dermatology Online Journal* 2008;14:9.

## Case 4. Skin Metastases

A 76-year-old man was referred with acute diarrhea. One year ago he was diagnosed with adenocarcinoma of the colon, went through anterior colonic resection, and received chemotherapy. Eight months later he was evaluated for cervical lymphadenopathy and swelling of the left upper and right lower extremities. Venous ultrasound of the affected limbs and CT angiography showed external compression of the left axillary and right ileac veins; there was massive enlargement of mediastinal and abdominal lymph nodes and a large tumor in the area of the colonic anastomosis. Fine needle aspiration of a cervical lymph node showed clusters of carcinoma cells consistent with metastatic adenocarcinoma. Biopsies of the inflamed mucosa in the narrowed area of the colonic anastomosis revealed adenocarcinoma. Two months before the present admission the patient observed the appearance of rapidly growing nodules on the chest wall.

On physical examination, the skin on the left side of chest, left arm and left flank had a tanned hue, felt infiltrated, and was dotted with nodules varying in size between a few millimeters to 2 cm, an appearance which is consistent with skin metastases (Figure 4).

Enlarged and firm lymph nodes were palpable in the left cervical, left axillary and inguinal areas. The left arm, the scrotum, and the right lower extremity were swollen.

Cutaneous metastases may be the first presentation of a malignant carcinoma, evidence of recurrence, or a late event during the course of a previously treated malignancy particularly in patients with melanoma, breast cancer, or mucosal cancers of the head and neck. The latter are tumors that invade veins and so cause metastases at sites distant from the primary tumor, inclusive the skin. Cutaneous metastases appear as skin-colored nodules, are discrete, firm, nontender and usually grow rapidly. Clinical diagnosis is easy, yet the diagnosis is often confused with cysts or benign fibrous tumors [1]. The rare presentation in a zosteriform distribution may be another source of confusion [2]. Development of cutaneous metastases from colon cancer is a rare occurrence, usually arising in the setting of diffusely-disseminated cancer and carrying a dismal prognosis.

Another pattern of cutaneous metastasis is a circumscribed skin inflammation with erythema, edema, warmth and tenderness, simulating erysipelas or cellulitis ('carcinoma erysipelatoides'); however, in contrast to erysipelas the patient is afebrile. The primary tumor is usually in the breast. The malignant cells invade and obstruct subepidermal lymphatic vessels, causing the inflammatory alterations in the skin in the vicinity of the primary tumor [3].

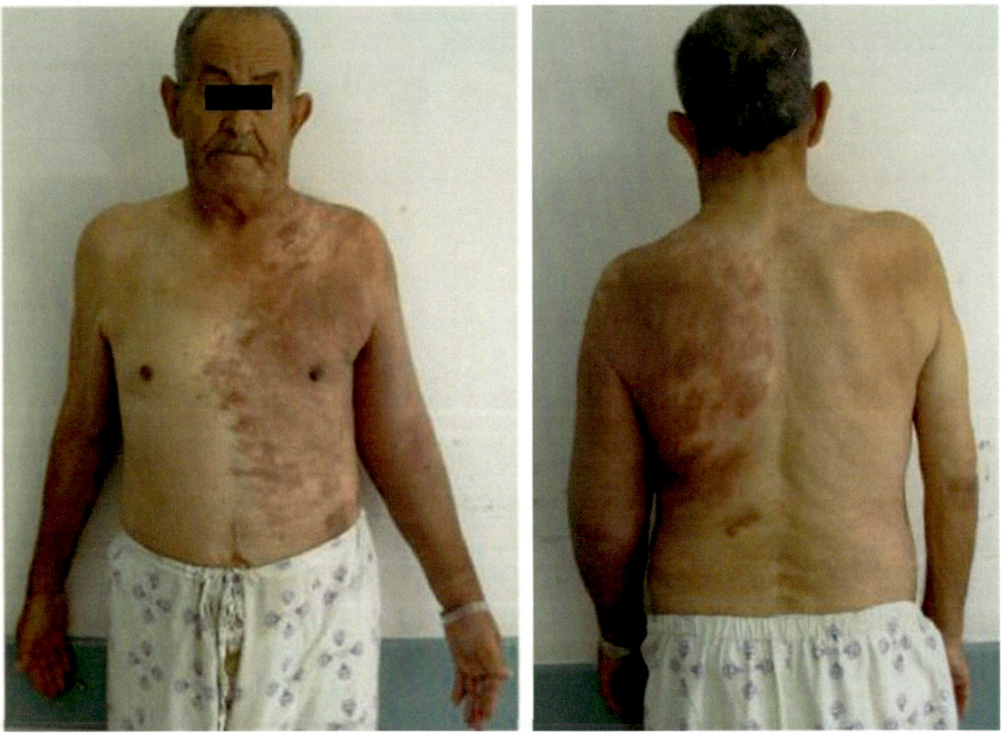

Figure 4. The skin on the left side of chest, left arm and left flank has a darker tone and is scattered with hard nodules. The left arm is swollen. The patient appears to be in good general health.

### Learning Points

- Skin-colored nodules that appear suddenly and grow fast should raise suspicion of cutaneous metastases; they may be the first presentation of a malignant carcinoma, evidence of recurrence, or a late event during the course of a previously treated malignancy.
- Carcinoma erysipelatoides, sometimes mistaken for erysipelas, most commonly originates from breast carcinoma. It denotes a poor prognosis.

## References

[1] Lookingbill DP, Spangler N, Helm KF. Cutaneous metastases in patients with metastatic carcinoma: a retrospective study of 4020 patients. *J. Am. Acad. Dermatol.* 1993;29(2 Pt 1):228-236.
[2] Bauzá A, Redondo P, Idoate MA. Cutaneous zosteriform squamous cell carcinoma metastasis arising in an immunocompetent patient. *Clin. Eperim. Dermatol.* 2002;27: 199-201.
[3] Singletary SE, Cristofanilli M. Defining the clinical diagnosis of inflammatory breast cancer. *Semin. Oncol.* 2008;35:7-10.

## Case 5. Acute Gouty Arthritis

A 93-year-old community-dwelling woman was referred from the emergency service with the diagnosis of arthritis of the first metacarpophalangeal joint. The onset was two weeks before admission with severe pain confined to the first metacarpophalangeal joint; the body temperature was normal. Nevertheless, the patient had received a 10-day course of oral cefuroxime 500 mg/day, without relief of arthritis. Her medical history was notable for arterial hypertension, myocardial infarction and hyperuricemia. There was no history of gout. The patient's current medications were aspirin 100 mg, Kaluril (containing hydrochlorothiazide 50 mg and amiloride hydrochloride 5 mg), diltiazem 120 mg, atenolol 50 mg/day, and allopurinol 150 mg/day (the latter was recently discontinued because of nausea attributed to this medication). On admission the patient was alert, her BP was 212/100 mmHg, the heart rate 61 bpm in sinus rhythm, the temperature 38.4$^0$C. Cardiac and pulmonary auscultation was unremarkable. The first toe on the left foot and the adjacent area were red-to-cyanotic, swollen and extremely tender. Laboratory tests showed 19,000 WBC, 75% neutrophils, and 8% band forms. The CRP was 237 mg/L, the serum creatinine 1.2 mg/dL and uric acid 14 mg/dL. The ECG showed sinus rhythm, right bundle branch block, a QR pattern in leads III and aVF consistent with an inferior wall scar. The chest x-rays showed mild enlargement of the cardiac silhouette.

The diagnosis of podagra was straightforward. Treatment with etodolac 800/day mg/day was started, subsequently supplemented with prednisone 30 mg/day, and transdermal fentanyl 25 mg/day. On the following morning, the skin overlying the first metatarso-phalangeal joint appeared eroded on several points with leakage of a whitish, thick, odorless liquid (Figure 5).

Microscopical examination of the discharge showed myriads of needle like crystals amongst numerous polymorphonuclear leukocytes, some containing similar crystals, confirming the diagnosis of gout. No bacteria were seen on direct examination or revealed on culture of the discharge. So, the impression on first glance of podagra, an easy to make diagnosis, was confirmed.

The patient's arterial hypertension was well controlled on diltiazem 180 mg. Intake of Kaluril and aspirin was discontinued. The body temperature returned to normal within 2 days. On day 9 in hospital, the pain and swelling had diminished and the discharge was minimal. On day 11 in hospital the patient complained of acute precordial pain and shortness of breath. The emergence of deep negative T waves in leads II, V4-V6 of the ECG and elevated troponin I 8.8 μg/L in the serum were consistent with acute myocardial infarction. The patient was transferred to the intensive coronary care. She died on the following morning.

*Podagra* is a term used to describe acute monoarthritis of the first metatarsophalangeal joint. Podagra is a typical bedside diagnosis and little more needs to be done before starting treatment. In younger patients, gout is often suspected on the basis of a typical attack of podagra or on the basis of tophi developing after many years of recurring attacks of monoarthritis. The common cause of podagra is gout. Infrequently, arthritis in the first metatarsophalangeal joint is caused by calcium pyrophosphate dihydrate, septic arthritis, traumatic conditions, and reactive arthritis [1]. The chief complaint associated with an acute gouty attack is unbearable pain accompanied by swelling, erythema, warmth and tenderness in the area of the first metatarsophalangeal joint. A low-grade fever may occur in conjunction with the inflammation. A rapid outburst of the symptoms from no pain to maximum pain over less than half a day and the symptoms limited to the typical joints (first metatarso-phalangeal joint, midfoot, or ankle) are consistent with a classical gout attack. If the patient has had similar acute attacks, which remitted on therapy over a 5 to 8 days, that too is typical and supports a presumptive diagnosis of gout. Pseudogout usually is slower in onset and slower to remit, lasting for weeks rather than days. Other joints that may be affected during a gouty attack are the ankle, knees, hands, and elbows [2-4].

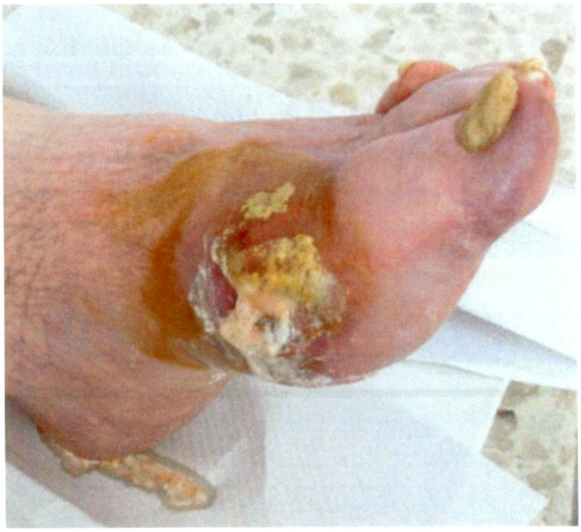

Figure 5. The area adjacent to the first toe is swollen and eroded with spill-over of a whitish, chalk-like fluid.

*Symptoms in the knee* are more problematic because septic arthritis and calcium pyrophosphate dihydrate crystal deposition disease (pseudogout) also commonly affect the knee.

*Bilateral olecranon bursitis* is a clinical clue to the diagnosis of gout.

*Tophi* are nodular masses of monosodium urate crystals deposited in the soft tissues. Tophy are late complications of hyperuricemia, occurring on average 12 years after the initial gouty attack. Rarely, tophi can develop without previous acute gouty arthritis. The most common sites of urate deposition are the base of the great toe, and the fingers, wrist, hand, olecranon bursae, Achilles tendon, and the helix of the ear. Complications of tophi include pain, soft tissue damage and deformity, joint destruction and nerve compression syndromes such as carpal tunnel syndrome.

*The three renal complications* of gout are nephrolithiasis, acute and chronic gouty nephropathy. Nephrolithiasis occurs in 10 to 25 percent of patients with primary gout.

*In elderly patients*, many symptoms often relied upon for diagnosing gout are lacking: elderly women are as often affected as males, a polyarticular onset is frequent, the upper extremities are often involved, tophi may be present before occurrence of arthritis, and renal insufficiency and diuretic use are common associated features.

*Radiographs* taken during initial episodes of gouty arthritis show soft tissue swelling but no bony abnormality. Radiological bony changes typically require a longer than 5 years course of gout. Late radiological findings include soft tissue tophi with or without calcification, chondrocalcinosis, osseous erosions with overhanging margins, geographic sclerotic margination to bony erosion, and intraosseous mineralization.

*Identification of crystals in the synovial fluid* from an inflamed joint is essential to endorse the diagnosis, by demonstrating the predominance of polymorphonuclear leukocytes in the synovial fluid and the presence of monosodium urate crystals in their cytoplasm. On microscopy, monosodium urate crystals appear needle-shaped and are negatively birefringent on polarized light. Occasionally, uric acid crystals are not found in the synovial fluid. However, aspiration repeated 6-24 hours later shows crystals in the synovial fluid in most of these patients. Identification of crystals in the synovial fluid or tissue is even more important in older patients, because the frequently atypical presentation of gout.

Examination of the joint fluid can also rule out disorders that mimic gout, such as septic arthritis and pseudogout. If the patient has had invasive procedures and has risk factors for bacteremia, it is imperative to get synovial fluid to rule out a septic arthritis. Furthermore, a chronically gouty joint is more susceptible to infection, so that patients who have well-established gout may still require joint aspiration to exclude secondary infection. The presence of cellulitis over an inflamed joint should not be an impediment of aspirating the joint or bursa since the reaction to crystals in a joint can produce an inflammation which resembles infectious cellulitis. Last but not least, if a patient says 'this is not like my previous gout attacks' the diagnosis is other than gout and aspiration of the involved joint should promptly follow [2, 3].

*Treatment of the acute gouty attack* presents the choice among three anti-inflammatory medications: colchicine, an NSAID, or a corticosteroid preparation [4, 5]. The sooner the drug is started with any of these agents, the more rapidly a complete response will be attained. *NSAIDs* are usually the preferred treatment for acute gouty attacks. Therapy for acute arthritis is ideally started fast, with high doses of an NSAID, given for the first 24 or 36 hours; this is important for getting the attack under control. While the analgesic dose of NSAIDs is rather low, e.g. for ibuprofen 400 mg three times daily, the anti-inflammatory dose is higher, e.g. ibuprofen 800 mg three times daily. For treatment of acute gouty arthritis naproxen is started with an initial dose 750 mg than followed by 250-500 mg twice daily. In head-to-head studies, various NSAIDs had similar benefits for acute gout. Even if a patient has a septic joint, which has been mistakenly diagnosed as gouty attack, an improvement can be witnessed but the benefit will be transient. So, if improvement is not maintained 1 to 2 days after therapy was started, the diagnosis becomes doubtful and the joint must be aspirated or re-aspirated. NSAID treatment should be continued for a few days after the symptoms have completely resolved. This may take in general 2 weeks. A common mistake is to discontinue NSAIDs when symptoms are still present, so attacks often recur. Gastric protection should be provided.

However, the need for such aggressive dosing is not a reason to use NSAIDs in patients with significant renal disease or other comorbidities for which NSAIDs are problematic. Many clinicians would avoid administration of NSAIDs when the patient's creatinine clearance is less than 60 mL/min, and would be very cautious if the patient has hypertension or congestive heart failure. If patients are on angiotensin-converting enzyme inhibitors, angiotensin receptor blockers, or beta-blockers, adding an NSAID may increase the risk for hyperkalemia to develop. Because the increased risk of adverse events in patients with diabetes or congestive heart failure, the duration of NSAID treatment might be shortened.

Treatment of a gouty attack is even more problematic in patients with ischemic heart disease. The quick resolution of arthritis is high priority and use of prednisone might be chosen, though steroids may increase the blood glucose, BP and cause fluid retention. NSAIDs could reduce the aspirin's platelet antiaggregant effect. The latter effect can be avoided by first taking aspirin and taking the NSAID two hours later, as demonstrated by co-administration of low dose aspirin and antiinflammatory dose naproxen [6]. The choice between selective COX-2 inhibitors versus nonselective COX inhibitors is important because of prostaglandins' effects on coronary blood flow. It well known that COX-2 is expressed in normal endothelial cells in response to shear stress and that inhibition of COX-2 is associated with suppression of prostacyclin synthesis. Major cardiovascular consequences of COX-2 inhibition include a shift in the prothrombotic/antithrombotic balance on endothelial surfaces toward thrombosis; an increase in sodium and water retention leading to edema, exacerbation of heart failure and hypertension; loss of the protective effects of COX-2 upregulation in the setting of myocardial ischemia and infarction may lead to a larger infarct size and an increased tendency to myocardial rupture. So, nonselective COX inhibitors like naproxen and ibuprofen might be preferred for the treatment of acute gout attacks in patients with ischemic heart disease. Some have argued that diclofenac is COX-2 selective. However, therapeutically relevant COX-2 selectivity will be difficult to attain, since the concentration of diclofenac necessary to achieve 80% inhibition of COX-2 is expected to cause a similar inhibition of COX-1. The estimated cardiovascular risks for all currently available NSAIDs were compared in a recent systematic review of controlled observational studies by McGettigan and Henry. They found that NSAIDs and selective COX-2 inhibitors confer dose-dependent elevated cardiovascular risk, with rofecoxib and diclofenac conferring the highest risk, and ibuprofen and naproxen the lowest [7]. Yet, many physicians prefer not to use NSAIDs in patients with significant heart disease.

*Prednisone* 20 to 40 mg per day or equivalent steroid may be useful, but a more aggressive dosing is preferred by many experts. In a randomized study, prednisolone was as effective as indomethacin in achieving pain relief, and caused fewer side effects [8]. Dividing the daily dose may prevent flares to occur during the night. Using a single daily steroid dose in the morning, primarily to spare the adrenal glands, is not considered necessary in gouty arthritis, where usually short courses of steroids are prescribed. The steroid doses needed to effectively treat an acute gout attack have a major effect on glucose levels in diabetic patients.

*Colchicine* is often preferred for patients in whom the diagnosis of gout is not confirmed, whereas NSAIDs are preferred when the diagnosis is confidently made. The relative efficacy of colchicine as compared with NSAIDs is unknown. Colchicine regimens of 0.5 mg to 1 mg three t.i.d. are the most popular and were found to be most often effective in a survey conducted by French rheumatologists. A traditional protocol, recommending hourly oral colchicine doses until onset of response or the occurrence of adverse effects (nausea, vomiting, diarrhea), is little in use today. Indeed, the number needed to treat before toxicity occurs is considerably less than the number for efficacy. An other concern in using colchicine relates to colchicine's drug interactions, with statins, some antibiotics, and some calcium channel blockers, which share drug transporters with colchicine.

If a patient cannot take medications by mouth or has active peptic ulcer disease, the choice is among intravenous colchicine, an intra-articular glucocorticoid, or parenteral glucocorticoids. Local application of ice packs may help control the pain of an acute attack. In some cases, narcotics may be added. Introduction of new treatments such as interleukin-1 antagonists for management of acute gout, and febuxostat and pegloticase for chronic gout might bring significant progress in the treatment of gout. Anti-inflammatory medications have no effect on uric acid levels.

*Drugs that affect serum urate concentrations* should neither been started nor stopped during an acute attack, since sudden fluctuations in serum urate levels may precipitate an acute attack. Hence, urate-lowering agents should not be started until an acute attack of gouty arthritis has ended. The goal of treatment with urate-lowering agents is to reduce the urate pool and achieve a target uric acid level ≤6 mg/dL. Allopurinol impairs the conversion of hypoxanthine to xanthine and the conversion of xanthine to uric acid. The effect of the drug depends on the dosage. Allopurinol in a dosage of 300 mg per day has been reported to reduce serum urate concentrations to <6 mg/dL in 70 percent of patients. The dose of allopurinol needs to be adjusted in patients with renal impairment: allopurinol should be started with a low dosage (50 to 100 mg/day) and titrated to appropriate levels while monitoring serum urate, CBC, and creatinine levels. Regardless of renal function, the correct dose of urate-lowering therapy is one that reduces the serum urate level to <6 mg/dL. Allopurinol is the drug of choice in patients with severe tophaceous deposits and in patients with a history of impaired renal function, uric acid nephropathy or nephrolithiasis. The drug is also preferred as a pretreatment agent to protect against uric acid nephropathy in patients with lymphoproliferative or myeloproliferative disorders. Allopurinol remains a first-line treatment for chronic hyperuricemia, but uricosuric agents may also be considered in some patients.

The patient should be informed that acute flares may occur following the initiation of urate-lowering agents. The frequency of such events can be reduced by continuing the anti-inflammatory treatment. Thus, colchicine 0.6 mg x 2/ day is indicated to prevent a flare of acute gout before starting allopurinol treatment and is discontinued usually 6 to 8 weeks after normalization of serum urate levels. According to other experts, anti-inflammatory prophylaxis should be continued for the first 6 to 12 months after the target serum uric acid level is achieved with urate-lowering therapy. Long-term colchicine 0.6 mg x 2/day may be necessary in patients with frequent gout attacks despite use of uricosuric agents. The side effects of allopurinol include Stevens-Johnson syndrome, leukopenia and gastrointestinal disturbances.

Febuxostat, a non-purine xanthine-oxidase inhibitor, is a new agent approved for the treatment of hyperuricemia in patients with gout. Febuxostat and allopurinol have similar safety profiles, although no cases of hypersensitivity syndrome have been reported with febuxostat. Patients with hypersensitivity reactions to allopurinol who were given febuxostat were able to tolerate the new drug [9].

Physical exercise, weight reduction, reduced alcohol consumption and discontinuation of certain medications if possible (low-dose aspirin, switching to losartan, and a lipid-lowering agent such as atorvastatin or fenofibrate) may help in lowering the uric acid level. Losartan, an angiotensin II receptor antagonist given as 50 mg/dL can be uricosuric. When given with hydrochlorothiazide it can blunt the hyperuricemic effect of the diuretic and potentiate its antihypertensive action.

There is more to be commented on our patient:

First, the gouty arthritis for the first time in life occurred after discontinuation of alopurinol treatment. Studies have shown that withdrawal of antihyperuricemic drugs may result after a variable period of time (several months or years in one study) in recurrence of acute gouty arthritis. Yet, we could not find in the literature reports on a first gouty attack upon discontinuation of alopurinol.

Second, myocardial infarction occurring during the course of acute gouty attack raises the question whether the acute arthritis was the trigger for the coronary event? One large scale study demonstrated that gouty arthritis is associated with an excess risk of acute myocardial infarction, and this is not explained by traditional cardiovascular risk factors. The underlying mechanism might involve the inflammation associated with gout, that might affect endothelial functions [10]. Yet, we could not find in the literature studies describing the time-lag between the onset of acute gouty arthritis and the subsequent occurrence of acute myocardial infarction.

Third, a detrimental effect of the NSAID etodolac should be considered. Etodolac is a preferential inhibitor of COX 2 and consequently it may cause a shift of the prothrombotic/antithrombotic balance on endothelial surfaces toward thrombosis.

Temporary discontinuation of administration of low-dose aspirin might also have predisposed to a coronary event. Indeed, it has been suggested that in patients at >3% risk of a vascular event the treatment of choice for acute gouty arthritis should be the combination of naproxen, low-dose aspirin and a proton pump inhibitor [6].

This case illustrates the ease of the diagnosis of typical podagra, the quick improvement of the gouty attack on treatment, occurrence of an unexpected complication, and the remaining of several unanswered questions.

## Learning Points

- Podagra describes acute monoarthritis of the first metatarsophalangeal joint. Its common cause is gout.
- Additional causes of monoarthritis of the first metatarsophalangeal joint are sepsis, traumatic conditions, and reactive arthritis.

- Identification of crystals in the synovial fluid from an inflamed joint is essential to endorse the diagnosis of gout, by showing the presence of polymorphonuclear leukocytes and intracellular monosodium urate crystals.
- In elderly patients, many of the clinical features often relied on for the diagnosis of gout are lacking, so identification of crystals in the synovial fluid or tissue is even more important.
- Treatment of the acute gouty attack presents the choice among an NSAID, a corticosteroid preparation, and colchicine.
- NSAIDs are usually the preferred treatment for acute gout attacks. The sooner the drug is started the more rapidly and complete will be the response.
- High doses of an NSAID should be given for the first 24 or 36 hours.
- NSAIDs should best be avoided in patients with creatinine clearance less than 60 mL/min, diabetes mellitus, arterial hypertension, ischemic heart disease, or heart failure.
- Gastric protection with a proton pump inhibitor should be provided.
- For patients at higher than 3% risk of a vascular event the choice should be naproxen together with low-dose aspirin and a proton pump inhibitor.

## References


[1] Boulman N, Slobodin G, Sharif D, Rozenbaum M, Rosner I. Pseudopodagra: A presenting manifestation of infective endocarditis. Clin Exp Rheumatol. 2005;23:251-253. 2.

[2] Wise CM. Crystal-associated arthritis in the elderly. *Rheum. Diseases Clinics N. Amer.* 2007;33:33-55.

[3] Baker JF, Schumacher HR. Update on gout and hyperuricemia. *Int. J. Clin. Pract.* 2010;64:371-377.

[4] Mandell BF, Edwards LN, Sundy JS, Simkin PA, Pile JC. Preventing and treating acute gout attacks across the clinical spectrum: A roundtable discussion. *Cleveland Clin. J. Med.* 2010; 77(Suppl 2):S2-S25.

[5] Schjerning Olsen A-M, Foesbol EL, Lindhardse J, Folkae F, Charlot M, Selmer C, Lamberts M, Olessen JB, Kober L, Hansen PR, Torp-Petersen C, Gislason GH. Duration of treatment with nonsteroidal anti-inflammatory drugs and impact on risk of death and recurrent myocardial infarction in patients with prior myocardial infarction. A nationwide cohort study. *Circulation* 2011;123:2226-2235.

[6] Patrignani P, Tacconelli S, Bruno A, Sostres C, Lanas A. Managing the effects of nonsteroidal antiinflmmatory drugs. *Expert Rev. Clin. Pharmacol.* 2011;4:605-621.

[7] McGettigan P, Henry D. Cardiovascular risk with non-steroidal anti-inflammatory drugs: systematic review of population-based controlled observational studies. *PLoS Med.* 2011;8:e1001098.

[8] Man CY, Cheung IT, Cameron PA, Rainer TH. Comparison of oral prednisolone/paracetamol and oral indomethacin/paracetamol combination therapy in the treatment of acute gout like arthritis: a double-blind, randomized, controlled trial. *Ann. Emerg. Med.* 2007; 49:670–677.

[9] Gaffo AL, Saag KG. Febuxostat: the evidence for its use in the treatment of hyperuricemia and gout. *Core Evid*. 2010;4:25-36.
[10] Krishnan E, Baker JF, Furst DE, Schumacher HR. Gout and the risk of acute myocardial infarction. *Arthritis Rheum*. 2006;54:2688-2696.

## Case 6. Digital Ischemia

An 87-year-old community-dwelling woman was referred from the emergency department with the diagnosis of right lower lobe pneumonia. Fever began on the same day, along with fatigue and dry cough. Notable in her medical history was essential thrombocytosis that was diagnosed on a routine check-up examination ten years ago. She was treated with hydroxyurea 1000 mg/day and aspirin 100 mg/day. There was no account of an ischemic or hemorrhagic event in the past. On admission to our ward, the patient's temperature was 39.4$^0$C, BP 122/50 mmHg, heart rate 92 bpm, and respiratory rate 26/minute. The distal two phalanges on fingers 2-5 on the patient's left hand were cyanotic and felt cold (Figure 6). Other areas were not affected by ischemia. The radial and cubital pulses were normal and on elevated arm stress test the patient did not develop symptoms. Dry crackles were heard at the base of the right lung field. The spleen felt slightly enlarged.

Laboratory tests showed hemoglobin 11.7 g/dL, WBC 11,000, polymorphonuclears 81%, platelets 760,000/mm$^3$, CRP 230 mg/L, creatine phosphokinase 120 U/dL (within the normal range), BUN 26 mg/dL, albumin 3.6 g/dL, globulin 3.2 g/dL. Chest x-rays showed a right lower lobe alveolar infiltrate; there was no cervical rib or deformity of the clavicle. Tests for cryoglobulin, cold agglutinin, anti hepatitis B and C virus antibodies, antinuclear and antiphospholipid antibodies were negative. There was no monoclonal spike on protein electrophoresis.

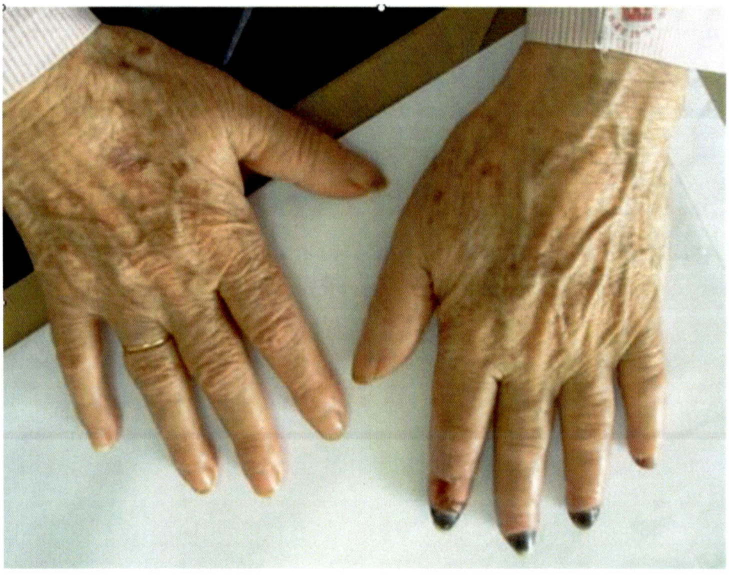

Figure 6. Digital ischemia on the left hand at the time of admission.

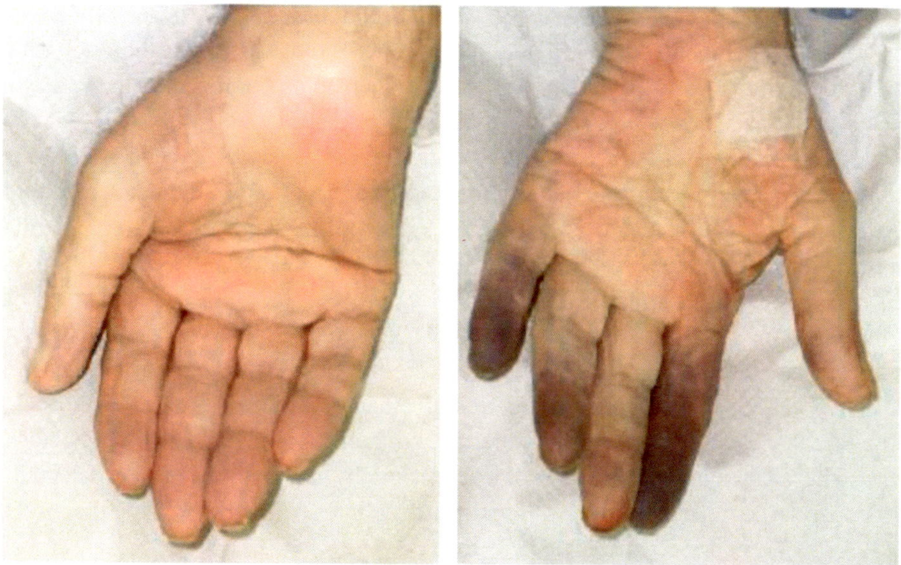

Figure 7. Digital ischemia without signs of gangrene two days later.

Antibiotic treatment with i.v. azithromycin and ceftriaxone was started, and hydration with isotonic saline. The hematologist consultant did consider treatment with platelet apheresis to be appropriate since there were no signs of life threatening thrombosis. The dose of hydroxyurea was increased to 2000 mg/day; aspirin 100 mg/day was continued. Two days later the digital ischemia had improved (Figure 7).

Critical digital ischemia and digital gangrene represent medical emergencies that require quick diagnosis and intensive treatment. The diagnosis of digital ischemia in our patient was straightforward; the supposed cause was the known predisposition of patients with essential thrombocytosis to develop thromboembolism. The latter being, however, a diagnosis of exclusion, additional etiologies were considered in the differential diagnosis. .

*Thoracic outlet syndrome* is defined by compression of the brachial plexus, subclavian vein, or subclavian artery at the superior opening of the thorax. The most reliable test in screening for thoracic outlet syndrome is *the elevated arm stress test*. With the patient sitting, the arms are abducted 90 degrees from the thorax and the elbows flexed 90 degrees, with the shoulders hold slightly behind the frontal plane, the patient is asked to open and close the fists slowly but steadily for 3 minutes and to describe any symptoms that develop. Normally, the patient performs this test without symptoms other than mild fatigue. In case of thoracic outlet syndrome the patient typically develops heaviness and fatigue of the involved limb, numbness of the hand, progressive aching through the arm and top of the shoulder, and drops the hand for relief [1]. Patients with carpal tunnel syndrome may experience dysesthesias in the fingers but do not have shoulder or arm pain. Patients with cervical disk syndromes may have pain in the neck and shoulder but have no arm or hand symptoms.

***Raynaud's phenomenon*** is a vasospastic disorder characterized by an exaggerated response to cold temperatures and/or emotional stress, resulting in transient digital ischemia. It manifests as a symmetric, sharply demarcated white or blue discoloration of the distal phalanges of the fingers or toes, followed by erythema after rewarming. Primary **Raynaud's** phenomenon usually occurs between the ages 15 and 25 years and is more likely to affect women than men. Secondary **Raynaud's phenomenon** has a later onset. Severe attacks, especially when accompanied by skin gangrene or ulceration warrants a thorough diagnostic evaluation for secondary causes. Secondary **Raynaud's phenomenon** occurs in more than 90% of patients with scleroderma or CREST syndrome, in approximately 30% of patients with systemic lupus erythematosus or Sjogren's syndrome, it may be associated with rheumatoid arthritis, carpal tunnel syndrome, ergotamine intake, vinyl chloride exposure, excessive smoking, trauma to the hands from vibrating tools, polycythemia, cryoglobulinemia, cold agglutinins, and paraproteinemia [2, 3].

*Atheroemboli* are microemboli consisting of cholesterol, calcium, platelet aggregates, and debris that break of from proximal atherosclerotic plaques or aneurysms and lodge in distal end arteries. The syndrome is seen more often in older men receiving warfarin treatment or after invasive vascular procedures. Atheroemboli produce a diversity of cutaneous findings, including acral petechiae, livedo reticularis, unilateral peripheral ulcers, cyanosis, and gangrene. The distal pulses are preserved. Occasionally the emboli can be detected in the retinal circulation as refractile interruptions in the column of arterial blood (the Hollenhorst plaques).

*Nonbacterial thrombotic endocarditis* may occur in patients with mucin-producing adenocarcinomas, more frequent in the elderly. Ischemic manifestations of the disorder are caused by embolization of cardiac vegetations to cerebral, renal, mesenteric, splenic, or peripheral arteries. Echocardiography reveals valvular vegetations in only a minority of patients. This is consistent with the variable size of the vegetations, from microscopic to several centimeters in diameter.

*Paraneoplastic digital gangrene* is a rare manifestation of the paraneoplastic hypercoagulability state. It may be thrombotic or embolic in nature, the latter originating from cardiac valvular vegetations or from venous thrombosis by 'paradoxical embolism'

*Symmetrical peripheral gangrene* of two or more extremities without large vessel obstruction or vasculitis is seen in sepsis, low output states, vasospastic conditions, myeloproliferative disorders and hyperviscosity syndrome.

*Paraproteinemia and hyperviscosity syndromes* may also complicate with digital ischemia.

*Cryoglobulinemia* is defined as the presence of circulating immunoglobulins that precipitate at temperatures below $37^0$C and redisolve on rewarming. Cryoglobulins are occasionally found in the blood of persons with multiple myeloma, leukemia, and certain forms of pneumonia. Mixed cryoglobulins are detectable in 40-50% of HCV-infected persons, whereas overt cryoglobulinemic vasculitis develops in less than 5%.

*Cold agglutinin disorders* are subdivided into primary and secondary. The latter are often associated with infections (Mycoplasma spp, Epstein-Barr virus, Cytomegalovirus, Legionella spp and Adenovirus), or with lymphoproliferative B-cell diseases. Up to 20% of community acquired pneumonia is caused by Mycoplasma pneumoniae and is considered a major cause in cold agglutinin-positive pneumonia. The classical clinical syndrome consists of hemolysis and Raynaud's phenomenon. Gangrene is an exceptional manifestation of cold agglutinin disease as agglutination is rapidly reversible on warming, almost never leading to permanent obstruction of blood vessels.

*Atherosclerosis* is the main cause of arm artery disease.

*Thrombangiitis obliterans* **(Buerger's disease)** is an inflammatory disorder of medium-sized small blood vessels and nerves affecting typically young male smokers.

*Takayasu's disease,* also known as pulseless disease, is a form of vasculitis of unknown cause that chiefly affects the aorta and its major branches, most frequently in young women.

*Cold injury* (frostbite, pernio) is a localized inflammatory lesion of the skin resulting from exposure to cold. Up to 50% of women developed pernio during wartime in northern Europe. Pernio is now uncommon, but is still seen in the temperate, humid climates of northwestern Europe and in the northern United States.

*Essential thrombocytosis and polycythemia vera* are myeloprolipherative disorders associated with a tendency for thromboembolism. Essential thrombocytosis is a clonal myeloproliferative disorder characterized by a sustained proliferation of megakaryocytes, which leads to increased numbers of circulating platelets, hyperplasia of bone marrow megakaryocytes, splenomegaly, and a clinical course interspersed with hemorrhagic or thrombotic episodes or both [4]. Many patients are asymptomatic and reach medical attention when extreme thrombocytosis is detected on a routine blood count. Others complain of having headaches, paresthesias of the extremities, or develop small or large vessel thrombosis, transient ischemic attacks, gangrene of toes, digital pain, erythromelalgia, or minor bleedings. Laboratory investigations show thrombocytosis, leukocytosis, and hyperuricemia.

Although thrombocytosis is the hallmark of essential thrombocytosis, more than 85% of cases with thrombocytosis seen in routine clinical practice represent reactive thrombocytosis associated with other conditions. The platelet count is a poor discriminator between essential and secondary thrombocytosis. The clinical scenario is often helpful in distinguishing essential from secondary thrombocytosis. In practice it is important to exclude the contribution of iron deficiency anemia or a hyposplenic state as possible causes of an otherwise unexplained thrombocytosis. The *JAK2* V617F mutation is found in 40%-60% of patients with essential thrombocytosis. Essential thrombocytosis remains a diagnosis of exclusion. Both secondary thrombocytosis and clonal thrombocytosis associated with other chronic myeloid disorders have to be ruled out before a diagnosis of essential thrombocytosis is made.

*A*symptomatic patients with essential thrombocytosis who are younger than 60 years old and do not have a history of thrombosis can be observed without cytoreductive therapy. The platelet count per se is not used as a guide to initiate cytoreductive therapy, as no direct correlation between platelet count and the incidence of thrombotic events has been demonstrated. Age greater than 60 years or a positive history of thrombosis are markers of increased thrombotic risk and are indications for cytoreduction. The treatment aims to reduce the platelet count to less than 400,000 $mm^3$ usually with the aid of hydroxyurea (starting dose 500 mg x 2 per day), or interferon alpha, anagrelide, and pegylated interferon. Low dose aspirin is indicated in patients with thromboses or erythromelalgia. For elderly persons, hydroxyurea is the primary cytoreductive agent. Only hydroxyurea has been shown prospectively to reduce the risk for thrombosis in patients with essential thrombocythemia, and in a randomized trial it was superior to anagrelide. Resistance to hydroxyurea has been reported in 11% to 17% of patients. In such situations, hydroxyurea can be combined with other platelet-lowering agents, such as anagrelide or interferon alpha.

Acute thrombosis in patients with essential thrombocythemia requires an immediate reduction of the platelet count to less than 400,000/ $mm^3$. If the platelet count is higher than 800,000/$mm^3$, platelet apheresis is indicated, usually combined with hydroxyurea. Use of aspirin or other NSAIDs should be avoided in patients with platelet counts greater than 1 million/$mm^3$ because of the risk of bleeding from acquired von Willebrand disease [5].

In our patient, the presence of essential thrombocytosis was not associated with symptoms for many years. The platelet count was maintained on hydroxyurea treatment in the range 400,000 to 500,000/mm3. Acute pneumonia might have complemented reactive thrombocytosis to background thrombocytosis of the chronic myeloproliferative disorder. Digital ischemia developed in the context of the saliently increased platelet count and acute infection. No cold agglutinins were detected, but might have been missed. A gamut of other possible etiologies of digital ischemia could be excluded with reasonable certitude.

The subsequent 14 days course in hospital was uneventful. Both pneumonia and digital ischemia remitted, and the platelet count decreased to 440,000/$mm^3$. On transthoracic echocardiography there was no evidence of valvular vegetation. A medical report six month later attested the favorable outcome with no further ischemic episode.

### Learning Points

- Digital ischemia is a first glance diagnosis, which cannot be missed.
- More demanding is to diagnose the etiology of digital ischemia that can be secondary to a gamut of vasospastic, vasculitic, thrombotic, embolic or mechanical disorders.
- The risk of digital gangrene is negligible in primary Raynaud's disease, but may be real in other disease states.
- The management of digital ischemia is tailored to specific etiologies.
- In elderly patients with essential thrombocytosis, chronic cytoreduction with hydroxyurea reduces the risk of vascular thrombosis.

## References

[1] Davidovic LB, Kostic DM, Jakovljevic NS, Kuzmanovic IL, Simic TM..Vascular thoracic outlet syndrome. *World J. Surg*. 2003; 27:545-550.

[2] Flavahan NA, Flavahan S, Mitra S Chotani MA.. The vasculopathy of Raynaud's phenomenon. *Rheum. Dis. Clin. North Am*. 2003; 29:275-291.

[3] Asherson RA, Cervera R, Shoenfeld Y. Peripheral vascular occlusions leading to gangrene and amputations in antiphospholipid antibody positive patients. *Ann. N. Y. Acad. Sci*. 2007;1108:515-529.

[4] Tefferi A, Thiele J, Orazi A, Kvasnicka HM, Barbui T, Hanson CA, Barosi G, Verstovsek S, Birgegard G, Mesa R, Reilly JT, Gisslinger H, Vannucchi AM, Cervantes F, Finazzi G, Hoffman R, Gilliland DG, Bloomfield CD, Vardiman JW.. Proposals and rationale for revision of the World Health Organization diagnostic criteria for polycthemia vera, essential thrombocytopenia, and primary myelofibrosis: recommendations from an ad hoc international expert panel. *Blood* 2007;110: 1092–1097.

[5] Elliott MA, Tefferi A. Thrombosis and haemorrhage in polycythaemia vera and essential thrombocythaemia. *Br. J. Haematol*. 2005;128:275-290.

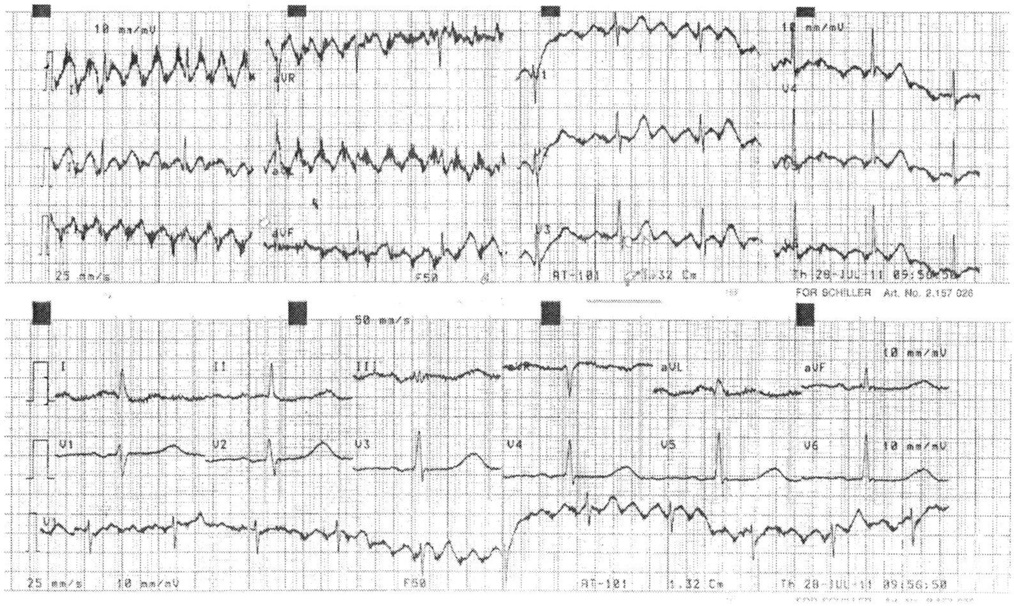

Figure 8. The upper tracing (A) shows abnormal waves, at a rate 300/minute, their amplitudes ranging between 0.4 mV in lead V1 and 0.8 mV in lead I; interspersed are narrow QRS complexes. This artifact was initially misinterpreted as atrial flutter. With the patient's hands at rest (tracing B) the abnormal waves disappeared in most leads.

## Case 7. Pseudo-Flutter

A 76-year-old woman was admitted with an acute urinary tract infection. She had resting and postural tremor that was ascribed to high dose quetapine and haloperidol she was receiving. Her admission ECG resembled atrial flutter (Figure 8), but could be correctly attributed to parkinsonian tremor.

Tremor is characterized by rhythmic oscillations of a body part. The regular cycle of motion differentiates tremor from chorea, tics and other movement disorders. In distinction from tremor, chorea is characterized by a restless, irregular activity that sometimes seems to jump from one area to another. Tics are repeated, brief, but more complex, stereotyped movements that are under some voluntary control. Genuine tremor can be classified on the basis of four clinical characteristics: anatomical pattern, the relative prominence of the tremor at rest or on maintaining a posture or with action, tremor frequency, and tremor amplitude. Tremor that is present at rest is usually parkinsonian. Tremor that appears only with posture as assessed by stretching out the pronated arms (postural tremor) is essential tremor or physiological tremor. Tremor that worsens with movement, e.g. when the patient is asked to perform finger–nose coordination testing, is often of cerebellar origin (action tremor).

The rate of the atrial flutter waves (F waves) is usually around 300 per minute, with a cycle frequency of 5 Hz. Typical atrial flutter results in a saw-tooth pattern in the inferior leads of the ECG and a positive F wave in lead $V_1$. The flutter waves may have variable appearances in different leads. Coincidentally, the frequency of the tremor in patients with parkinsonian syndrome is also around 5 Hz. The tremor-induced artifact in the ECG may mimic atrial flutter (Figure 8A leads V1-V5) or ventricular tachycardia if the artifact has large amplitude (Figure 8A leads I and aVL). The correct diagnosis is made on observing that the suspected arrhythmia occurs only during the patient's tremor. To avoid misinterpretation, physicians should have the knowledge of motion-related ECG artifacts and know the means to eliminate them by holding the tremulous limb.

### Learning Points

- Typical atrial flutter results in a saw-tooth pattern in the inferior leads of the ECG and a positive F waves in lead $V_1$.
- The flutter waves may have variable appearances in different leads. It is important not to rely on a single lead, particularly a limb lead, in making the diagnosis.
- Parkinsonian tremor has a frequency around 5 Hz, similar to the cycle frequency of atrial flutter. That's why parkinsonian tremor can cause an artifact in the ECG which resembles atrial flutter waves, a misinterpretation important to be avoided.

## References

[1] Alty JA, Kempster PA. A practical guide to the differential diagnosis of tremor *Postgrad. Med. J.* 2011;87:623-629.

[2] Márquez MF, Colín L, Guevara M, Iturralde P, Hermosillo AG. Common electrocardiographic artifacts mimicking arrhythmias in ambulatory monitoring. *Am. Heart J.* 2002 Aug;144:187-197.

[3] Patel SI, Souter MJ. Equipment-related electrocardiographic artifacts: causes, characteristics, consequences, and correction. *Anesthesiology.* 2008;108:138-148.

[4] Patel S. Electrocardiographic artifact mimicking ventricular tachycardia during high-frequency oscillatory ventilation: A case report. *Am. J. Crit. Care* 2006;15:310-311.

*Chapter II*

# Erysipelas, Cellulitis and Other Calf Dermatitides – A Bedside Diagnosis but not so Simple

Skin infections of the legs are common in the elderly. Abscesses, furuncles and wounds are culturable sources for microbiota. Erysipelas, cellulitis and infections of the deep subcutaneous tissues are 'nonculturable'. The types of cutaneous infection differ by their clinical features, epidemiology, risk factors, causative organisms, prognosis, and the treatment required. Yet, in the initial stages it may be difficult to distinguish between superficial and deep skin infections. Moreover, it may not be easy to discriminate an infectious from a non-infectious cellulitis. The diagnosis may be even more challenging in the case of a coexisting chronic skin disorders. Hence, apparently the simplest bedside diagnosis might be not as simple.

## Case 8. Erysipelas or Acute Lipodermatosclerosis?

A 70-year-old woman was admitted to hospital with fever and painful swelling of the right calf. For many years she suffered of swollen feet, varicous veins and repeated episodes of erysipelas of the right calf. She was currently not taking medications and neglected to wear compression stockings. On physical examination, her temperature was 38.9$^0$C, the BP 166/82 mmHg, heart rate 92 bpm, respirations 18/minute. There were grade 2 edema of the ankles and the dorsum of the feet, abundant perimaleolar reticular veins, and engorged calf veins with downward-going impulse on coughing. Her right calf was swollen. The skin in the distal part of the right calf was shiny-pink, tender and felt warm on palpation. There was no distinct demarcation between the erythematous and the normal skin, but two days later the demarcation line became clear. On both calves, the skin and subcutaneous tissues were thickened and indurated in a sleeve-like distribution beginning about 10 centimeters distal to the knees; the indurated areas were not exactly matching the congested or hyperpigmented areas. Remarkable among ancillary laboratory tests were WBC 18,100/mm$^3$ and CRP 153 mg/L. Duplex ultrasonography with the patient supine showed engorged deep and superficial veins in the thighs and calves and venous reflux; the veins were easily compressible; no luminal clots or anatomic causes of external compression were apparent.

The clinical diagnoses were acute cellulitis of the right calf, bilateral lipodermatosclerosis of the calves, and chronic venous insufficiency. Empirical treatment with cloxacillin 500 mg every 6 hours was started. Leg elevation and compression stocking with a gradient of 30-40 mmHg were recommended, but not tolerated by the patient. After 4 days the body temperature returned to normal; there was some fading of the erythema and swelling of right calf. Blood cultures were negative. After 10 days on antibiotic treatment the swelling and erythema were still evident (Figure 9) while the patient was comfortable except for pruritus and a dull discomfort in the right calf.

This case brings in focus several issues of practical importance:

*Infectious cellulitis may be confused with a flare of lipodermatosclerosis* [3]. Lipodermatosclerosis is a form of chronic non-infectious cellulitis that complicates venous insufficiency. It is the consequence of prolonged high pressure in veins, the deposition of fibrin around capillaries, and the resultant impaired $O_2$ diffusion and inflammatory reaction. The inflammatory and fibrosing alterations involve the subcutaneous adipose layer, superficial fascia and perimysium and are similar to the inflammatory and fibrosing process present in eosinophilic fasciitis and its variants. Lipodermatosclerosis comprises a broad spectrum of clinical and pathological manifestations, ranging from an acute inflammatory phase to a chronic fibrotic phase.

Chronic phase lipodermatosclerosis is characterized by induration, a permanent brown-red to violet discoloration of the skin, and an 'inverted wine bottle' configuration of the calf. The diagnosis is easily established on clinical examination and there is usually no need for histological confirmation. In general, biopsies should not be taken because lipodermatosclerosis can lead to poor healing of wounds.

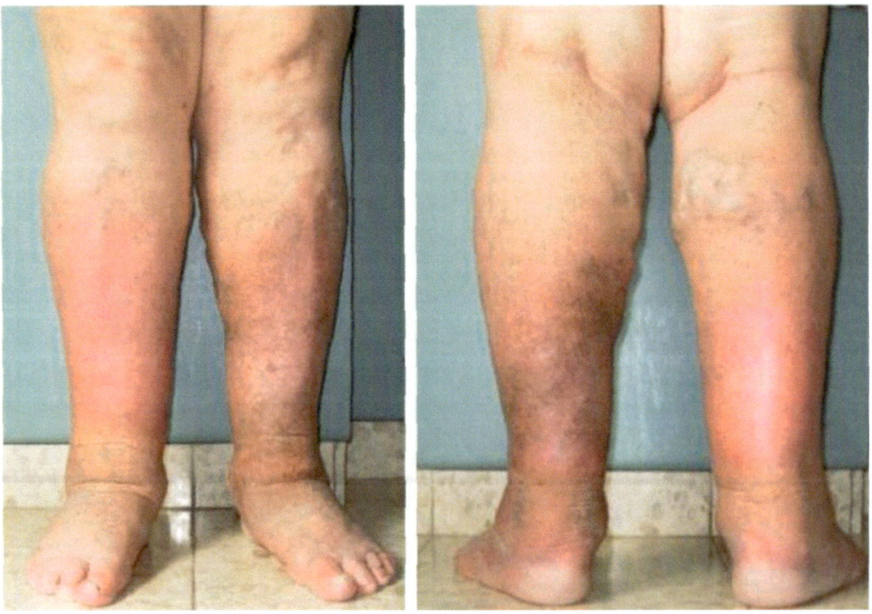

Figure 9. Large varicous veins in the calves, numerous perimaleolar reticular veins, chronic lipodermatosclerosis and acute cellulitis of the right calf.

Acute lipodermatosclerosis and acute exacerbations of chronic lipodermatosclerosis emerge with erythema, warmth, tenderness and swelling of the calf that can easily be confused with infectious cellulitis. Severe pain is a leading symptom in patients with acute lipodermatosclerosis; the patients are often unable to tolerate compression therapy, as in the present patient. Proper diagnosis is important to avoid unnecessary diagnostic procedures, unnecessary treatments, and because acute lipodermatosclerosis responds rapidly to stanozolol.

Yet, the discrimination between acute lipodermatosclerosis and infectious cellulitis is uncertain. We could not find in the literature studies on this topic. In facing such dilemma, clinicians often prescribe a course of antibiotic treatment and, if remission of fever occurs within 2 to 4 days, the favorable response is ascribed by right or not to antibiotic effect. Such quick response to antibiotic treatment was observed in the patient described in this report. For acute lipodermatosclerosis, use of compression gradient stockings or an intermittent pneumatic pump may be helpful if tolerated. Nonsteroidal anti-inflammatory agents are sometimes of benefit and safer than corticosteroids. Stanozolol, an anabolic steroid given over 8 weeks, effectively alleviates pain and reduces dermal thickness in patients with acute lipodermatosclerosis [4]. More recently, dapsone has also been found to be effective for this purpose. Sclerotherapy is efficient for the treatment of acute lipodermatosclerosis. Usually, skin inflammation decreases within a week after sclerotherapy.

*Infectious cellulitis may be confused with* an acute *deep venous thrombosis,* a true dilemma in the early hours after onset of symptoms. Both disorders present with unilateral leg edema, warmth or erythema. Fever may sometimes precede local signs of cellulitis by up to 24 hours, thus adding to the difficulty in making an early diagnosis [1]. In the patient described in this report, chills and high fever occurring from the beginning made deep venous thrombosis unlikely, rather sepsis was suspected.

*Concurrent onset of cellulitis and deep vein thrombosis* is a difficult diagnosis that should not be missed. A true association between deep vein thrombosis and cellulitis has been reported with frequencies ranging from 0 to 15%. On methodical search, only 3 cases of deep vein thrombosis out of 431 consecutive patients with cellulitis of the leg were revealed [2]. The authors concluded that a systematic search for deep vein thrombosis is not warranted in patients with leg cellulitis. However, when prothrombotic risk factors are present in a patient with leg cellulitis, such as immobilization, previous thromboembolism, intravenous injection of illicit drugs, septic phlebitis, chemotherapy through central venous lines, or endovenous laser treatment, it may be reasonable to perform a Doppler ultrasound examination in search of deep vein thrombosis in the affected limb. The accuracy of Doppler ultrasound may be suboptimal in certain settings: venous insufficiency is a common cause of false-negative ultrasound results in the presence of acute venous thrombosis. Therefore, repeated examinations of the lower extremities by ultrasound should be considered for superior diagnostic accuracy.

*Various other disorders can masquerade as cellulitis:* contact dermatitis, especially in the acute form; insect stings which may trigger an extensive regional reaction; eosinophilic cellulitis (Wells syndrome) characterized by acute pruritic dermatitis and eosinophilia; erythema nodosum when presenting as a large solitary erythematous lesion; panniculitis of various etiologies ($\alpha_1$-antitrypsin deficiency, lupus panniculitis, postirradiation panniculitis, Weber–Christian disease, cytophagic histiocytic panniculitis, post-steroid panniculitis, and nodular panniculitis); cutaneous lymphoma; lymphedema; sarcoidosis; subcutaneous plaques in polyarteritis nodosa; pyoderma gangrenosum and Sweet's syndrome.

*Lesions closely resembling erysipelas* may occur in familial Mediterranean fever, inflammatory carcinoma of the breast, early facial herpes zoster, contact dermatitis and giant urticaria. The typical clinical context in each enables to make the diagnosis.

In the present case we diagnosed acute cellulitis of the right calf, occurring on the background of bilateral lipodermatosclerosis of the calves and chronic venous insufficiency. The patient was treated with cloxacillin and leg elevation. The fever and local signs of acute inflammation remitted. She was advised to wear compression stockings and to consult a phlebologist in considering ablation of the varicous veins. Oral penicillin for prophylaxis of erysipelas recurrence was prescribed.

## Learning Points

- Chronic venous insufficiency predisposes to infectious complications, prominent among them being erysipelas and cellulitis of the calves.
- Chronic venous insufficiency also predisposes to development of a chronic, low-grade, non-infectious cellulitis called 'lipodermatosclerosis'.
- Chronic venous insufficiency also predisposes to occurrence of an acute noninfectious cellulitis called 'acute lipodermatosclerosis'.
- The differential diagnosis between acute lipodermatosclerosis and erysipelas is empirical and unsure.

# References

[1] Kennedy D, Setnik G, Li J. Physical examination findings in deep venous thrombosis. *Emerg. Med. Clin. North Amer.* 2001;19:869-876.

[2] Bersier D, Bounameaux H. Cellulitis and deep vein thrombosis: a controversial association. *J. Thromb. Haemost.* 2003;1:867-868.

[3] Bruce AJ, Bennett DD, Lohse CM, Rooke TW, Davis MD. Lipodermatosclerosis: review of cases evaluated at Mayo Clinic. *J. Am. Acad. Dermatol.* 2002;46:187-192. Greenberg AS, Hasan A, Montalvo BM, Falabella A, Falanga V. Acute lipodermatosclerosis is associated with venous insufficiency. *J. Am. Acad. Dermatol.* 1996; 35:566-568.

[4] Vesić S, Vuković J, Medenica LJ, Pavlović MD. Acute lipodermatosclerosis: an open clinical trial of stanozolol in patients unable to sustain compression therapy. *Dermatol. Online J.* 2008;14:1.

# Case 9. Acute Cellulitis and Chronic Stasis Dermatitis

A 72-year-old man presented with high fever, painful swelling of the left calf, leukocytosis and elevated CRP. He had chronic venous insufficiency and a many years long history of eczema of the calves. On physical examination, a chronic, poorly demarcated, scaly, itchy rash was noticed on the calves and the dorsum of the feet, more prominent on the left side. The right calf was swollen, erythematous, and felt warmer than adjacent segments. This poorly defined erythematous area involving the distal 2/3 of the right calf was suggestive either of erysipelas or acute stasis dermatitis. Treatment with cefazolin 1g x 3/day was started, followed by remission of fever within 48 hours and subsequent resolution of the acute inflammatory changes. A diagnosis of infectious cellulitis was proposed. Topical corticosteroid treatment was applied to the eruption on the left calf and foot. The photography shown in the Figure 10 was taken 6 days after beginning antibiotic treatment. This case illustrates acute cellulitis on the right calf occurring on the background of chronic stasis dermatitis.

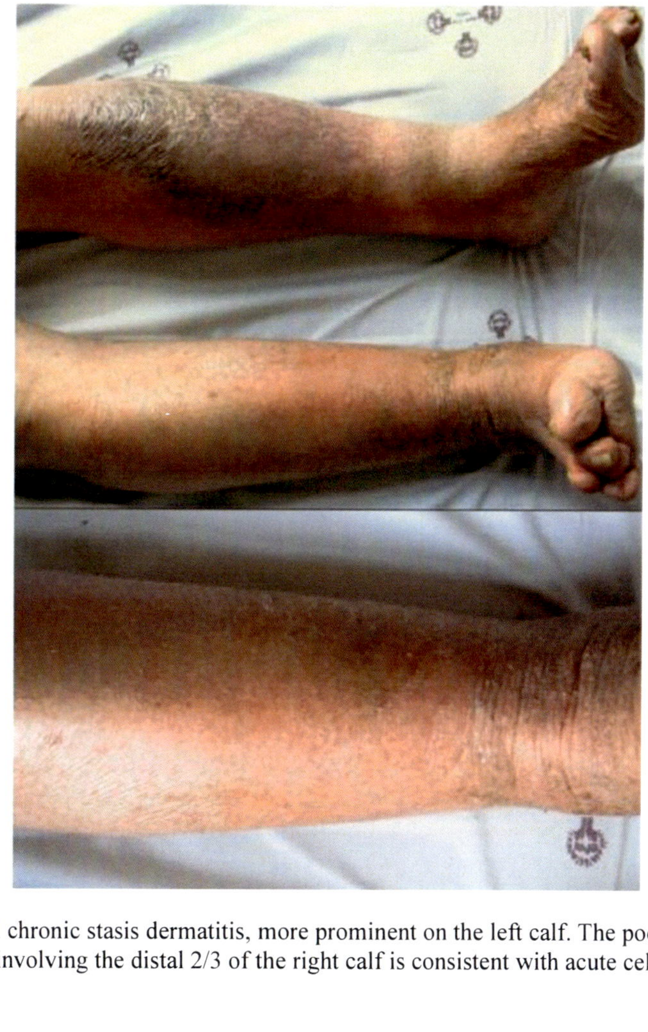

Figure 10. Bilateral chronic stasis dermatitis, more prominent on the left calf. The poorly defined erythematous area involving the distal 2/3 of the right calf is consistent with acute cellulitis.

Stasis dermatitis is heterogeneous group of pruritic inflammatory disorders, stigmatized a 'wastebasket diagnosis'. Some authors suggested that stasis dermatitis represents an allergic response to an epidermal protein antigen generated through increased hydrostatic pressure. Other authors gave emphasis to the role of an increased susceptibility of the skin to irritation and trauma. In agreement with either hypothesis is the fact that calf eruptions similar to stasis dermatitis may be observed in patients with chronic leg edema but without venous insufficiency, or under the influence of vasodilator drugs such as amlodipine [1]. Patients with stasis dermatitis have significantly more positive reactions when patch tested with components of previously used topical agents. Topical medications that contain potential sensitizers such as lanolin, benzocaine, parabens, calamine, and neomycin should be avoided by patients with stasis dermatitis. Propylene glycol is a ubiquitous component of many topical medications, including corticosteroid creams. Propylene glycol is known to cause allergic contact dermatitis, and when considering this possibility topical agents should be replaced with an agent free of propylene glycol. Allergy to corticosteroids in topical medications is also possible.

This case illustrates chronic stasis dermatitis on the left calf and acute cellulitis on the right calf, the latter occurring on the background of chronic stasis dermatitis.

### Learning Point

- The differential diagnosis between acute stasis dermatitis and erysipelas is empirical and unsure.

## References

[1] Barron GS, Jacob SE, Kirsner RS. Dermatologic complications of chronic venous disease: medical management and beyond. *Ann. Vasc. Surg*. 2007;21:652-662.

[2] Weeden D. Skin pathology. 2nd ed. Churchill LivingstoneEdinburgh 2002. p. 112.

[3] Gosnell AL Stasis dermatitis as a complication of amlodipine therapy. *J. Drugs Dermatol.* 2009; 8:135-137.

## Case 10. Acute Stasis Dermatitis

An 84-year-old woman presented with a 10-day history of a burning sensation in the distal part of the calves and an emerging shallow ulcer on the left calf. The body temperature was normal. A swab culture from the skin ulcer grew pseudomonas aeruginosa. Treatment with ciprofloxacine was started and the patient was referred to the Acute Care for Elderly Unit. Her medical history was remarkable for recurrent erysipelas of the calves, aortic stenosis and regurgitation, chronic atrial fibrillation, moderate pulmonary hypertension, tricuspid regurgitation, hiatal hernia, hyperthyroidism, osteoporosis, and atypical ductal hyperplasia on a recent breast biopsy. She was a non-smoker and abstained from alcohol. She was regularly treated with warfarin, propafenone hydrochloride 450 mg/day, propilthiouracil

50 mg/day, hydrochlorothiazide 25 mg/day, omeprasol 20 mg/day, raloxifene 60 mg/day, calcium carbonate 600 mg/day, and penicillin V 500 mg/day (for secondary prophylaxis after recurrent erysipelas).

Her height was 156 cm, weight 65 kg, BMI 27, temperature 36.7$^0$C, BP 132/64 mmHg while standing, and heart rate 77 bpm. A grade 3/6 systolic ejection murmur and a grade 2/4 regurgitant murmur were perceived over the aortic focus. The jugular veins were not engorged and there was no hepato-jugular reflux. Extensive areas of bright red inflammation were noticed in the distal part of the calves and dorsa of the feet, with distinct demarcation between the involved and the normal skin. A number of reticular veins were seen adjacent to the maleoli. No varices were apparent. Two shallow ulcers were present on the antero-lateral aspect of the left calf, 2 x 2 cm in diameter, as well as several tiny exulcerations covered with a sero-sanguinolent exudate. The toe web spaces contained a macerated scale consistent with tinea pedis infection (Figure 11A). The pulsations of the tibialis posterior and dorsalis pedis arteries were normal. In the standing position, the skin color changed almost instantaneously becoming cyanotic, and a substantial swelling of the distal part of the calves occurred within minutes (Figure 11B).

Laboratory studies revealed WBC 11,000/mm$^3$ with 68% neutrophils, and CRP 88 mg/L. The chest x-rays showed an enlarged cardiac silhouette. The ankle brachial indices were 1 and 1.1, respectively. Venous Doppler ultrasonography showed reflux in the femoral vein and in the great saphenous vein. The diagnosis of venous insufficiency was established based on results of the ultrasound examination. Treatment with oral ciprofloxacin was continued for 10 days, topical 10% zinc oxide cream [1] was applied to the erythematous areas, compression bandages to the calves, and antifungal paste to the interdigital spaces. Regular walking was recommended. There was slow and continual improvement of the calf erythema; the serous exudation came to an end.

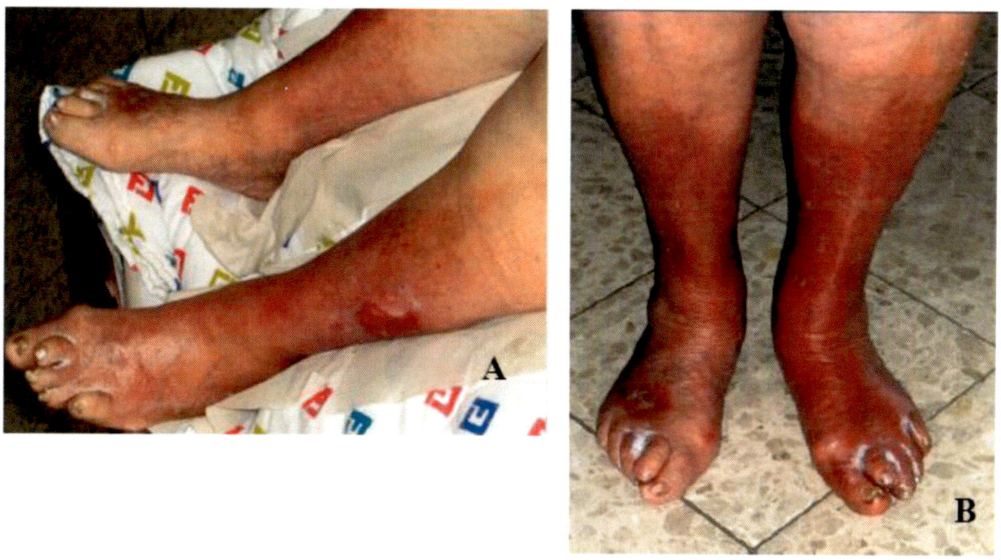


Figure 11. Dermatitis appearing as wide areas of bright red inflammation on the distal parts of the calves and the dorsa of the feet, with distinct demarcation between the involved and the normal skin (A). Two shallow ulcers are visible on the antero-lateral aspect of the left calf. On standing up the skin color changed to cyanotic (B).

In summary, this patient presented with an acute dermatitis resembling erysipelas on both calves, but without associated fever and systemic symptoms. The disorder developed while the patient was taking penicillin V prophylaxis. Isolation of pseudomonas aeruginosa from the base of the skin ulceration was the reason for ciprofloxacin treatment, started before admission to hospital and continued on ward. Several questions were raised:

Is *the surface microflora in leg wounds pertinent* in distinguishing infection from contamination? The ideal method for sampling the microflora of wounds remains controversial. Swabbing alone fails to provide information on the bacteria invading the deep tissue of the wounds. In a prospective study, only 22% of venous ulcers with a positive smear developed a clinical infection. Therefore, distinction between wound colonization and wound infection relies mainly on clinical judgment. In our patient, the growth of proteus in the specimen obtained by swabbing the shallow skin ulceration may signify contamination, since the patient had neither fever, nor debries or purulent discharge [2, 3]. On the other hand the possibility of genuine infection could not be discarded.

*If not erysipelas, what is the nature of the patient's dermatitis*? Easily excluded were contact dermatitis, atopic dermatitis and xerosis. Allergic contact dermatitis rarely occurs with modern wound dressings and is exceptional with zinc oxide topical application. 'Venous eczema' also called chronic stasis dermatitis is a poorly demarcated, scaly eruption that responds well to topical corticosteroid treatment [4] Our patient's dermatitis was clearly different from chronic stasis dermatitis. Acute stasis dermatitis is an appropriate consideration in this case. Acute stasis dermatitis appears as a red, superficial, itchy plaque suddenly emerging on the lower leg. Weeping and crusts may appear. Skin biopsy of stasis dermatitis, although rarely indicated, shows an acute or subacute dermatitis. This acute process can easily be confused with an infectious cellulitis [4]. Even more, stasis dermatitis is often the first manifestation of venous insufficiency that has not been diagnosed previously and needs to be evaluated and treated.

*Acute stasis dermatitis* responds to treatment with systemic antibiotics, wet compresses, and topical steroids [4]. Topical treatment for stasis dermatitis does not differ from treatment of other forms of acute eczematous dermatitis. Weeping lesions can be managed with wet-to-damp gauze dressings soaked with water or with a drying agent, such as aluminum acetate. Topical corticosteroids are frequently used for reducing inflammation and itching in acute flares; triamcinolone 0.1% ointment is usually effective. But, using topical corticosteroids makes the patient more susceptible to infection. Open excoriations and erosions are treated with a topical antibiotic, such as mupirocin. Superficial impetiginization is treated with topical mupirocin or a systemic antibiotic. Our final diagnosis was acute stasis dermatitis as the presenting feature of chronic venous insufficiency.

*The significance of instantaneous cyanosis and edema* that occurred upon assuming the erect position is not a characteristic feature of erysipelas or cellulitis. The diagnosis of acrocyanosis could easily be discarded. Acrocyanosis is characterized by persistent cyanosis of the hands, feet or face. The extremities are cold and clammy and may exhibit some swelling. An other differential is erythromelalgia, characterized by an episodic painful burning sensation, erythema and swelling in the extremities, a disorder very different from the features noticed in our patient. The vasodilatory effect of raloxifene may have contributed to hyperemia in this patient. To explain the instantaneous dependent cyanosis and edema we submit that the increased inflow to the calves (the conjoint effect of dermatitis, raloxifene, and augmented arterial inflow upon assuming the standing position) in addition to diminished outflow (due to venous insufficiency) may have resulted in a substantial engorgement of the microcirculation. The proof to this hypothesis is lacking because plethysmography, with and without proximal venous occlusion, with and without raloxifene administration, was not available.

### Learning Points

- Chronic stasis dermatitis is a persistent, poorly demarcated, scaly and itchy rash occurring on the lower legs usually in patients with venous disease, but also in conjunction lymph stasis and edema due to other disorders.
- Chronic stasis dermatitis is clinically distinct from erysipelas.
- In contradistinction, acute stasis dermatitis appears as a red, superficial, itchy plaque emerging swiftly on leg on the background of venous insufficiency. This acute process can easily be confused with an infectious cellulitis.
- Acute stasis dermatitis may be the first manifestation of an occult venous insufficiency. In such circumstances the diagnosis may be even more challenging.
- Although most cases are diagnosed clinically, a skin biopsy may be indicated when there is no clear history and when physical findings are atypical.

## References

[1] Lansdown AB, Mirastschijski U, Stubbs N, Scanlon E, Agren MS. Zinc in wound healing: theoretical, experimental, and clinical aspects. *Wound Repair Regen.* 2007;15:2-16.

[2] Robson MC, Cooper DM, Aslam R, Gould LJ, Harding KG, Margolis DJ, Ochs DE, Serena TE, Snyder RJ, Steed DL, Thomas DR, Wiersma-Bryant L. Guidelines for the treatment of venous ulcers. *Wound Repair Regen.* 2006;14:649-662.

[3] Lorentzen HF. Clinical assessment of infection in nonhealing ulcers analyzed by latent class analysis. *Wound Repair Regen.* 2006; 14: 350-353.

[4] Barron GS, Jacob SE, Kirsner RS. Dermatologic complications of chronic venous disease: medical management and beyond. *Ann. Vasc. Surg.* 2007;21:652-662.

[5] Weeden D.: Skin pathology. 2nd ed. Churchill LivingstoneEdinburgh 2002. p. 112.

[6] Gosnell AL Stasis dermatitis as a complication of amlodipine therapy. *J. Drugs Dermatol.* 2009; 8: 135-137.

## Case 11. Bilateral Erysipelas-<br>The Differential Diagnosis

A 93-year-old male residing in a nursing home was admitted with vomiting, fever and an eruption involving the calves. Remarkable in his medical history were ischemic heart disease and Alzheimer type dementia. There was no account of heart failure, leg edema or cellulitis. The patient's regular medications were aspirin 100 mg/day and simvastatin 10 mg/day. On admission, the temperature was 39.3°C, heart rate 82 bpm, BP 132/68 mmHg. Erythematous, sharply demarcated plaques were noticed on both calves (Figure 12). A whitish, dry and scaly interdigital eruption was seen on the web between the toes on both feet and extended onto the dorsum of the feet. The physical examination was otherwise unremarkable.

The WBC was 25,300/mm$^3$ and the CRP 128 mg/L. He was treated with intravenous cefazolin and topical clotrimazole in the areas between the toes. The fever resolved and the eruption faded within 4 days. Blood cultures were negative. Bilateral erysipelas of the calves and interdigital tinea pedis was diagnosed.

*The diagnosis of erysipelas* is based on the characteristic appearance of the calf eruption and the clinical setting. The area of inflammation is typically bright red, edematous and distinctly demarcated, and its occurrence is associated with high fever. Bacteriological examination from blood cultures and needle aspiration focused on the erythematous skin lesion rarely provides positive results and is thought unnecessary. The first choice of treatment is antibiotics aimed at streptococci; improvement is expected to occur within a few days [1], as was noticed in this patient. Erysipelas is confined in 70% of patients to one lower extremity, less frequently to the face, but concomitant erysipelas of both legs is probably rare. We could not find in the Medline database a report of bilateral lower extremity erysipelas.

A differential diagnosis was mandatory [2]. Bilateral infectious cellulitis of the lower extremities is an acute infection extending more deeply than erysipelas and lacking the distinctive anatomical features described for erysipelas. The plaque-like erythema nodosum of familial Mediterranean fever may resemble erysipelas, but the clinical context and response to treatment are different. Contact dermatitis or giant urticaria may resemble erysipelas, but are distinguished from the latter by normal body temperature and accompanying pruritus. Chronic venous insufficiency predisposes to uni- or bilateral acute lipodermatosclerosis, which may resemble erysipelas but lasts for several months [3]. Acute stasis dermatitis is usually a complication of venous insufficiency; it presents as red, superficial, itchy plaques emerging on the lower leg; however, there was no evidence of venous insufficiency in our patient [4]. Lymphoma, panniculitides, pyoderma gangrenosum and Sweet's syndrome may masquerade as cellulitis or erysipelas [2].

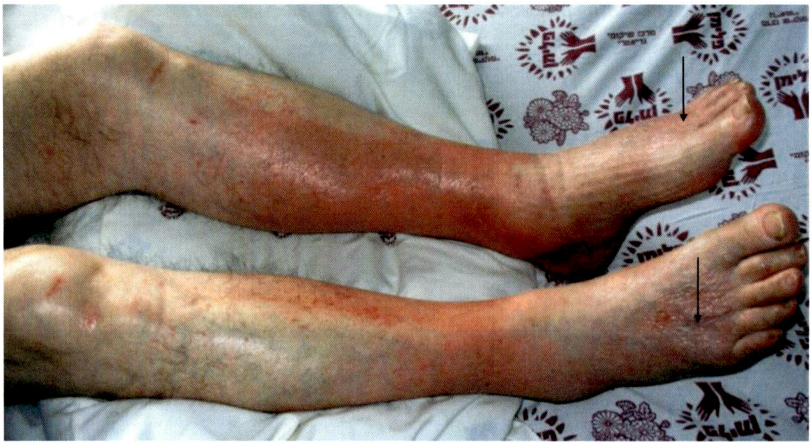

Figure 12. Sleeve-like, bright red, sharply demarcated plaques with irregular borders, extending from below the maleoli to the proximal third of the calves. Notice the scaly eruption spreading from the interdigital web to the dorsum of the feet consistent with tinea (arrows).

In the present case a diagnosis of coincident bilateral erysipelas in association with interdigital tinea was suggested, based on the typical clinical features and the fast response to antibiotic treatment. Pathogens may enter the skin at the site of tinea lesions. It appears that bilateral interdigital tinea was complicated in this patient by bilateral erysipelas of the legs, an unusual but possible occurrence.

### Learning Points

- The diagnosis of erysipelas is based on the clinical appearance of the lesion (bright red, edematous, with distinct demarcation) and the clinical context. Typically, erysipelas is unilateral.
- Predisposed are patients with disrupted skin barrier by trauma, eczema, tinea, impetigo or edema.
- Incidentally, erysipelas may occur simultaneously on both lower extremities.

## References


[1] Stevens DL, Bisno AL, Chambers FE, Dale FE, Everett D, Dellinger P, Goldstein EJC, Gorbach SL, Hirschmann JW, Kaplan EL, Montoya JG, Wade JC. Practice guidelines for the diagnosis and management of skin and soft-tissue infections. Practice guidelines for the diagnosis and management of skin and soft-tissue infections. *Clin. Infect. Dis.* 2005;41:1373-1406.

[2] Falagas ME, Vergidis PI. Narrative Review: Diseases that masquerade as infectious cellulitis. *Ann. Intern. Med.* 2005;142:47-55.

[3] Greenberg AS, Hasan A, Montalvo BM, Falabella A, Falanga V. Acute lipodermatosclerosis is associated with venous insufficiency. *J. Am. Acad. Dermatol.* 1996;35:566-568.

[4] Barron GS, Jacob SE, Kirsner RS. Dermatologic complications of chronic venous disease: medical management and beyond. *Ann. Vasc. Surg.* 2007;21:652-662.


# Case 12. Erysipelas - Three Cycles of Fever

An 80-year-old male nursing home resident presented with 2-day history of aching in the left calf associated with chills and $39^0$C fever. Treatment with amoxicillin/clavulanate was started and the patient was referred to the ward of Acute Care for Elderly. The patient's medical history was remarkable for type 2 diabetes mellitus, ischemic heart disease, arterial hypertension, and mild chronic renal failure. His current medications were clonidine 0.075 x 2/day, propranolol 40 mg x 2/day, furosemide 40 mg/day, aspirin 100 mg/day, simvastatin 20 mg/day, and metformin 1900 mg/day. At the time of admission the patient was alert, the body temperature was $39.3^0$ C, BP 151/67 mmHg, heart rate 66 bpm, SaO2 on ambient air 92%. The left calf was swollen, tender and felt warmer than the adjacent segments.

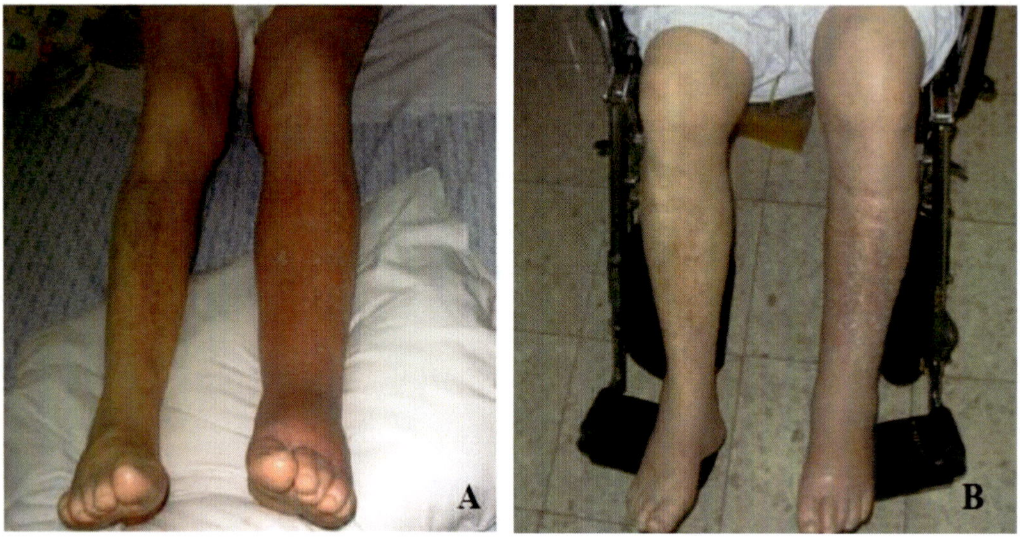


Figure 13. Bright erythema and swelling confined to the patient's left calf and distal aspect of the thigh (A); fading of the erythema on the left calf with concomitant swelling of the right ankle (B).

There was no cutaneous erythema or pitting edema. Otherwise, the examination was unremarkable. Laboratory studies revealed WBC 20,000/mm$^3$ with 86% neutrophils, CRP 274 mg/L, and serum creatinine 2 mg/dL. Treatment with i.v. amoxicillin/clavulanate 1g x 3/day was continued.

Two days on antibiotic treatment, the temperature had decreased to 37.4$^0$ C, while the left calf and distal 10 cm on the left thigh became bright red, the erythematous area being clearly demarcated (Figure 13A). This appearance was consistent with the diagnosis of erysipelas.

Unexpectedly, on the fifth day in hospital, the temperature had risen to 39.2$^0$C. No crepitations were felt over the inflamed area on the leg. The WBC increased to 27,000 with 20% band forms and 66% neutrophils, the serum creatinine was 1.7 mg/dL, the creatinine kinase 44 U/L (within the normal range). Duplex scan of the lower extremities showed normal compressibility and flow in the popliteal and femoral veins; no subcutaneous or deep collection was revealed. At this point in time, clindamycin 600 mg x 3/day i.v. was added and ampicillin/clavulanate was replaced with i.v. cefazolin 1g x 3/day. The temperature returned soon to normal. However, after four days of combined clindamycin – cefazolin treatment the fever relapsed. The recurrence of fever was associated with pain and swelling of the contralateral ankle, mild edema of the contralateral foot, sharp pain in the right wrist, while the erysipelas of the left leg had almost resolved (Figure 13B). The unusual course of fever occurring in three successive cycles was challenging.

*The treatment of choice for erysipelas* had been penicillin for many years. With early treatment the prognosis is excellent [1]. Rarely, however, the process may spread to deeper levels of the skin and soft tissues. If staphylococcal infection is suspected, a penicillinase-resistant semisynthetic penicillin or cephalosporin should be selected. Because the distinction between erysipelas and cellulitis is sometimes impossible the management of both, erysipelas and cellulitis, may benefit from a similar approach. Results of a recent large, prospective study in the USA are reassuring by showing that diffuse nonculturable skin infections (erysipelas and cellulitis) are caused mainly by beta-hemolytic streptococci, even so during the recent MRSA epidemic. For this infection treatment with beta-lactam antibiotics is still effective showing an overall 95% response rate [2]. Treatment with cefazolin or oxacillin is often the initial treatment of choice for both erysipelas and cellulitis. Clindamycin or vancomycin may be used in patients who manifest hypersensitivity to β-lactam antibiotics.

*The expected time to response to antibiotic treatment* of either erysipelas or cellulitis is 1-2 days: time to defervescence 12-16 hours, median time to cessation of erythema advancement 22 hours, median time to improvement of patient-reported pain 40 hours [3]. Lack of clinical response to antibiotic treatment may be due to unusual organisms, resistant strains of staphylococcus or streptococcus, or extension of the infection to deeper tissues (abscess, septic phlebitis, deep vein thrombosis, necrotizing fasciitis or myonecrosis). The lack of lasting resolution of fever on antibiotic treatment in our patient was intriguing. Yet, blood cultures did not grow microbiota, the serum creatinine kinase was repeatedly within the normal range, and ultrasound did not reveal venous occlusion or a collection in the deeper tissues.

*A Herxheimer type reaction* may rarely develop early on antibiotic treatment, characterized by high fever and worsening of the cutaneous inflammation after initiation of a new antibiotic. This type of reaction is probably caused by an enhanced release of enzymes by the pathogen under the effect of bactericidal antibiotics. In the present case, the late relapse of fever on day 5 of treatment is not consistent with a Herxheimer type reaction.

*Several noninfectious disorders* might masquerade as infectious cellulitis or erysipelas [4]. When cellulitis does not respond to conventional antimicrobial treatment, clinicians should consider, among other explanations: *contact dermatitis*, especially in the acute form; *insect stings* which may trigger an extensive regional reaction that may resemble infectious cellulitis; *eosinophilic cellulitis* (Wells syndrome) characterized by acute pruritic dermatitis and eosinophilia; *erythema nodosum* which may sometimes present as a large solitary erythematous lesion resembling infectious cellulitis; *lipodermatosclerosis* which is a form of panniculitis that complicates venous insufficiency and its acute form could masquerade as cellulitis; *panniculitis of various etiologies* ($\alpha_1$-antitrypsin deficiency, lupus panniculitis, postirradiation panniculitis, Weber–Christian disease, cytophagic histiocytic panniculitis, post-steroid panniculitis, and nodular panniculitis); in rare cases, *cutaneous lymphoma* presents as cellulitis. In the case of this patient, the fast progression of skin inflammation at onset, its look typical of erysipelas, and the quick resolution of skin inflammation on antibiotic treatment were consistent with an infectious cause and against other etiologies. Drug fever became a main consideration to explain the first recurrence of fever.

*Drug fever* is diagnosed by revealing the link between the initiation of a drug treatment and the onset of fever (the typical time lag is 5 - 10 days), followed by resolution of fever within 1-2 days of discontinuing the causative drug. Antibiotics are the most frequent cause of drug fever. Drug fever is a diagnosis by exclusion that can be confirmed only after other causes of fever have been discarded. Follow-up is mandatory to attest that the fever subsided spontaneously [5]. Drug fever induced by amoxicillin was the proposed explanation for the patient's second cycle of fever.

*Serum sickness* was considered when a third cycle of fever occurred together with articular pain, while cutaneous symptoms were fading. Serum sickness is a clinical syndrome characterized by fever, arthralgia, urticarial eruption, gastrointestinal disturbances, lymphadenopathy, often proteinuria or nephritis, and sometimes neurological symptoms. Discontinuation of the offending drug and symptomatic treatment with antihistamines and topical corticosteroids is recommended. A short course of oral corticosteroids may be required in patients with severe symptoms. If more than one drug is listed among the possible causes, it is usual to discontinue one drug at one time and a second drug another time. The culprit drug should be avoided in the future.

*Cross-allergy* between cefamezin and amoxicillin was considered in the present case. Indeed, cefamezin, a first-generation cephalosporin, has a modest risk of cross-allergy with penicillins [6]. The patient being treated at this time with cefamezin and clindamycin, cefamezin was discontinued first, while continuing clindamycin treatment. Within 2 days the temperature returned to normal, within 3 days the articular pain and swelling remitted and the WBC decreased. Subsequently, clindamycin treatment was also terminated. Two months after his discharge from hospital there was no recurrence of fever, eruption and arthritis.

Cross-allergy reactions should be distinguished from so-called flare-up reactions. The latter are due to massive immune stimulation during a drug allergy. Because of drug hypersensitivity, in changing one drug with another, the second drug may cause a transient aggravation of preexisting symptoms. The reaction is often misinterpreted as allergy to the second drug; however, this second drug is well tolerated when given later again, in contrast to genuine drug allergy.

Three cycles of fever occurred during the patient's present hospital stay. The first febrile episode was caused by erysipelas and remitted on treatment with ampicillin/clavulanate. The second episode was drug-fever caused by amoxicillin/clavulanate. The third was serum sickness attributed to cefamezin, in suspecting that the patient had cefamezin - amoxycillin cross sensitivity.

## Learning Points

- An important clue to the diagnosis a drug hypersensitivity reaction is the temporal association between initiation of a drug treatment and the onset of the symptoms and signs, as well as the waning of the clinical manifestations upon discontinuation of the drug.
- Drug hypersensitivity reactions account for approximately 15% of adverse drug reactions, and antibiotics are among the most common causes.
- The symptoms of drug hypersensitivity reactions are diverse, nonspecific, and of variable severity.
- Drug fever is a difficult diagnosis because it is confirmed only after other causes of fever are eliminated. Follow-up of patients is mandatory to confirm that the fever subsided spontaneously.
- If more than one drug is listed among the possible causes of drug fever it is recommended to discontinue one drug at one time and a second drug another time.
- When the offender drug is identified, the patient should be provided instruction on avoidance, including a written list of cross-reactive drugs.
- When ambiguity exists which drug induced a severe immunologic reaction, plans should be made to pursue a definitive diagnosis after the patient's convalescence.

- Skin tests, such as patch, prick, and intracutaneous tests are the most readily available form of allergy testing, but often do not yield positive reactions, even in patients with well documented histories.
- Provocation tests are considered to be the gold standard, but carry the risk of severe hypersensitivity reactions.
- In vitro tests are safe. One important limitation of these tests is that they can be performed not earlier than 3 weeks after remission of the drug hypersensitivity reaction; so in vitro tests have no value for taking decisions in real time.

## References

[1] Kroshinsky D, Grossman ME, Fox LP. Approach to the patient with presumed cellulitis. *Semin. Cutan. Med. Surg*. 2007;26:168-178.

[2] Jeng A, Behesti M, Li J, Nathan R. The Role of [beta]-hemolytic streptococci in causing diffuse, nonculturable cellulitis: a prospective investigation. *Medicine* (Baltimore) 2010;89:217-226.

[3] Pertel PE, Eisenstein BI, Link AS, Donfrid B, Biermann EJA, Bernardo P, et al. The efficacy and safety of daptomycin vs. vancomycin for the treatament of cellulitis and erysipelas. *Int. J. Clin. Pract*. 2009;63:368-375.

[4] Falagas ME, Vergidis PI. Narrative Review: Diseases that masquerade as infectious cellulitis. *Ann. Intern. Med*. 2005;142:47-55.

[5] Patel RA, Gallagher JC. Drug fever. Pharmacotherapy. 2010;30:57-69. 6. Pichichero ME. Use of selected cephalosporins in penicillin-allergic patients: a paradigm shift. *Diagn. Microbiol. Infect. Dis*. 2007;57(3 Suppl):13S-18S.

## Case 13. Bullous Disease of Diabetes

A 79-year-old community dwelling man was referred to our ward for difficult to treat dermatitis and edema involving the calves and thighs. The onset has been three months earlier. The patient has been treated with furosemide and topical Aflumycin (prednisolone and gentamicin) and later Diprogenta (bethametasone diproprionate) but without improvement. Remarkable in the patient's history were diabetes mellitus type 2, arterial hypertension, diastolic heart failure (the left ventricular ejection fraction on recent transthoracic echocardiography was 55%), ischemic stroke four years ago with secondary convulsive disorder, cervical spinal stenosis, spondylosis, peripheral obstructive arterial disease, peripheral neuropathy, and chronic renal failure. The medications during the preceding month included glibenclamide 5 mg/day, simvastatin 80 mg, bezafibrate 400 mg, diltiazem 120 mg, clopidogrel 75 mg, aspirin 100 mg, furosemide 80 mg, paroxetine 20 mg, bethahistine 32 mg, brotizolam 0.25 mg, phenytoin 300 mg, propranolol 80 mg, omeprazole 20 mg and folic acid 5 mg/day.

At the time of admission the patient was alert, his body temperature was $36.6^0$C, supine BP 120/60 mmHg, heart rate 72 bpm; after 2 minutes of sitting the BP decreased to 91/45 mmHg. Pulse oxymetry showed SaO2 92%. The body mass index was 33. Pitting edema +++

extended over the buttocks, thighs and calves. Cardiac and pulmonary auscultation was unremarkable. There was no lymphadenopathy, hepatomegaly or splenomegaly. On the extensor aspects of the calves there were several, discrete, erythematous nodules, 0.5 to 2 cm in diameter, and a few larger plaques; several superficial skin ulcers and a few bullae containing a clear fluid were noticed on the calves (Figure 14). Relevant laboratory data were hemoglobin 10.4 g/dL, MCV 97, WBC 10,700/mm$^3$, neutrophils 76%, eosinophils 2%, HbA1C 6.4%, serum creatinine 2.3 mg/dL, BUN 54 mg/dL, albumin 4 g/dL, thyroid-stimulating hormone 4.1 μIU/L. Chest x-rays and the ECG were unremarkable.

The diagnosis focused on possible causes of bilateral, severe leg edema, and on causes of calf dermatitis. A dermatology consultant limited the differential to bullosis diabeticorum, pemphigoid, and contact dermatitis.

*Contact dermatitis* is an inflammation of the skin, caused by getting in direct touch with a specific allergen, and resulting in edema and erythema, usually with superimposed vesicles or bullae. Contact dermatitis may be further categorized as allergic or irritant. Allergic contact dermatitis is a cell-mediated type IV hypersensitivity reaction involving T-cells and arising after a characteristic sensitization step. Sensitization takes approximately one week before the local reaction is induced. During the elicitation phase, re-exposure to the sensitized antigen triggers swiftly the clinical reaction after 24 to 48 hours, the time expected for a type IV hypersensitivity reaction to manifest itself. Detailed history of hygiene habits often reveals the causative agent. Propylene glycol is a ubiquitous substance, known to cause allergic contact dermatitis. It is found in many topical medications, such are moistering lotions and crèmes, electrode gels, and even shaving crème, and also in corticosteroid creams. If dermal allergy to propylene glycol is suspected, the topical agent should be stopped and replaced with an agent not containing propylene glycol.

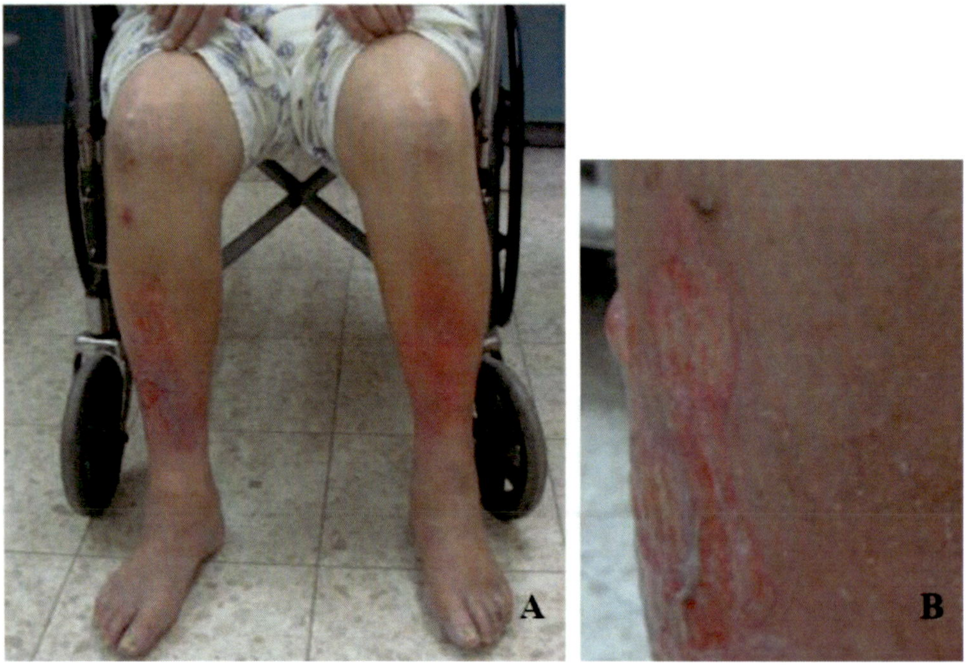


Figure 14. Erythematous nodules and plaques on the anterolateral aspect of the patient's swollen calves (A). Bulla and adjacent shallow skin ulcer (B).

*Bullous pemphigoid* is a relatively benign, autoimmune subepidermal bullous disease, most cases occurring after age 60 years and the frequency increasing with advancing age. Coexistence with other disorders is probably coincidental and there is little evidence of an association with internal malignancy. Drug allergy is often suspected to cause pemphigoid; stopping medications or changing to a different drug may help. Bullous pemphigoid is mediated by autoantibodies that bind to the bullous pemphigoid antigens 230 (BP230) and 180 (BP180). These IgG autoantibodies are found both circulating and bound in the lamina lucida region of the basement membrane zone of the epidermis.

Pemphigoid begins with a localized area of erythema or with pruritic urticarial plaques that gradually become more edematous and extensive. Itching is usually moderate to severe. In most cases the plaques turn dark red or cyanotic in 1 to 3 weeks, as vesicles and bullae appear on their surface. The eruption is usually generalized, but localized variants of bullous pemphigoid have been reported. Bullous pemphigoid may occur at sites of trauma and with little spread of the condition outside such areas. Firm pressure on the blister will not result in the blister's extension into normal skin (Nikolsky's sign is negative) as distinctive feature from pemphigus. Most bullae rupture within a week, leaving an eroded base that, unlike the situation with pemphigus does not spread and heals rapidly. Oral blisters, if present, are mild and transient. The patients remain afebrile, relatively comfortable, and ambulatory. The diagnosis is confirmed with histological studies and direct and/or indirect immuno-fluorescence.

Untreated pemphigoid may remain localized and undergo spontaneous remission, or may become generalized. Treatment with topical corticosteroid is effective; it is superior to oral corticosteroid therapy. Nevertheless, systemic steroids combined with immunosuppressive agents have long been the mainstay of treatment. Antibiotics, dapsone, and topical steroids may be a safe and effective alternative for some patients. Generalized pemphigoid has a poor prognosis in older patients and those in bad general condition. Increase mortality may be related to old age. Among 369 patients hospitalized for bullous pemphigoid, mortality within 1 year was 29%; risk factors for death within 1 year were age >80 years, corticosteroid dose >37 mg at the time of discharge, serum albumin level <3.6 g/dL, and ESR erythrocyte sedimentation rate >30 mm/hour [1].

*Bullous disease of diabetes* (bullosis diabeticorum) is considered a rare disorder. Most reports are limited to a few cases. Affected are mostly elderly persons; Most patients have a background peripheral neuropathy. The lesions are tense blisters evolving rapidly, mostly on the feet. Specific treatment is unnecessary because the condition is self-limiting. The blister should be left intact whenever possible to serve as a sterile dressing and to avoid secondary infection. Staphylococcal superinfections may occur, requiring antibiotic therapy. Aspiration of fluid from bullae may be beneficial to prevent accidental rupture. The median time to healing was 2.5 months (range 0.5-23 months) in one study. The correct diagnosis was often missed and patients were often treated inadequately [2, 3].

*The cause of bilateral leg edema* in our patient was obscure. Four factors may be may be involved in the pathophysiology of bilateral leg edema: increased venous pressure, decreased plasma oncotic pressure, capillary hyperpermeability, and decreased lymphatic drainage. Bilateral leg edema may pose a diagnostic challenge because it is shared by a number of diseases [4]. In distinction, unilateral leg edema may be easily attributed to a local disorder: insect bile, bee sting, contact dermatitis, erysipelas, venous thrombosis, or Baker's cyst. A systematic approach to the patient with bilateral leg edema allows for cost-effective evaluation and treatment. First, leg edema should be distinguished from the expansion of subcutaneous layers by other disease processes: ‘lipedema’, cutaneous myxedema, eosiniphilic fasciitis and the related fasciitis-panniculitis syndrome.

*Lipedema* is a disorder of the adipose tissue that occurs almost exclusively in women, and is characterized by excessive expansion of the adipose tissue symmetrically, usually from the waist to a distinct line just above the ankles, a pattern unlike the common distribution of the adipose tissue in obesity. A distinguishing feature of lipedema is the lack of involvement of the feet. Stemmer’s sign, i.e. squaring of the toes caused by edema in the digits, characterizes lymphedema and is not present in lipedema.

*Pretibial myxedema* is characterized by bilateral, firm, pink or purple-brown nodules and plaques and nonpitting edema, involving the lateral or anterior aspects of the calves, and representing a cutaneous manifestation of thyroid disease.

*Eosinophilic fasciitis* is characterized by swelling and induration of the skin that extends into deeper subcutaneous tissues, and is associated with chronic inflammation and fibrosis. The etiology and pathogenic mechanisms remain elusive. Often, symmetrical limb segments are affected. At the beginning, there is edema and erythema of the involved areas, followed by 'peau d'orange' appearance and in a later phase by woody skin induration. The toes and fingers are spared. The skin induration can lead to joint contractures with limited mobility. Laboratory tests may show peripheral eosinophilia and an elevated erythrocyte sedimentation rate, but these are not mandatory for the diagnosis. Confirmation of the clinical diagnosis is made by surgical skin-to-muscle biopsy, showing swelling and induration of the skin that extends into deeper subcutaneous tissues and is associated with fibrosis and chronic inflammation. Similar pathological findings may be encountered in other disorders, such as morphea profunda, lupus panniculitis, lipodermatosclerosis of chronic venous insufficiency, eosinophilia-myalgia syndrome induced by ingestion of *L*-tryptophan, chronic lymphedema, graft-versus-host reaction, postirradiation injury, chronic Lyme disease, erysipelas, systemic infections and malignant neoplasms. All these disorders share the finding of an indurated skin due to chronic inflammation and fibrosis of the subcutaneous septa and muscular fascia [5].

*Bilateral leg edema secondary to increased venous pressure* may be caused by chronic venous insufficiency, deep venous thrombosis, inferior vena cava thrombosis or compression, compartment syndrome; it may be the remote effect of right heart failure, pulmonary hypertension, constrictive pericarditis, restrictive cardiomyopathy, or tricuspid valvular disease. Transmission of the hydrostatic pressure along the venous colomn extending from the right atrium down to the foot, in the absence of competent venous valves, elicits standing venous pressure up to 100 mmHg. High pressures also can result from external compression or internal occlusion of a large vein. In any case, hyperfiltration in the terminal circulation will result in edema if not compensated by increased lymph drainage. It is often hold that clinical examination in good light provides nearly all the information necessary for the diagnosis of chronic venous insufficiency. However, in one study the predictive value of clinical signs of venous disease did not exceed 0.76 [6]. To increase the accuracy of diagnosis, physical examination should be combined with non-invasive hemodynamic assessment of the venous circulation. Challenging may be a situation, when bilateral leg edema is the presenting sign of constrictive pericarditis or restrictive cardiomyopathy. Echocardiography can allow the differentiation of restrictive cardiomyopathy from pericardial constriction based o different respiratory patterns of ventricular filling [7].

*Bilateral leg edema secondary to increased capillary permeability* may be due to local inflammation, infection, contact dermatitis, burns, vasodilator drugs, or may be idiopathic in case of cyclic edema. Vasodilatory edema is a common adverse effect of antihypertensive therapy. In decreasing order of power, the use of the following drugs may be associated with vasodilatory edema: minoxidil, hydralazine, amlodipine, lercanidipine, doxazocine, antiadrenergic drugs, verapamil, and diltiazem [8]. Vasodilatory edema is dose-dependent. The addition of an angiotensin-converting enzyme inhibitor or an angiotensin receptor blocker to a dihydropyridine calcium antagonist significantly reduces vasodilatory edema. In contrast, giving a diuretic has little effect on vasodilatory edema. Thus, low-dose combination therapy of a dihydropyridine calcium antagonist with either an angiotensin-converting enzyme inhibitor or an angiotensin receptor blocker may be preferred over high-dose monotherapy. Other medications that cause peripheral edema are antidepressants, corticosteroids, estrogens, testosterone, NSAIDs, rosiglitazone, pioglitazone and troglilatazone.

*Edema due to decrease plasma oncotic pressure often* appears in the context of generalized edema. Decreased plasma oncotic pressure may be secondary to malnutrition, liver cirrhosis, nephrotic syndrome, malabsorption, advanced cancer, or beriberi.

In our patient, the findings on physical examination permitted to exclude lipedema, lymphedema, pretibial myxedema, eosinophilic fasciitis and variants of the fasciitis panniculitis syndrome. The plasma albumin level was in the normal range. He was not receiving medications known to increase vascular permeability. Diuretic treatment 180 mg/day furosemide in continuous i.v. perfusion and spironolactone 12.5 mg/day did not result in improvement of edema and in weight loss, but unfortunately caused the serum creatinine to increase from 1.5 to 3.1 mg/dL. Under topical treatment with saline compresses there was no improvement of cutaneous eruption and new bullae emerged. Additional diagnostic work-up comprised spirometry showing severe restrictive lung disease, echocardiography showing normal cardiac anatomy and function, and abdominal CT which was unremarkable, in particular there was no evidence of compression or thrombosis of abdominal veins. Because emergence of prerenal azotemia the diuretic medication was tapered to furosemide p.o. 80 mg/day. A second dermatology consultant gave low priority for taking a skin biopsy.

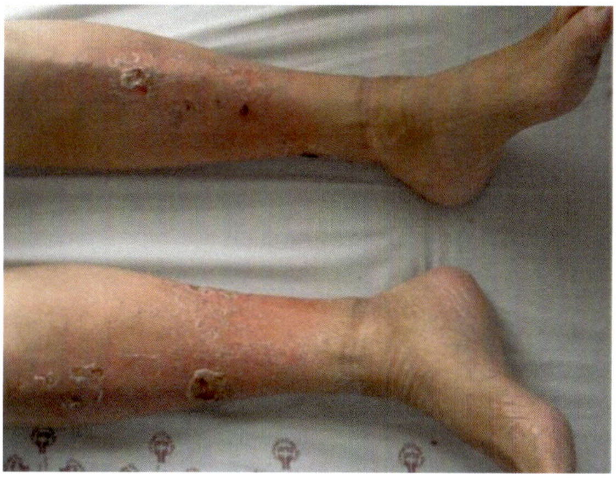

Figure 15. Three weeks later the edema, plaques, bullae and ulcers regressed. Dry crusts cover some of the lesions.

While tapering medications, unexpectedly, the diuresis increased and there was a striking improvement of leg edema and dermatitis (Figure 15). Thus, bilateral leg edema unresponsive to high dose i.v. furosemide surprisingly remitted on half dose oral furosemide.

Bullous dermatitis of the calves in this diabetic person, being refractory to treatment with topical steroids but remitting spontaneously, matches the diagnostic criteria for bullosis diabeticorum. The etiology of bilateral leg edema, however, remains obscure: maybe increased fluid exudation due to dermatitis contributed to the deleterious effects of renal failure on water and electrolyte balance. The pathophysiological link between vesiculo-bullous disorders and leg edema has not been adequately studied; no evidence based recommendations on management can be proposed.

### Learning Points

- Among inflammatory vesiculo-bullous disorders confined to the calves in an elderly person, the main diagnostic alternatives are pemphigoid, contact dermatitis and bullosis diabeticorum. Consultation with a dermatologist may be warranted.
- The blisters should be kept close unless their content becomes turbid and an infection has probably occurred.
- Wet compresses should be applied to the involved area, removed after 30 minutes, and replaced with a freshly immersed cloth. The wet cloth macerates the vesicles and, when removed, mechanically debrides the area and prevents crusts from accumulating.
- Antibiotic treatment is recommended for the treatment of bullous pemphigoid, but is unnecessary and may be harmful in contact dermatitis or bullosis diabeticorum.

## References

[1] Rzany B, Partscht K, Jung M, Kippes W, Mecking D, Baima B, Prudlo C, Pawelczyk B, Messmer EM, Schuhmann M, Sinkgraven R, Büchner L, Büdinger L, Pfeiffer C, Sticherling M, Hertl M, Kaiser HW, Meurer M, Zillikens D, Messer G. Risk factors for lethal outcome in patients with bullous pemphigoid: low serum albumin level, high dosage of glucocorticosteroids, and old age. *Arch. Dermatol.* 2002;138:903-908.

[2] Lipsky BA, Naker PD, Aharoni JH. Diabetic bullae: 12 cases of a purportedly rare cutaneous disorder. *Int. J. Dermatol.* 2000; 39:196-200.

[3] Larsen R, Jensen T, Karlsmark T, Holstein PE. Incidence of bullosis diabeticorum--a controversial cause of chronic foot ulceration. *Int. Wound J.* 2008;5:592-596.

[4] Cho S, Atwood JE. Peripheral edema. *Amer. J. Med.* 2002;113:580-586.

[5] Naschitz JE, Boss JH, Misselevich I, Yeshurun D, Rosner I. The fasciitis-panniculitis syndromes. Clinical and pathologic features. *Medicine* (Baltimore) 1996;75:6-16.

[6] Nelzén O, Bergqvist D, Lindhagen A. Venous and non-venous leg ulcers: clinical history and appearance in a population study. *Br. J. Surg.* 1994;81:182-187. 7.
[7] Khandaker MH, Espinosa RE, Nishimura RA, Sinak LJ, Hayes SN, Melduni RM, Oh JK. Pericardial disease: diagnosis and management. *Mayo Clinic Proceedings* 2010;85: 572-593.
[8] Messerli FH. Vasodilatory edema: a common side effect of antihypertensive therapy. *Cur. Cardiol. Rep.* 2002;4:479-482.

*Chapter III*

# Skin Ulcers

There are four common types of skin ulcers: pressure ulcers, venous ulcers, ischemic and neuropathic ulcers. Numerous uncommon skin ulcers are classified as follows: 1) vasculitic ulcers (thrombangiitis obliterans, microscopical variant polyangiitis nodosa, cryoglob-uninemia, rheumatoid arthritis, Wegener's granulomatosis, systemic lupus erythematosus, nodular vasculitis, cholesterol embolism, antiphospholipid antibody syndrome, calci-phylaxis); 2) ulcers complicating hematological disorders (sickle cell anemia, warfarin-induced skin necrosis, heparin-induced thrombocytopenia, disseminated intravascular coagulation, essential thrombocythemia, therapy with hydroxyurea); 3) ulcers induced by trauma (burns, cold, factitial, stings, bites, skin aging); 4) ulcers complicating metabolic disorders (diabetes mellitus, necrobiosis lipoidica diabeticorum, gout); 5) panniculitides (Weber Christian disease, pancreatic fat necrosis, alpha1-antitripsin deficiency); 6) neutrophilic dermatoses (pyoderma gangrenosum, Sweet's syndrome);7) infections (ecthyma gangrenosum, furuncle, mycobacterial Burundi ulcer, erythema induratum Bazin, septic emboli, cutaneous leishmaniasis, cutaneous antrax, syphilis, leprosy, fungal infection, trichophytin granuloma, cryptococcus neofomans, coccidioides immitis);8) exulcerated neoplasia (cutaneous T cell lymphoma, basal cell carcinoma, metastatic tumors, Kaposi sarcoma, squamous cell carcinoma, Merkel cell tumor, malignant transformation of a benign ulcer or scar).

The common etiologies of skin ulcers - pressure sores, trauma, ischemic, venous, and neuropathic ulcers - are easily diagnosed. Atypical skin ulcers may pose challenging diagnostic problems. This chapter is dedicated to the latter.

## Case 14. Dissecting Hematoma of the Skin

A 72-yr-old woman was suffering from progressive disability due to heart failure and chronic obstructive pulmonary disease. She was treated with furosemide, enalapril, pravastatin, verapamil, alopurinol and warfarin. Echocardiography showed severe pulmonary hypertension, mild aortic regurgitation, mild mitral stenosis and regurgitation; the diameter of left atrium was 48 mm; left ventricular contractility was preserved. Recently, she was admitted to the department of internal medicine with exacerbation of chronic obstructive pulmonary disease. Treatment with prednisone was instituted, initially 40 mg/day than tapered to 20 mg/day; ciprofloxacin was added. She was transferred to our ward for subacute care and reconditioning, receiving furosemide 120 mg/day, enalapril 20 mg, pravastatin 20 mg, verapamil 120 mg, alopurinol 100 mg, prednisone 20 mg/day, warfarin 2.5 mg/day, and ciprofloxacin 1 g/day. At the time of her arrival to our ward she was confused. The body temperature was 36.8$^0$C, BP 120/72 mmHg, heart rate 86 bpm, respiratory rate 32 /min, arterial oxygen saturation 76% while breathing ambient air and 93% on nasal oxygen mask. The jugular veins were engorged. The thorax showed a barrel type deformity. Dry crackles were perceived over the lower half of the lung fields, and a grade 4/6 systolic murmur and 2/4 diastolic murmur at the cardiac apex.

The skin in the distal areas on the calves showed a mix of brown and violet shades. Fourteen shallow skin lesions were counted over the distal areas of the left thigh and left calf; these lesions measured 0.5 – 1 cm in diameter, were well demarcated, round, with slightly irregular borders; the lesions were covered by crusts of apparently different ages. Laboratory tests were remarkable for CRP 30 mg/L, serum creatinine 1.6 mg/dL, albumin 3.3 g/L, PT-INR 2.4, and activated partial prothrombin time 32 seconds. Results of CBC, liver function tests and urinalysis were within the normal range. Chest x-rays showed an alveolar infiltrate confined to the lower lobe of the left lung. The patient's previous medications were continued except for ciprofloxacine that was replaced by piperacillin-tazobactam 4.5g x 3/day intravenously, and oxygen administered continuously by nasal mask.

The disease course was complicated by a succession of events: delirium that remitted after tapering the dose of prednisone to 5 mg/day; watery diarrhea clostridium toxin negative that remitted on oral metronidazole treatment; and a difficult to achieve warfarin therapeutic goal (PT-INR was in the range 1.3 to 1.7). While still receiving 20 mg of prednisone/day, two echymoses emerged on the extensor aspect of the patient's left forearm, which subsequently evolved into hemorrhagic blisters. The larger of the two blisters reached 5 cm in diameter, had peripheral red borders and a violaceous liquid center. The content of the blister was aspirated and grew methicillin-resistant Staphylococcus aureus. Skin punch biopsies were taken from the peripheral rim of the lesion. Treatment with vancomycin was administered intravenously and hydrogel dressings were applied locally. A few days later, the lesion had transformed into a well demarcated ulcer with violaceous undermined borders and a clean basis (Figure 16).

Histological examination of the skin biopsy specimen showed a mixed cellular infiltrate in the epidermis, dermis and subcutaneous layers. No granulomas or intracellular microbiota were seen. The patient's general state was improving, the body temperature was normal, there was neither purpura nor mucosal bleeding, and results of ancillary laboratory tests remained essentially unchanged. Results of tests for antinuclear antibodies, C3 and C4 complement fractions, rheumatoid factor, anti-neutrophil cytoplasmic antibodies, antiphospholipid antibodies, lupus anticoagulant, immune globulins IgG, IgA and IgM were unremarkable.

*The differential diagnosis* concentrated on a gamut of dermatological disorders, cutaneous manifestations of systemic diseases, and iatrogenic effects of corticosteroids and warfarin treatment. A 'pattern diagnosis' was attempted based on the appearance of the smaller skin lesions (that went through evolutionary stages of shallow skin necrosis covered by a crust) and the larger lesion (that went through evolutionary stages of a hemorrhagic blister to deep skin ulcer). The latter lesion was reminiscent of pyoderma gangrenosum.

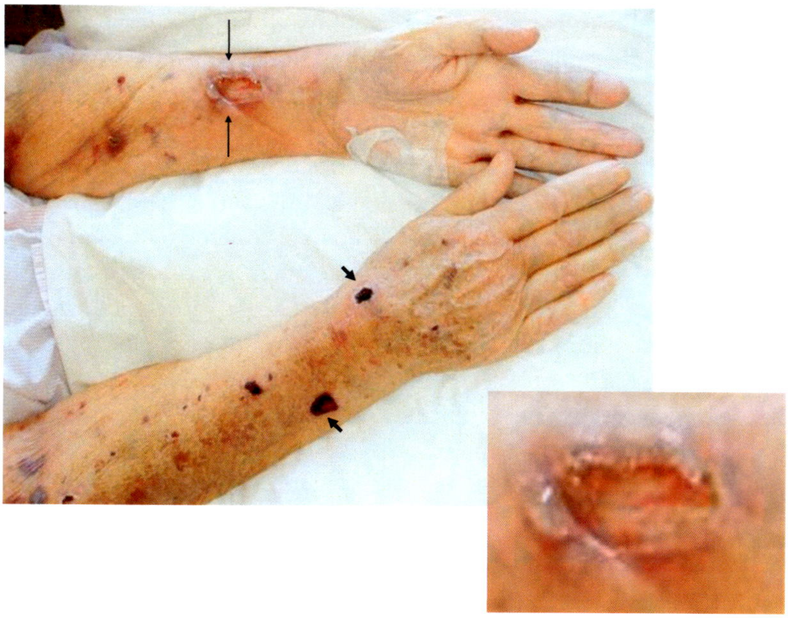

Figure 16. A skin ulcer is seen on the volar aspect of the left forearm (thin arrows). A magnification of the ulcerated area is shown in the inset. A scaling crust surrounded by ecchymosis is seen 10 cm proximally to the ulcer. These two lesions represent different outcomes of hemorrhagic blisters, which proceeded by 7-10 days to the findings seen in the photograph. Numerous small lesions covered by brownish-violet crusts are seen on the dorsal aspect of the right forearm (thick arrows).

*Pyoderma gangrenosum* may occur as a primary disorder or in association with another disease, most often ulcerative colitis, regional enteritis, leukemia, preleukemic states or monoclonal gammopathies. Patients with pyoderma gangrenosum usually describe the initial lesion as a small, red papule or pustule changing into a larger ulcerative lesion. Lesions may occur singly or in groups, most commonly on the lower extremities, although they may appear anywhere on the body. The lesions have a liquefying center, purple undermining borders and may be covered by hemorrhagic blisters. Pathergy, the phenomenon whereby lesions of a disease can be induced at sites of skin trauma, occurs in up to 50% of patients. Pain is a common complaint of patients with pyoderma gangrenosum [1]. Pain was not present in our patient. The two primary variants of pyoderma gangrenosum are the classical ulcerative form usually occurring on the legs, and the more superficial variant known as atypical pyoderma gangrenosum that often occurs on the upper extremities.

The histopathologic findings in pyoderma gangrenosum are not specific. Nevertheless, taking a biopsy is recommended in almost all affected patients in being useful to exclude other diseases. Microscopic features of pyoderma gangrenosum are a massive neutrophilic infiltration associated with hemorrhage and necrosis of the overlying epidermis. Neutrophils may be observed around and within the vessel walls but the full picture of vasculitis is usually absent. In view of the nonspecific features on histological examination, the diagnosis of pyoderma gangrenosum rests on the constellation of clinical and pathologic features and on exclusion of other conditions that may cause skin ulcers. [1]

Therapy of pyoderma gangrenosum is based on corticosteroids and immunosuppressants. The smaller early lesions may be treated with intra-lesional injection of triamcinolone. Systemic corticosteroids are recommended for larger active or fully evolved lesions.

Prednisone 40 to 80 mg daily is required for initial control of the disease, followed by later down-tapering the dose. If there is no response after 10 days the dose is increased to 100 to 120 mg/day. Wound dressings are useful to minimize the pain and the risk of secondary infection. The lesions heal without eschar formation.

Overall, the appearance of the patient's larger lesion was consistent with the superficial variant of pyoderma gangrenosum known as atypical pyoderma gangrenosum, provided all other etiologies of skin ulceration could be excluded. The numerous minute lesions on the patient's extremities but sparing the trunk could be explained as manifestations of pathergy. However, there were several inconsistencies with the diagnosis of pyoderma gangrenosum. First, the skin lesions had appeared while the patient was receiving prednisone, initially 40 mg and later 20 mg/day. The emergence of pyoderma gangrenosum under pharmacologic-dose prednisone treatment is unusual. Later in the course of hospitalization, under the impression that prednisone might be the cause of the patient's confusional state, the dose was tapered to 5 mg/day. The delirium remitted and at the same time the skin lesions improved. The relatively fast improvement under physiological doses of the glucocorticoid is inconsistent with the typical course of pyoderma gangrenosum. Pyoderma gangrenosum being a diagnosis by exclusion, other entities were considered in the differential diagnosis.

Easily excluded based on clinical findings, histology and results of laboratory tests was a spectrum of ischemic ulcers, vasculitides, infectious ulcers (ecthyma gangrenosum, furuncle, mycobacterial and fungal ulcers), and ulcerated neoplasms.

*Dissecting hematoma of the skin* is a complication due to mechanical fragility of the skin. It occurs predominantly in the lower extremities of old persons suffering from skin aging ('dermatoporosis'). There is a female predisposition to dermatoporosis in general and dissecting hematoma of the skin in particular. Dissecting hematomas of the skin may be precipitated by anticoagulant or corticosteroid therapy (as this patient was receiving). Minimal trauma may cause massive bleedings into the virtual space between the dermis and subcutaneous adipose tissue or the subcutaneous adipose layer and the muscle fascia. The evolving hematoma can compromise the blood supply to the skin and cause necrosis. In such situation immediate surgical evacuation of the hematoma and necrotic tissues should be performed to avoid extensive skin damage [2].

The final diagnosis in this patient was dissecting hematoma of the skin, predisposed by dermatoporosis, anticoagulant and corticosteroid treatment. Three months later the ulcer and the minute skin lesions were healed.

## Learning Points

- Common skin ulcers in the elderly are due to ischemia, venous insufficiency, neuropathy or trauma; they are easily diagnosed.
- Atypical skin ulcers may pose challenging diagnostic problems: a spectrum of vasculopathies, infections affecting the skin, ulcerated neoplasms, panniculitis and neutrophilic dermatoses should be considered in the differential diagnosis.
- Among the clinical manifestations of skin aging, dissecting skin hematomas cause significant morbidity needing hospitalization and urgent surgical procedures.

## References

[1] Callen JP, Jackson JM. Pyoderma gangrenosum: an update. *Rheum. Dis. Clin. North Am.* 2007;33:787-802.

[2] Saurat H. Dermatoporosis. The functional side of skin aging. *Dermatology* 2007;215: 271-272.

# Case 15. Ischemic Leg Ulcers on Typical and on Unusual Sites

A 60-year-old community dwelling man with mild mental retardation and type II diabetes mellitus developed painful ulcers on the right knee, heel, and first toe. He was until recently well and not taking medications. On physical examination, the body temperature was normal, the heart rate was 72 bpm, and the brachial BP was 134/72 mmHg comparable on both sides. The radial and carotid pulses felt normal, but the femoral and distal leg pulses were not palpable. Round and well demarcated skin ulcers were noticed on the right knee, heel and big toe, their bases being covered by a brownish fibrin deposit (Figure 16). The ankle brachial indices were 0.19 on the right and 0.36 on the left side, consistent with severe ischemia. The serum creatinine was 0.9 mg/dL, total cholesterol 155 mg/dL, triglycerides 116 mg/dL, TSH 1.4 mIU/L; levels of cadiolipin, homocystein, vitamin B12 and folic acid were within the normal range.

On CT angiography, the lumen of the abdominal aorta was irregular and narrowed, both iliac arteries exhibited extensive stenoses, and there were segmental successive stenoses along the right superficial femoral artery; more distal arterial segments were not narrowed (Figure 18).

The patient's clinical and angiographic findings were consistent with aortoiliac occlusive disease (Leriche syndrome). The patient was referred to vascular surgery. Following the stenting of the iliac arteries the distal pulses became at once palpable. The good result observed immediately after revascularization was confirmed on follow-up by the healing of the ischemic leg ulcers.

*Ulcers due to arterial insufficiency* typically occur on the toes, heels or anterior shin, are round or punched-out and well demarcated, their base is covered by a yellow fibrin layer or necrotic eschar. Affected patients complain of intermittent claudication and ischemic rest pain. On physical examination, chronic limb ischemia is characterized by hair loss, skin atrophy, nail dystrophy, and decreased or not palpable pulses. The ankle-brachial index is usually <0.7. Peripheral obstructive arterial disease is the common cause of ischemic leg ulcers [1]. Infrequent causes of ischemic ulcers are thrombangiitis obliterans (typically a disease of young male smokers), vasculitis (microscopical variant polyangiitis nodosa, cryoglobuninemia, rheumatoid arthritis, Wegener's granulomatosis, systemic lupus erythematosus, nodular vasculitis), cholesterol embolism, antiphospholipid antibody syndrome, and calciphylaxis.

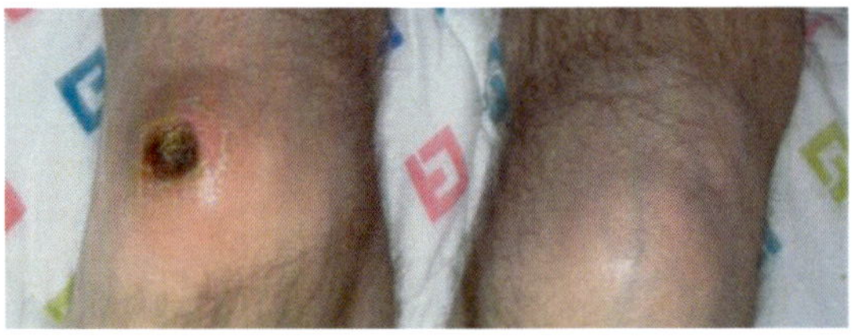

A.

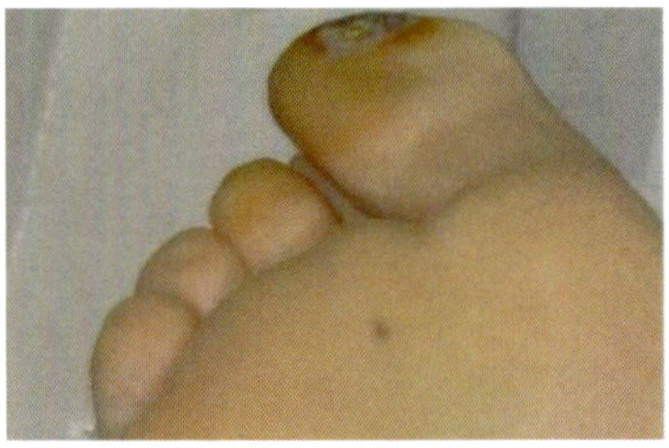

B.

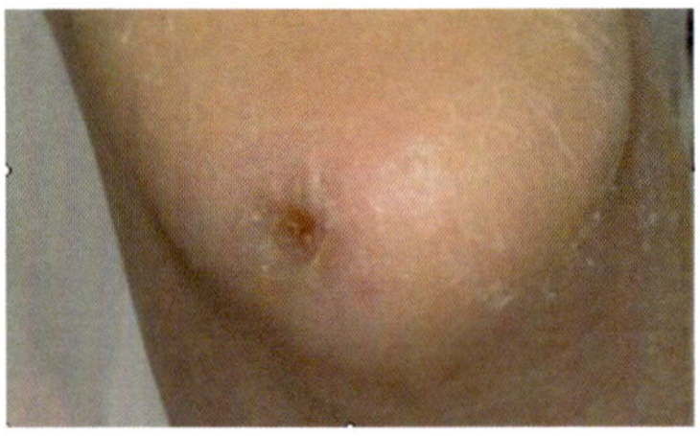

C.

Figure 17. Ischemic skin ulcers on the right leg: the right knee (A), first toe (B) and heel (C).

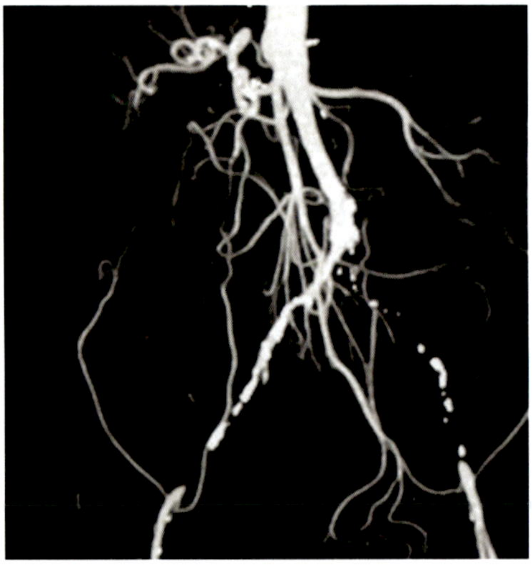

Figure 18. CT angiography showing severe aorto-iliac disease.

*Absent femoral pulses* in the patient under discussion focused the differential diagnosis on diseases of large arteries: congenital aortic coarctation, aortic dissection or occlusive aorto-iliac disease. The latter diagnosis was established on CT angiography. Patients with aortoiliac occlusive disease (Leriche syndrome) complain of buttock or thigh claudication or, occasionally, rest pain. Impotence in men may also point to aortoiliac occlusive disease. Femoral pulses are absent or markedly reduced. Pulse volume recordings show damped or monophasic signals over the femoral arteries. Rarely, aortoiliac occlusive disease is a source of peripheral atheroemboli. Leriche syndrome often necessitates angioplasty. Lesions at the aortic bifurcation and proximal common iliac arteries can be safely stented. However, surgery is often required: aorto-bifemoral bypass, endarterectomy of the aorta and iliacs, or extra-anatomic bypass (axillo-bifemoral bypass or femoro-femoral bypass). Mortality rates for aorto-bifemoral bypass are 4% to 6% [2].

### Learning Points

- Ischemic ulcers typically occur on the toes, heels or anterior shin, are round or punched-out and well demarcated.
- Peripheral obstructive arterial disease is the common cause of ischemic ulcers; one of its uncommon variants is aortoiliac occlusive disease (Leriche syndrome)
- Leriche's triad comprises claudication in the thighs or buttocks, absent or diminished femoral pulses, and impotence.
- Leriche syndrome often necessitates angioplasty or vascular surgery, in distinction from standard management of peripheral obstructive arterial disease which usually is non-invasive.

## References

[1] Olin JW, Sealove BA. Peripheral artery disease: current insight into the disease and its diagnosis and management. *Mayo Clin. Proc.* 2010;85:678-692.

[2] Krankernberg H, Schlüter M, Schwencke C, Walter D, Pascotto A, Sandstede J, Tübler T. Endovascular reconstruction of the aortic bifurcation in patients with Leriche syndrome. *Clin. Res. Cardiol.* 2009;98:657-664.

## Case 16. Unusual Pressure Ulcer

A 69-year-old man was referred in March 2011 with the diagnosis of urinary tract infection. His medical history was remarkable for fibrous histiocytoma in the left thigh diagnosed in 1987; the tumor was resected and radiation therapy was administered. In 2000 a pathological fracture of left femur occurred, without evidence of tumor recurrence, and was treated by nailing. In 2006 there was loosening of the femoral nail. A lytic lesion in the femoral shaft was exposed and turned out to be caused by osteosarcoma. Combined chemo-therapy and radiation therapy were administered. More recently, a solitary pulmonary nodule was revealed on chest x-rays, and left femoral vein thrombosis on venous ultrasound. The patient's latest medications were enoxaparin 120 mg/day, pregabalin, oxycontin and levothyroxine.

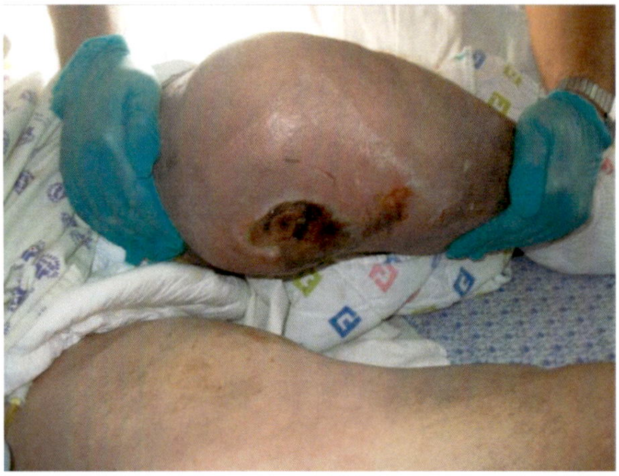

Figure 19. Large grade 4 skin ulcer adjacent to the knee.

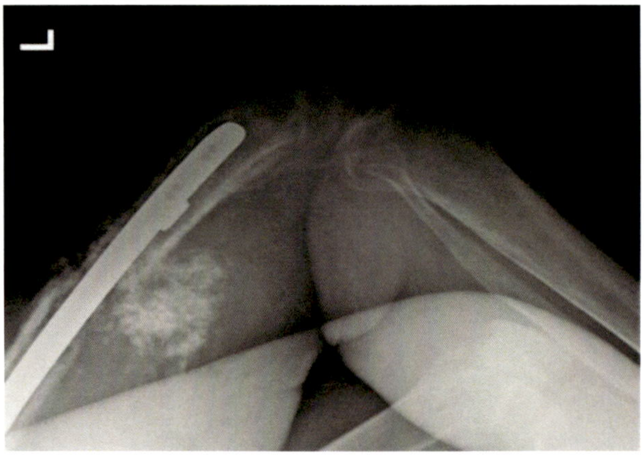

Figure 20. Extensive destruction of the femoral shaft, prominent periosteal reaction, and adjacent large radio-dense mass with cloudy appearance.

His vital signs were within normal limits, except for a temperature of 38.8°C.

On physical examination there was severe lymphedema of the left thigh and calf, flexion-contracture of the left thigh and calf, several grade 2 to 4 pressure sores on the left thigh, right buttock, and both heels. The large ulcer on the medial aspect of the left knee had irregular margins and a maximal diameter of 6 cm; it was 3 cm deep; a few islands of necrotic tissue were noticed on ulcer's base (Figure 19). A plain x-ray of the left thigh exhibited dense tumor-bone formation, a sunburst pattern of periosteal reaction, and severe resorption of the femoral shaft (Figure 20).

The patient received empirical treatment with ciprofloxacine and the fever and urinary symptoms subsided. Topical treatment of the skin ulcer was of no perceptible benefit.

*To identify infection of a chronic wound*, most practitioners rely solely on the presence of purulent exudate, heat, edema, and erythema. Yet, the latter signs may be absent in the presence of wound infection. The current reference standard for diagnosis of infection is a deep tissue biopsy culture. A search of multiple databases aimed to determine the accuracy of clinical symptoms and signs to diagnose infection in chronic wounds and to determine whether there is a preferred noninvasive method for culturing chronic wounds [1]. Analysis of the data showed that an increase in the level of pain (likelihood ratio range, 11-20) made infection more likely, but its absence (negative likelihood ratio range, 0.64-0.88) did not rule out infection. Other items in the history and physical examination, in isolation or in combination, appeared to have limited utility when infection was diagnosed in chronic wounds. The appearance of the wound exudate, serous exudate versus purulent, is not useful to predict infection when the reference standard is a deep tissue biopsy culture. Routine laboratory studies had uncertain value in predicting infection of a chronic wound. Evidence suggests that the swab culture provides no information (likelihood ratio range CI crosses 1.0), unless Levine technique is used. Levine's technique consists in rotating the swab over a 1x1-cm area for 5 seconds with sufficient pressure to extract fluid from within the wound tissue. Yet, if the physician assesses the probability of infection as 90% because of the presence of pain, a negative swab result with Levine technique still confers a probability of 81% for infection.

*Neoplasias are uncommon causes of skin ulcers.* Several types of skin tumors may exulcerate: cutaneous T cell lymphoma, basal cell carcinoma, metastatic tumors, Kaposi sarcoma, squamous cell carcinoma, Merkel cell tumor. Tumor in scar may result from the malignant transformation of a benign ulcer or scar (Marjolin's ulcer). Basal cell carcinoma, squamous cell carcinoma, and Marjolin's ulcer may have an appearance similar to a chronic or an acute wound. Diagnosis of 'wound malignancy' is of particular concern in the geriatric population as the average age for presentation of squamous cell cancer is 70 years. Hence, a biopsy should be obtained from all ulcers and wounds that do not respond to appropriate protocols of care. An accurate diagnosis is essential for positive treatment outcomes [2].

*Osteosarcoma*, previously diagnosed in this patient, is characterized by the production of osteoid by malignant cells. Primary osteosarcomas occur at the sites of the most rapid bone growth, including the distal femur, the proximal tibia, and the proximal humerus. Secondary osteosarcomas occur most often at the site of another disease process, such as previous radiation treatment as in this patient. The time to presentation of secondary osteosarcomas averages 10 to 15 years after radiation exposure. Plain radiographs are valuable tools for the diagnosis. The most common appearance is that of an aggressive lesion in the metaphysis of a long bone, with areas of bone production and bone destruction. With rapidly growing processes, the periosteum cannot produce new bone as fast as the lesion is growing. Therefore, rather than a solid pattern of new bone formation, one sees an interrupted pattern. This interrupted pattern can manifest as a thin shell of calcified new bone, a lamellated or 'onion-skin' reaction, or a pattern called 'sunburst' or 'hair-on-end' periosteal reaction [3]. With multiagent chemotherapy and appropriate surgical treatment most studies report long-term survival in 60% to 75% of patients with high-grade osteosarcoma without metastases at initial presentation and 90% for low-grade lesions.

The large ulcer in our patient's thigh was not caused by direct extension of the tumor to the skin. We thought that it was an atypical pressure sore. The unusual location of the pressure sore in this case could be explained by the combined effects of the sustained pressure exerted by the bony mass on the surrounding soft tissues, knee-to-knee friction, venous and lymphatic stasis, leading to repeated and difficult to treat infections.

### Learning Points

- Skin ulcers on unusual sites may be due to unusual causes.
- Malignant tumors originating in the skin or secondarily invading the skin may cause atypical skin ulcers.
- A biopsy should be obtained from skin ulcers that do not respond to care; an accurate diagnosis is essential for positive treatment outcomes

## References

[1] Reddy M, Gill SS, Wu W, Kalkar SR, Rochon PA. Does this patient have an infection of a chronic wound? *JAMA* 2012;307:605-611.
[2] Snyder RJ. Skin cancers and wounds in the geriatric population: a review. *Ostomy Wound Manage*. 2009;55:64-76.
[3] Craft AW. Osteosarcoma: the European Osteosarcoma Intergroup (EOI) perspective. *Cancer Treat Res*. 2009;152:263-74.

## Case 17. Skin Ulcers in a Patient with Chronic HCV Infection

A 64-year-old woman was referred on June 21$^{st}$ 2011 for treatment of chronic skin ulcers. She was living until recently independently in the community. Remarkable in the patient's medical history were diabetes mellitus type 2 diagnosed in 1984, chronic HCV hepatitis diagnosed in 1994, piecemeal necrosis and bridging fibrosis shown on liver needle biopsy in 1998. Subsequently she had received a course of interferon alpha and ribavirin treatment. She suffered from arterial hypertension and ischemic heart disease. In December 2010 she underwent coronary artery bypass surgery with a venous graft collected from her right leg, as well as aortic valve replacement with a biologic graft. Echocardiography showed diastolic impairment and preserved systolic left ventricular systolic function.

The site on the right calf wherefrom the vein had been harvested did not heal and advanced into a progressively growing ulcer. Purpura, also noticed in December 2010, was the reason for taking skin biopsies from the left calf; the biopsy sites evolved also into growing ulcers (Figure 21A). Topical wound treatment and systemic antibiotics were of no avail. In April 2011 the patient was admitted to the department of plastic surgery with the diagnosis of infected calf wounds and adjacent cellulitis; debridement, topical wound management and systemic antibiotics did not prevent further deterioration. The patient's regular medications were aspirin 100 mg, valsartan 80 mg, bisoprolol 10 mg, insulin glargine 28 U, insulin actrapid 10 U x 3/day, and vitamin D3 600 mg/day.

At the time of admission to our ward in June 2011 the patient was alert, the temperature was 36.5$^0$C, BP 118/56 mmHg, heart rate 68 bpm, respirations 16/min, SaO2 in ambient air 98%. The skin was pale. A maculo-papular eruption was noticed on the patient's chest and buttocks, with a few lesions covered by crusts, others were exulcerated, and one lesion had the appearance of a round punched-out ulcer (Figure 21B). The salient pathology was confined to the calves, were livedo reticularis, large ulcers with undermined borders, and several superficial ulcers were present (Figure 21C). The spleen was palpable 4 cm below the costal margin. The remainder of the physical examination was unremarkable.

The hemoglobin was 10 g/dL, MCV 72 fL, serum iron 23 mcg/dL, transferin saturation 5.8%, serum creatinine 1.8 mg/dL (prior to cardiac surgery the serum creatinine was 0.98 - 1.1 mg/dL). Other laboratory tests yielded the following results: HCV antibodies +, HBsAg -, C3 normal, C4 fraction of complement 3.2 mg/dL (normal >14 mg), rheumatoid factor 368 IU/mL (+++), citrulinated peptide 0.3 U/mL (normal), cryoglobulin ++. The following tests were negative or within the normal range: cANCA, pANCA, ANA, anti dsDNA, SSA, SSB, IgG, IgM, IgA. The CRP was 5 mg/L (pseudo normal?) and the ESR 32 mm/1hour (normal or pseudo normal?). The urinalysis was unremarkable. The surgical skin biopsy taken from the left calf showed leukocytoclastic vasculitis.

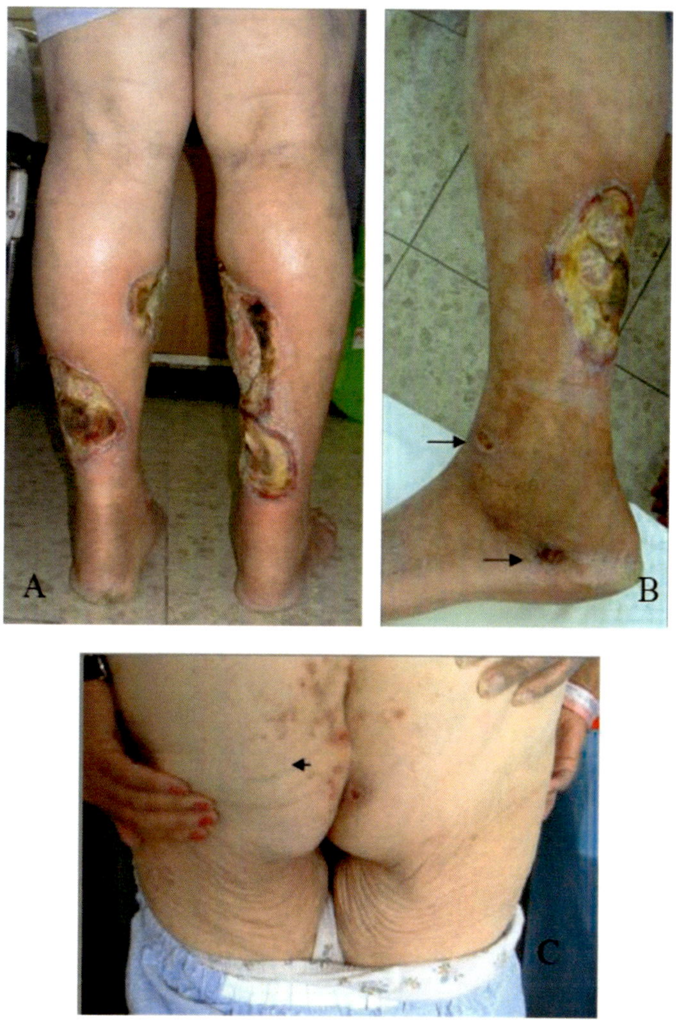


Figure 21. Grade 3 skin ulcers with undermined borders partly covered by escars (A); livedo reticularis, large ulcers, and small superficial ulcers (arrows) (B); maculo-papular eruption, lesion covered by a tiny crust, exulcerated lesions and punched-out ulcer (arrow) (C).

In summarizing, the following features were representative of the patient's present illness: post-traumatic skin ulcers with fast progression and very painful; disseminated small shallow ulcers and disseminated skin eruption; small vessel vasculitis; cryoglobulinemia, low C4 complement, elevated rheumatoid factor; hepatitis C virus associated chronic liver disease; and renal failure of recent onset. The parsimony diagnosis, which can contain all these findings, is cryoglobulinemic vasculitis secondary to chronic hepatitis C virus disease. The main differential diagnosis is pyoderma gangrenosum.

*Cryoglobulinemia* is defined by the presence of circulating immunoglobulins that precipitate at temperatures below $37^0$C and redisolve on rewarming. Type II cryoglobulinemia is the one most commonly associated with chronic hepatitis C (HCV) infection. This type is called 'mixed' because the antibodies found in the cryoprecipitate are of two kinds: one antibody is a polyclonal IgG and the other antibody is a monoclonal IgM directed against the IgG. Rates of HCV infection among patients with mixed cryoglobulinemia range from 30 to 96 percent; among patients with HCV infection 29 to 54 percent have cryoglobulins [1, 2]. The causal determinism between HCV and mixed cryoglobulinemia is supported also by the presence of anti-HCV antibodies and HCV RNA in the cryoprecipitate at concentrations higher than they are found in the serum. Mixed cryoglobulinemia appears to result from the interaction between HCV and lymphocytes, which causes activation and expansion of B cells, the latter producing IgM with rheumatoid-factor activity. Cryoglobulins can precipitate in the walls of small and medium sized vessels, causing vasculitis. On histopathology, thrombi are found in the lumen of small and medium sized vessels. The thrombi are positive for IgG and IgM. The clinical course of cryoglobulinemic disease varies: about half of patients have chronic disease with no involvement of vital organs, a third have moderate-to-severe disease with chronic renal failure or cirrhosis, and nearly 15% present with life-threatening disease.

Cutaneous manifestations of cryoglobulinemic vasculitis include palpable purpura, livedo reticularis, leg ulcers (all three were present in the propositus), acrocyanosis, cold urticaria, and Raynaud's phenomenon. These ulcers can be extremely painful (as in our patient who necessitated opiates). Extracutaneous symptoms include arthralgia, asthenia, peripheral neuropathy, and membrano-proliferative or membranous glomerulonephritis. In testing for cryoglobulins the blood must be kept at body temperature until it has clotted and the serum has been drawn off, because these proteins precipitate from the serum as it is cooled; then the serum is tested for the abnormal proteins. If this precaution is not observed, the test may be spuriously negative [1].

A definite diagnosis of mixed cryoglobulinemia syndrome is established when the following criteria are met: 1. serum mixed cryoglobulins + purpura + leukocytoclastic vasculitis ± low C4, or 2. serum mixed cryoglobulins + two minor clinical symptoms (chronic hepatitis , membranoproliferative glomerulonephritis, peripheral neuropathy, skin ulcers) + two minor serological or pathological findings (rheumatoid factor, HCV+, HBV+, clonal B cell infiltrates) ± low C4 [1]. According to the above criteria a diagnosis of mixed cryoglobulinemic syndrome was endorsed in our patient. The main differential diagnosis was pyoderma gangrenosum, a topic discussed in detail under Case 14. The diagnosis of pyoderma gangrenosum is based on characteristic clinical features, response to corticosteroid therapy and, notably, on exclusion of other disease entities [3, 4]. Though pathergy and non-healing surgical wounds in the patient under discussion are features consistent with pyoderma gangrenosum, the diagnosis of mixed cryoglobulinemic syndrome was favored by overall evidence.

*Treatment of cryoglobulinemic vasculitis* dependents on the severity of the disease and on the etiology. Any underlying infection, malignant condition, hematologic disorder, or autoimmune disease should be treated specifically. Arthralgias often respond to nonsteroidal anti-inflammatory drugs. Low-dose glucocorticoids can be used for minor or intermittent symptoms in the skin, joints, and in sensory neuropathy. Rapidly progressive vasculitis or glomerulonephritis requires high-dose glucocorticoids, cytotoxic agents, and plasmapheresis. Interferon plus ribavirin are the mainstay of treatment for mixed cryoglobulinemia in all HCV genotypes. Clearance of the virus correlates well with reduction of CD5-positive B-cells and circulating cryoglobulins. Unfortunately relapse rates are high after discontinuation of therapy. The use of the anti-CD20 drug rituximab to target B-cells has recently shown efficacy in controlling mixed cryoglobulinemia in selected patients. Two protease inhibitors, telaprevir and boceprevir, were recently approved by the Food and Drug Administration for the treatment of HCV infection. Telaprevir combined with peginterferon plus ribavirin significantly improved rates of sustained virologic response in patients with previously treated HCV infection [1, 2].

In having diagnosed in our patient mixed cryoglobulinemic vasculitis associated with chronic HCV infection, and after exclusion of other possible nosologies, the patient was referred to a tertiary care center for treatment. Further evaluation revealed high titers of hepatitis C RNA, the cryoglobulin was IgM/K, and an abdominal CT showed an enlarged micronodular liver along with a 20 cm large spleen. Treatment was limited to prednisone 60 mg/day, in considering contraindications to antiviral agents. Later rituximab was added. However overwhelming sepsis developed that did not respond to antibiotic treatment and the patient expired.

## Learning Points

- Ischemic skin ulcers may be the consequence of cryoglobulinemic vasculitis, especially in patients with chronic HCV or HBV hepatitis.
- Skin ulcers secondary to cryoglobulinemic vasculitis not always exhibit the characteristic features of ischemic ulcers, i.e. punched-out and well demarcated ulcers usually located on toes, heels or anterior shin.
- Therefore, the presence of skin ulcers in a patient with chronic hepatitis C or B makes screening for cryoglobulins mandatory. If screening is positive, additional work-up is recommended.
- Therapy of vasculitic skin ulcers differs from the routine management of pressure sores, venous, ischemic atherosclerotic and neuropathic ulcers.
- Interferon plus ribavirin are the mainstay of treatment for mixed cryoglobulinemia associate with HCV infection.

# References


[1] Pietrogrande M, De Vita S, Zignego AL, Pioltelli P, Sansonno D, Sollima S, Atzeni F, Saccardo F, Quartuccio L, Bruno S, Bruno R, Campanini M, Candela M, Castelnovo L, Gabrielli A, Gaeta GB, Marson P, Mascia MT, Mazzaro C, Mazzotta F, Meroni P, Montecucco C, Ossi E, Piccinino F, Prati D, Puoti M, Riboldi P, Riva A, Roccatello D, Sagnelli E, Scaini P, Scarpato S, Sinico R, Taliani G, Tavoni A, Bonacci E, Renoldi P, Filippini D, Sarzi-Puttini P, Ferri C, Monti G, Galli M. Recommendations for the management of mixed cryoglobulinemia syndrome in hepatitis C virus-infected patients. *Autoimmun. Rev.* 2011;10:444-454.

[2] Rosen HR. Chronic hepatitis C infection. *N. Engl. J. Med.* 2011;364:2429-2438.

[3] Bennett ML, Jackson JM, Jorizzo JL, Fleischer AB Jr, White WL, Callen JP. Pyoderma gangrenosum. A comparison of typical and atypical forms with an emphasis on time to remission. Case review of 86 patients from 2 institutions. *Medicine.* (Baltimore) 2000;79:37-46.

[4] Callen JP, Jackson JM. Pyoderma gangrenosum: an update. *Rheum. Dis. Clin. North Am.* 2007;33:787-802.

*Chapter IV*

# Gastointestinal Disorders - Red Flags

The choice of the topics in this chapter reflects the author's experience, for good and bad. The selection of cases is deliberately eclectic.

## Case 18. Pseudomembranous Colitis with Leukemoid Reaction

An 83-year-old woman was transferred for subacute care from the department of internal medicine with the diagnoses acute clostridium difficile diarrhea, Alzheimer's type dementia, arterial hypertension and obesity. Clostridium toxin B has been found in the patient's stool by enzyme immunoassay. She was treated with intravenous fluids and oral metronidazole 500 mg t.i.d. under contact precautions. The fever had resolved and she had passed one formed stool on the day before her transfer to our ward. One month before admission the patient's had received a ten-day course of ciprofloxacine treatment for E. coli urinary infection.

On examination, the patient was drowsy but could be easily waken up, the oral temperature was 36.8$^0$C, BP 124/70 mmHg, heart rate 88 bpm, respirations 22/minute, and SaO2 in ambient air 92%. The abdomen was slightly distended with normal bowel sounds. The WBC was 42.000 with 72% neutrophils, 11% band forms, and hematocrit 52%. A plain abdominal film showed dilation of the entire colon, thickening of the colonic walls and loss of haustral markings. The diameter of the cecum was 12 cm. In suspecting imminent colonic perforation the patient was referred to surgery. On arriving the BP had decreased to 70/50 mmHg. Emergency colectomy was proposed but agreement was not granted by the patient's family. She died on the same day.

*Severe pseudomembranous colitis* is diagnosed in only 3% to 5% of patients with *C. difficile* infection, but is associated with a mortality rate of up to 65%. Severe colitis may present with abdominal pain, peritoneal signs, colonic dilatation, leukocytosis, and a progressive sepsis; infarction and perforation of the colon are frequently found on surgery [1]. Clinical symptoms and signs may be discrete or absent in the elderly patient. Contrary to common belief, diarrhea may be minimal or absent at this point of the disease course because of ileus. In such situations the diagnosis is even more challenging and important since early diagnosis and treatment of fulminant clostridial colitis might improve the outcome. Early colectomy before vasopressor therapy is required may improve the chance of survival. Yet, mortality from fulminant C. difficile colitis was 48% in one series of patients in spite of surgical intervention [2].

*Predictors of severe disease* that could serve as alerts include immunosuppression, hypotension, hypoalbuminemia, and pronounced leukocytosis (mean 27,000/mm$^3$ with 12% band forms in the series of Longo). Abdominal computed tomography correctly identified 98% of cases of fulminant colitis. In patients with a marked leukocytosis or bandemia, as observed in the present case, early referral to surgery is recommended since severe leukocytosis frequently heralds hypotension and impending perforation.

*C. difficile disease* was thought to be mainly a nosocomial infection associated with administration of broad-spectrum antibiotics, and the disease was usually not life threatening. Emergence of the epidemic strain BI/NAP1/027, which produces a binary toxin in addition to the 2 classic C. difficile toxins A and B, is associated with high rates of mortality [3]. Recently, C. difficile has been reported also in nonhospital-based settings, such as community-acquired cases. Furthermore, in recent years there is increasing resistance of C. difficile to metronidazole treatment.

*Prophylactic* probiotic administration by consumption of an Actimel drink containing L. casei, L. bulgaricus, and S. thermophilus can reduce the incidence of antibiotic associated diarrhea including C. difficile associated diarrhea. This has the potential to decrease morbidity, healthcare costs, and mortality if used routinely in patients older than 50 years. In one study, the estimated average cost of one course of probiotic treatment in 2006 was $20 (assuming an average antibiotic course of 10 days plus a further seven days of probiotics, and using current retail prices for Actimel, about $0.60). The cost to prevent one case of antibiotic associated diarrhea would be $100 for and $120 for one case of C. difficile diarrhea [4]. Yet, the utility of probiotic prophylaxis for antibiotic associated diarrhea and clostridial diarrhea remains controversial.

## Learning Points

- Severe pseudomembranous colitis occurs in 3% to 5% of patients with C. difficile infection and is associated with a mortality rate of up to 65%.
- Early predictors of severity, which could serve as 'red flags' are immunosuppression, hypotension, hypoalbuminemia, and pronounced leukocytosis.
- Patients with clostridial colitis who present marked leukocytosis or bandemia are candidates for surgery.
- Prophylactic administration of a probiotic in elderly patients during and following a course of broad spectrum antibiotics has the potential to decrease morbidity, mortality and healthcare costs.

# References

[1] Adams SD, Mercer DW. Fulminant Clostridium difficile colitis. *Curry Opin. Crit. Care*. 2007;13:450-455.

[2] Longo WE, Mazuski JE, Virgo KS, Lee P, Bahadursingh AN, Johnson FE. Outcome after colectomy for Clostridium difficile colitis. *Dis. Colon Rectum*. 2004; 47: 1620-1626.

[3] McFarland LV, Beneda HW, Clarridge JE, Raugi GJ. Implications of the changing face of Clostridium difficile disease for health care practitioners. *Am. J. Infect. Control.* 2007; 35:237-253.

[4] Hickson M, D'Souza AL, Muthu N, Rogers TR, Rajkumar C, Bulpitt CJ. Use of probiotic Lactobacillus preparation to prevent diarrhoea associated with antibiotics: randomised double blind placebo controlled trial. *BMJ* 2007;14;335:80.

## Case 19. Rectal Perforation – Red Flag too Late

A 93-year-old man was admitted to our ward in an attempt to improve the control of severe chronic heart failure. Records from a recent admission to another hospital notified pulmonary congestion, left ventricular ejection fraction 18%, frequent ectopic atrial beats, and an estimated glomerular filtration rate 42 mL/min/1.73 $m^2$. He was treated with furosemide 60 mg/day, ramipril 2.5 mg/day, micropirin 100 mg/day, simvastatin 20 mg/day, and vitamin D 600 mg/day. The patient was dyspneic at rest, the sitting BP was 90/45 mmHg, there was +2 bilateral calf edema, wet rales were perceived over the lower lung fields, and there was severe adipose tissue and muscle wasting. The BUN was 48 mg/dL and the serum creatinine was 1.6 mg/dL. On the ward, the patient received a course of continuous i.v. furosemide drip 120 mg/day, oxygen through nasal prongs, vitamin B1, along with his usual medications. The patient was repeatedly administered microenemas because of refractory constipation.

During the two weeks course of treatment his condition stabilized and discharge was scheduled, when the nurse reported having seen a small amount of blood on the patient's diaper. Digital rectal examination revealed external hemorrhoids; no tumoral mass or fecal impaction was felt. The examination was not particularly painful. Although the patient's BP, temperature and general condition were unchanged, the discharged was postponed. Six hours later the patient complained of severe pain in the lower abdomen. The BP had dropped to 67/46 mmHg and the bowel sounds were no longer audible. Emergency CT imaging showed air pockets adjacent to the rectum. Traumatic rectal perforation was diagnosed. In the operating room fecal diversion was performed with a temporary loop colostomy, along with repair of the mucosal defect. The subsequent course was marked by sepsis, deterioration of heart failure, and shock. The patient died 9 days later.

*Rectal perforation* may be the result of direct trauma, apart from carcinoma or the rectum. Perforation has bee described in complicating rectal temperature measurement, enema, transanal irrigation, colonoscopy, sclerotherapy for hemorrhoids, anal rape, and transverse fracture of the sacrum without any other injury to the pelvis [1]. The clinical presentation depends on the site of perforation [2]. The columnar mucosa above the pectinate line is insensate and therefore it is unusual that patients develop pain immediately after rectal perforation; pain is felt hours later when fecal contamination occurs. Rectal perforation above the peritoneal reflection carries the risk of peritonitis; these patients usually present with typical acute abdomen.

Low-rectal perforations often have occult presentations with diagnosis delayed for many hours or even several days. The diagnosis may be particularly difficult in the oldest old because of barriers to communication (likely), atypical presentation of illness (often), and multiple co-morbidities (usually). Sometimes the patients have no complaint at all. Late diagnosis results in greater tissue soilage and the risk of pararectal abscess and sepsis. Rectal perforation below the peritoneal reflection does usually not cause peritonitis.

Rectal bleeding and the late onset of pain in the patient presented herein were confusing for the beginning. Painless rectal bleeding may occur with internal hemorrhoids, cancer, or precancerous lesions; we could not find in a scrutiny of the literature rectal bleeding mentioned in the context of traumatic rectal perforation.

*To prevent iatrogenic rectal perforation*, several rules should be respected. The anorectal angle is such that most perforations will involve the anterior wall of the rectum. Hence, after insertion of the finger or the enema nozzle, the direction should point slightly posteriorly to keep within the center of the rectal lumen. Special caution should be exercised in patients with proctitis, rectal diverticula, anorectal strictures, or masses that might angulate or compress the rectum (fibroid uterus or enlarged prostate).

*For management of rectal perforation below the peritoneal reflection* surgical debridement is imperative together with parenteral antibiotics, presacral drainage, and distal bowel irrigation. Primary repair of rectal perforation and fecal diversion is considered according to the clinical context. For the management of iatrogenic rectal perforation that occurred during prostate surgery or during a pre-procedural bowel preparation, the primary repair of large rectal defects may be adequate without temporary colonic diversion, as well as conservative management of small perforations [3].

### Learning Points

- Perforation of the rectum may occur as a result of direct trauma by the nozzle of enemas.
- In real time, perforation may not be associated with pain, so the complication can go unsuspected for several hours or days.
- Rectal perforation above the peritoneal reflection complicates with peritonitis: these patients present with typical acute abdomen.
- Rectal perforation below the peritoneal reflection does usually not cause peritonitis but complicate with pararectal abscess: the diagnosis is often delayed.
- The diagnosis of rectal perforation relies on CT imaging.
- To prevent iatrogenic rectal perforation insertion of the enema nozzle should point slightly posteriorly to keep within the center of the rectal lumen.

## References

[1] Handley DV, Rieger NA, Rodda DJ. Rectal perforation from colonic irrigation administered by alternative practitioners. *MJA* 2004; 181: 575-576.

[2] Nolan JF. Delayed presentation of rectal perforation. *R. Soc. Med.* 1990; 83: 744–745.

[3] Madhala O, Greif F, Cohen M, Leicuk S. Major rectal perforations caused by enema: is surgery mandatory? *Dig. Surg.* 1998;25:270-272.

# Case 20. Dysphagia

An 82-year-old woman was referred for evaluation of dysphagia for solid food and liquids of more than one year duration. She felt that food was stuck in her throat. Attempted endoscopy had failed to enter the esophagus. A proposed barium swallow was declined by the patient. During the preceding months she had lost 7 kg of weight. Her medical history was remarkable for arterial hypertension, Alzheimer's disease with grade 1 dementia, and depressive disorder. She had suffered a stroke 9 years ago followed by good functional recovery. The patient's current medications were lercanidipine 10 mg/day, atenolol 50 mg/day and citalopram 20 mg/day. Physical examination on admission and results of ancillary laboratory tests were unremarkable. CT imaging exhibited a large Zenker's diverticulum posterior to the cervical esophagus and extending into the thorax (Figure 22). The patient was recommended to undergo an endoscopic stapling procedure for the treatment of Zenker's diverticulum but she refused any intervention.

*Swallowing* involves activity of muscles of the oropharynx, laryngeal, and esophageal regions coordinated at a brainstem level. In the oral phase, the food is taken into the mouth and chewed if needed; saliva is secreted to provide lubrication and digestive enzymes; the food bolus is formed and shaped by the tongue. The tongue then propels the bolus to the pharyngeal inlet and delivers it into the pharynx. During the pharyngeal phase of swallowing, coordinated movements seal off the nasal passages and protect the trachea while the crico-pharyngeal muscles relax and allow the bolus to enter the pharynx. The bolus then progresses to the esophagus propelled by peristaltic contractions; on relaxation of the lower esophageal sphincter it enters into the stomach. Dysphagia can originate from disturbances in the mouth, pharynx, or esophagus and can involve mechanical, musculoskeletal, or neurogenic mechanisms. Dysphagia is considered to be an alarm symptom, indicating the need for immediate evaluation to define the cause and initiate appropriate therapy.

*Age-related alterations of deglutition* are caused by changes in head and neck anatomy as well as by neural mechanisms which support the swallowing. These changes contribute to alterations in swallowing in healthy older adults, a phenomenon called 'presbyphagia'. However, presbyphagia is rarely symptomatic and dysphagia in elderly persons should not be attributed to normal aging [1].

*Mechanical dysphagia* is caused by structural abnormalities within or adjacent to the mouth, pharynx, and esophagus, that can interfere with swallowing despite fully intact nervous and musculoskeletal systems. Macroglossia, temporomandibular joint dislocation, intraoral tumors, retropharyngeal tumor or abscess, cervical anterior osteophytes, Zenker's diverticulum, or thyroid gland enlargement can cause dysphagia. The esophageal transit can be impaired by esophageal tumors, esophageal stricture, vascular abnormalities such as aortic aneurysm or an aberrant origin of the subclavian artery, by hiatal hernia or gastroesophageal reflux.

*Neuromuscular dysphagia* is caused by certain muscular dystrophies, inflammatory myopathies, myasthenia gravis, and processes affecting the cerebral cortex, subcortical white matter, subcortical gray matter, brainstem, spinal cord, or peripheral nerves. Dysphagia develops in 45% to 57% of patients following stroke causing pulmonary aspiration in 48% and malnutrition in 65% of patients. Dysphagia after stroke often indicates brainstem localization, primarily affecting the pharyngeal phase of swallowing. Impaired swallowing also occurs in strokes involving cortical and subcortical structures. In hemispheric strokes the predominant abnormality may be a delay in initiation of voluntary swallowing. Swallowing often improves spontaneously in the days and weeks after the stroke. Improvement is more likely to occur after cortical strokes compared with those of brainstem origin; the improvement is probably the result of compensatory reorganization of undamaged brain areas [2, 3]. Dysphagia is a potential complication of carotid endarterectomy, not on the basis of stroke, but due to laryngeal or cranial nerve injury; most deficits are mild and transient. Dysphagia occurs in 30% to 82% of patients with Parkinson's disease; treatment with levodopa has inconsistent effects on parkinsonian dysphagia. Dysphagia is also frequently noticed in the parkinsonism-plus syndromes, such as progressive supranuclear palsy, multiple system atrophy, corticobasal degeneration, and dementia with Lewy bodies.

*Clinical examination* can provide clues to the diagnosis:

- Difficulty when initiating swallowing or repeated attempts to succeed at swallowing suggests an oropharyngeal source for the dysphagia. Patients who have difficulty transferring food from the mouth to the pharynx will often reposition their body to optimize alignment of the bolus for presentation to the pharynx. Such patients may extend their arms and neck during swallowing, and will often use their finger to move food into proper position.
- Oral dysfunction can lead to food spillage, sialorrhea, little by little swallows, and dysarthria.
- Pharyngeal dysphagia is characterized by a sensation of 'food getting stuck' immediately upon swallowing, postnasal regurgitation, coughing or choking during food consumption, and dysphonia. Patients with oropharyngeal dysphagia point toward the cervical region when asked to identify the site of their symptoms.
- Retrosternal dysphagia usually corresponds with the location of the lesion in the esophagus.
- Dysphagia for solid food but not for liquids is more likely to be caused by a mechanical obstruction.
- Dysphagia for both solids and liquids is more typical for an esophageal motility disorder.
- A history of dry mouth or eyes may indicate inadequate saliva production. It is important to obtain a detailed review of medications which can reduce salivary flow: anticholinergics, antihistamines, and certain antihypertensive agents. Sjögren's syndrome is a consideration.
- Changes in speech often implicate neuromuscular dysfunction.
- A malignant cause should be considered in older patients presenting with oropharyngeal dysphagia, particularly those with a history of alcohol abuse, smoking, or weight loss.
- Pain upon swallowing (odynophagia) can result from inflammation, infection or neoplasia.

*Examination* of the oral cavity, head and neck, and supraclavicular regions may reveal lymphadenopathy, a mass, facial muscle weakness, poor dentition, or other abnormalities potentially causing dysphagia. Neurologic examination should include testing of cranial nerves, especially those involved in swallowing (sensory components of cranial nerves V, IX and X, and motor components of cranial nerves V, VII, X, XI and XII). Lip and tongue function can be easily assessed during routine neurological examination, and both palatal and gag reflexes can be evaluated. Halitosis and regurgitation of indigested food suggest Zenker's diverticulum. The presence of cough on swallowing water is predictive of aspiration.

*The modified barium swallow* test has become a standard method for assessing oropharyngeal dysphagia. Patients are observed on videofluoroscopy whilst swallowing barium-impregnated food of differing consistencies (thin liquid, pudding, and cookie). By this method, oral and pharyngeal functions can be characterized and the presence of aspiration accurately documented; the response to corrective measures, such as positioning techniques, can also be evaluated. Videoendoscopy of the pharynx allows direct visualization of the pharyngeal component of swallowing before and after passage of the food bolus. Its primary value is to demonstrate the presence of residual material in the pharynx after a swallow, indicating an increased risk of aspiration.

*Therapy for oropharyngeal dysphagia* depends on the etiology. Neoplasms usually are treated by surgery. Following stroke, nasogastric tube feeding can temporarily provide adequate nutrition until swallowing improves sufficiently to allow oral feeding. For individuals in whom significant dysphagia persists after stroke, percutaneous endoscopic placement of a gastrostomy tube may become necessary. Partially dentulous elderly patients who have difficulty masticating may benefit from prosthetic teeth.

Swallowing rehabilitation depends on the cause of oropharyngeal dysphagia. When specific swallowing training is required, referral to a specialist in swallowing disorders is helpful. Several maneuvers during swallowing may reduce oropharyngeal dysphagia, and their use should be based upon the specific defect. Dietary modifications may improve swallowing and help avoid aspiration. Some patients are more tolerant of solid food or soft consistencies. For patients with intolerance to liquids, commercially available food additives that thicken liquids may be helpful, since increasing bolus viscosity can improve swallowing function. Other patients benefit from a reduction in the volume of their mouthfuls, or an alternation of solid and liquid boluses, which can facilitate transfer. In some cases, feeding with a particular implement, such as a cup, straw or spoon, may improve swallowing. Assistance provided by a caretaker during meals can be helpful. For patients whose dysphagia is related to neurologic dysfunction, giving meals during times of maximal attentiveness may be beneficial.

*Zenker's diverticulum* was probably the cause of dysphagia for solid foods and liquids in the present case. Zenker's diverticulum is a posterior outpouching of the mucosa through an area of muscular weakness in the cervical esophagus, between the transverse fibers of the cricopharyngeus and the oblique fibers of the lower inferior constrictor. The etiology is controversial and is probably due to elevated upper esophageal pressure, cricopharyngeus dysfunction and reflux. Over time, the diverticle tends to enlarge and to cause progressive swallowing disability. The pouch alongside the esophagus may accumulate food or liquid. As the pouch fills, the contents are regurgitated into the throat, leading to symptoms of dysphagia and/or aspiration. Zenker's diverticula are typically found in older individuals, and are often problematic because they may interfere with proper dietary intake or may complicate with aspiration pneumonia. Symptoms include difficult swallowing, coughing, choking sensations, halitosis, and regurgitation of food .The diagnosis of a Zenker's diverticulum is made through the findings on a barium swallow showing an outpouching posterior to the cervical segment of esophagus; there is usually a prominent muscular bar at the level of the upper esophageal sphincter, which causes an indentation.

Treatment of a Zenker's diverticulum has traditionally involved an open surgical approach to resect the diverticulum and incise the cricopharyngeus muscle. The open surgical approach may be the safest alternative for patients with diverticula more than 5 cm in diameter that extend into the thorax. Endoscopic techniques are suitable for patients with diverticula 2 to 5 cm in diameter. An alternative endoscopic approach involves the use a stapling device to divide the common party wall located between the sac and the esophagus [4]. With the latter technique the patients are able to be discharged on the same day or on the day following surgery. Resection of small diverticula is not required.

## Learning Points

- Dysphagia can originate from disturbances in the mouth, pharynx, or esophagus and can involve mechanical, musculoskeletal, or neurogenic mechanisms.
- The modified barium swallow test is the gold standard method for assessing oropharyngeal dysphagia.
- Difficulty swallowing, coughing, choking sensations, bad breath, and regurgitation of food should call attention to a possible Zenker's diverticulum.
- An open surgical approach is usually preferred for treatment of Zenker's diverticula larger than 5 cm that extend into the thorax.
- Endoscopic techniques are suitable for patients with medium-sized diverticula, 2 to 5 cm in diameter.
- Resection of small diverticula is not required.

# References

[1] Ney DM, Weiss JM, Kind AJ, Robbins J. Senescent swallowing: impact, strategies, and interventions. *Nutr. Clin. Pract.* 2009;24:395-413.

[2] Teasell R, Foley N, Fisher J, Finestone H. The incidence, management, and complications of dysphagia in patients with medullary strokes admitted to a rehabilitation unit. *Dysphagia* 2002;17:115-120.

[3] Terre R, Mearin F. Oropharyngeal dysphagia after the acute phase of stroke: predictors of aspiration. Neurogastroenterol Motil. 2006;18:200-205. 4. Lara LF, Tang S-J. Flexible endoscopic clip-assisted Zenker's diverticulotomy. *Gatrointestinal Endoscopy* 2008;67:704-708.

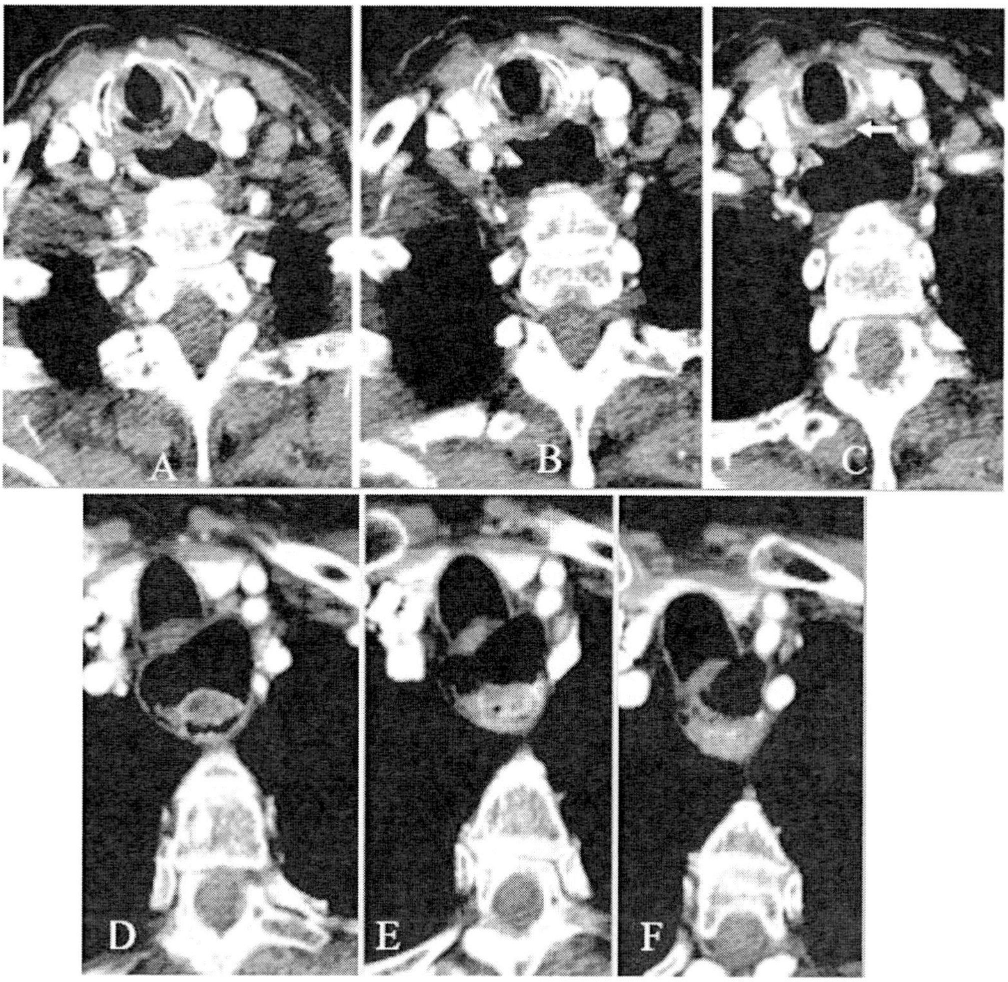


Figure 22. Axial contrast-enhanced CT shows a large Zenker's diverticulum posterior to the cervical esophagus extending into the thorax. The arrow in figure C points to the esophagus. The diverticulum contains air, food products and oral contrast, seen in D-E.

## Case 21. Dysphagia and Pulmonary Aspirations, Zenker's Diverticle

A 73-year-old man was admitted with malnutrition, secondary to severe dysphagia, and pulmonary aspirations. A large Zenker's diverticulum was diagnosed and resected two years ago by an open approach. The patient's symptoms remitted and he gained 20 kg in weight. Recently there was recurrence of the difficulty in swallowing, coughing, and choking sensations. He was referred to our ward when high fever had occurred associated with a dry cough. Bilateral basal pulmonary infiltrates were noticed on chest x-rays. On CT a collection of air and contrast material adjacent to the left cricopharyngeus muscle indicated recurrence of Zenker's diverticulum (Figure 23). Bilateral basal pulmonary infiltrates contained beads of aspirated contrast material (Figure 24). The patient was treated with i.v. antibiotics and subsequently referred for endoscopic surgery of Zenker's diverticulum.

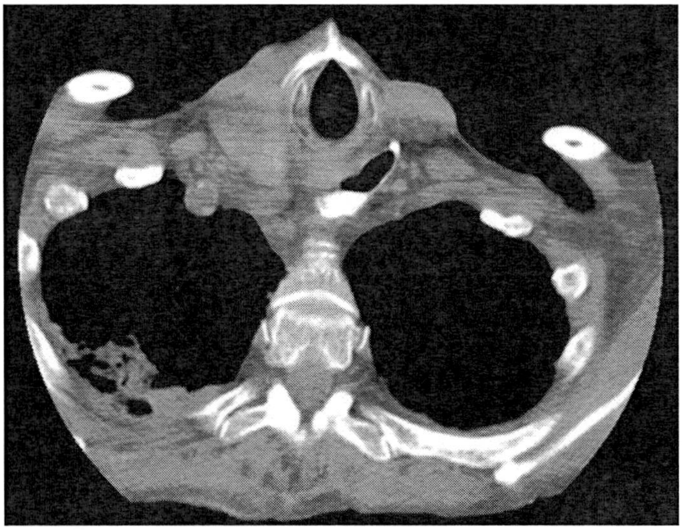

Figure 23. Collection of air and contrast adjacent to the left side of the cricopharyngeus muscle contained in a Zenker's diverticle.

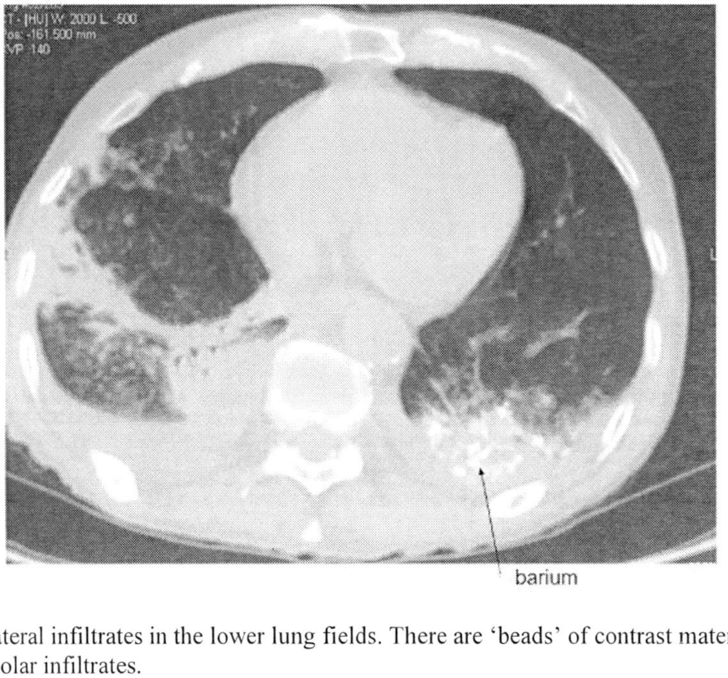


Figure 24. Bilateral infiltrates in the lower lung fields. There are 'beads' of contrast material scattered within the alveolar infiltrates.

*Aspiration-related disorders* include aspiration bacterial pneumonia, aspiration chemical pneumonitis, lung abscess, lipoid pneumonia, airway obstruction, and chronic pulmonary fibrosis. Advanced age, neurologic disorders and gastroesophageal reflux disease are common risk factors for aspiration. Zenker's diverticulum is also a recognized risk factor for pulmonary aspiration.

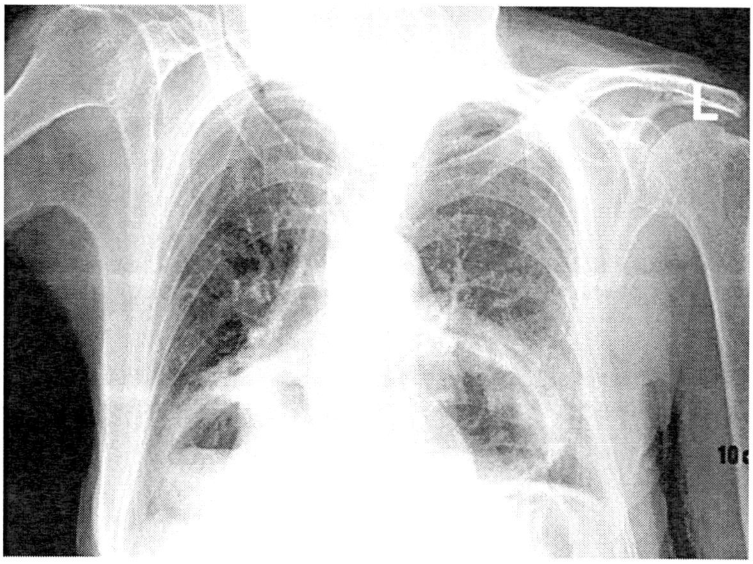


Figure 25. Large diaphragmatic hernia.

## Case 22. Surgical Gastrostomy or PEG?

A 79-year-old man with cerebrovascular disease was malnourished because of severe oropharyngeal dysphagia. He was referred for percutaneous endoscopic gastrostomy (PEG), but the procedure could not be performed because the inability to transilluminate the anterior abdominal wall. Inspection of the chest x-rays showed a large diaphragmatic hernia that contained almost the entire stomach (Figure 25). Subsequently, surgical gastrostomy was performed.

*PEG is indicated* for patients who will be unable to consume sufficient nutrition over a period of more than 30 days, despite a functioning gastrointestinal tract. The procedure involves the placement of a percutaneous gastrostomy tube after endoscopic transillumination of the abdominal wall such as to find an appropriate site for gastrostomy. The main indications are neurological disorders, anatomical impediment, and radiation injury. PEG placement in patients with advanced dementia is controversial as studies showed that PEG does not prolong the patient's life [1].

*Contraindications to PEG* include peritonitis, abdominal wall infection, abdominal burns, high aspiration risk, atypical abdominal anatomy, and a short expected life span. Also, inability to trans-illuminate the anterior abdominal wall and ineffective digital intrusion of the abdominal wall to locate a safe gastric access site are absolute contraindications to PEG. Relative contraindications for PEG are gastric varices, severe obesity, prior partial gastric resection, ascites, and coagulopathy.

The inability to trans-illuminate on gastroscopy the anterior abdominal wall may be due to the stomach being contained in the thorax within a large diaphragmatic hernia. Diaphragmatic hernias are usually discovered incidentally on chest x-ray, on upper gastrointestinal studies or on endoscopy. Many patients are asymptomatic or have vague symptoms of epigastric or substernal pain, postprandial fullness, nausea, and retching.

Occasionally, complications occur such are gastric volvulus, bleeding (from gastric ulceration, gastritis, or erosions), and respiratory complications resulting from mechanical compression of the lung by organs protruding through the diaphragmatic defect. An upright radiograph of the thorax may be diagnostic, revealing a retrocardiac air-fluid level within a paraesophageal hernia or showing an intrathoracic stomach. Type I or sliding hiatal hernia accounts for more than 95 percent of cases. Most small hiatal hernias are asymptomatic and, even with larger type I hernias, the main clinical implication is the propensity to develop gastroesophageal reflux disease. The likelihood of symptomatic gastroesophageal reflux increases with the size of the hiatal hernia. Type II, III, and IV are paraesophageal hernias.

*Laparoscopic gastrostomy* is an accepted alternative to PEG. Altered anatomic relationship of the stomach to other intra-abdominal organs or with the abdominal wall may prevent safe endoscopic placement of the tube. Visualizing and manipulating the stomach during laparoscopy enables the surgeon to complete the procedure and reduces the risk of injury to the adjacent organs [2].

*Surgical hernia repair* is rarely indicated for an isolated, asymptomatic type I hiatal hernia. If symptoms of GERD occur in association with a large hiatus hernia, either medical or surgical treatment is indicated to control the reflux. Surgical approaches to type II hiatal hernias comprise reduction of the herniated stomach into the abdomen, excision of the hernia sac, closure of the hiatal defect, an antireflux procedure, and gastropexy to prevent reherniation. Laparoscopic repair is also possible. The prognosis is excellent following surgical repair of a type II hiatal hernia.

### Learning Points

- A chest x-rays showing a large diaphragmatic hernia containing much of the stomach may indicate inability to trans-illuminate the anterior abdominal wall during endoscopy and precludes safe performance of PEG.
- In patients with large diaphragmatic hernias surgical gastrostomy may be indicated.

## References

[1] Freeman C, Ricevuto A, Delegge MH. Enteral nutrition in patients with dementia and stroke. *Curr. Opinion Gastroenterol.* 2010;26:156-159.

[2] Xenos ES. Percutaneous endoscopic gastrostomy in a patient with a large hiatal hernia using laparoscopy. *JSLS.* 2000;4:231-233.

# Case 23. Clogged Gastrostomy Tube

A 90-year-old man was admitted with the diagnosis of urosepsis and made an uneventful recovery on antibiotic treatment. His medical history was notable for dementia following several cerebrovascular events, dysphagia and pulmonary aspirations. A gastrostomy tube has been placed endoscopically eight months ago. On the 6$^{h}$ day in hospital the attending nurse reported difficulty to administer liquids through the gastrostomy tube and oozing of the feeding formulation around the tube. The nurse also reported that she felt a hard knob within the abdominal wall at the tube's entry site, which she was not aware of its presence before. There were no signs of abdominal wall infection, dermatitis or bleeding. A presumptive diagnosis of buried bumper syndrome was made; this diagnosis was confirmed on CT showing that the internal bumper of the feeding tube was located within the layers of the abdominal wall. The clogged and buried tube was removed under local anesthesia and another gastrostomy tube was inserted through the same entry.

*The buried bumper syndrome* is a rare but serious late complication of PEG tubes. It occurs as a result of excessive traction on the tube that causes undue tension and leads to gastric ulceration at the internal bumper site. The bumper than becomes lodged between the gastric wall and the skin along the track of the gastrostomy tube. Common manifestations of this inadvertent event are the inability to infuse the feeding solution through the tube, peritubular leakage of food, and abdominal pain. Trying to administer feeding by force in this situation may result in abscess formation within the abdominal wall. Emergency evaluation by abdominal ultrasound or CT will show the subcutaneous location of the bumper. Early endoscopy will show a small irregular gap in the gastric mucosa; however, delaying the endoscopy may permit re-epithelisation and closure of the internal orifice of the gastrostomy track and the diagnosis can be missed [1, 2].

In diagnosing this condition, the gastrostomy tube should be removed because it may continue to migrate until it is completely impacted in the abdominal wall and may cause perforation of the stomach into the peritoneum. Endoscopic ultrasound of the gastric wall provides valuable information in deciding whether a surgical or endoscopic approach should be attempted to remove the PEG tube. In order to prevent this complication, during daily cleaning of the external PEG site the tube should be pushed inside approximately 1 cm and rotated prior to repositioning the external bolster. External traction on the tube should be avoided, as well as placement of gauze pads beneath the external bolster.

*Other PEG complications* occur often, the most common being infection at the site of tube entry which happens in up to 30% of cases. These infections are usually of minor importance and can be treated with antibiotics, but can occasionally they can lead to necrotizing fasciitis which requires surgical debridement. Pre-procedure antibiotics have been shown to reduce the frequency of minor wound infections after PEG. Other complications include bleeding during PEG usually due to puncture of an artery in the gastric wall (minor and self-limited or requiring endoscopic therapy in 1% of cases), premature tube dislodgement that can lead to peritonitis, inadvertent puncture of the liver and colon, and seeding of the gastrostomy site with tumor implants.

## Learning Points

- Difficulty to administer liquids through the gastrostomy tube, or presence of any leak around the tube, or pain in the abdominal wall should alert the clinician to the possibility of buried bumper.
- Trying to administer feeding by force in this situation may lead to abscess formation in the abdominal wall.

- The migrated internal bumper can usually be palpated in the abdominal wall indicating the diagnosis.
- Abdominal ultrasound, CT or endoscopy establishes the diagnosis.
- Once the diagnosis is confirmed, the gastrostomy tube should be removed either by external traction or by surgery under local anesthesia; another tube is inserted in place.

## References

[1] McClave SA, Jafri NS. Spectrum of morbidity related to bolster placement at time of percutaneous endoscopic gastrostomy: buried bumper syndrome to leakage and peritonitis. *Gastrointest. Endosc. Clin. N. Am.* 2007;17:731-746.

[2] Anagnostopoulos GK, Kostopoulos P, Arvanitidis DM. Buried bumper syndrome with a fatal outcome. Presenting early as gastrointestinal bleeding after percutaneous endoscopic gastrostomy placement. *J. Postgrad. Med.* 2003; 49: 325-327.

# Case 24. Colonic Obstruction versus Pseudoobstruction

An 89-year-old woman was referred for subacute care with the diagnosis of colonic pseudoobstruction. Her medical history was remarkable for arterial hypertension, chronic normocytic anemia, chronic constipation, and severe dementia of Alzheimer's type, the latter diagnosed two years ago. She was living in the community together with a caregiver under 24-hours supervision. Abdominal distension, nausea, and refusal to eat began three weeks ago and she was admitted to another hospital in April 2011, with the suspicion of volvulus of the sigmoid colon versus colonic pseudoobstruction. Abdominal CT examination showed severe distension of the colon without mural thickening, a lesion or volvulus. Attempted colonoscopy failed twice because of poor bowel preparation. During a three weeks hospital stay there was no improvement. An intercurrent febrile disease was diagnosed as E. coli septicemia and remitted on ciprofloxacin treatment. Eventually a nasogastric feeding tube was inserted and the patient received enteric feeding. The patient's regular medications were continued including aspirin 100 mg and folic acid 5 mg/day.

On admission to our ward she was alert, cooperative but refusing to eat and unwilling to tolerate the nasogastric tube. Her body temperature was normal, the BP 125-180/80 mmHg, heart rate 80 bpm, and SaO2 in ambient air 93%. The abdomen was tense and tympanitic. Bowel sounds were hyperactive and high pitched. Laboratory examination showed hemoglobin 10.2 g/dL, WBC 6100/mm3; the levels of thyrotropin, serum sodium, potassium, calcium, magnesium, vitamin B12 and folic acid were within the normal range. Plain abdominal radiographs showed a dilated colon, to a greater degree in the sigmoid segment, with normal haustral markings, and filled with air from the cecum to the rectum, (Figure 26).

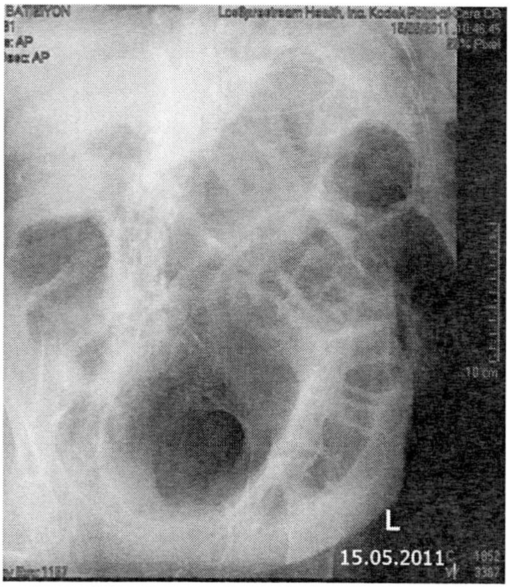


Figure 26. Markedly distended air filled sigmoid colon with effacement of haustra. Other colonic segments are distended to a lesser degree.

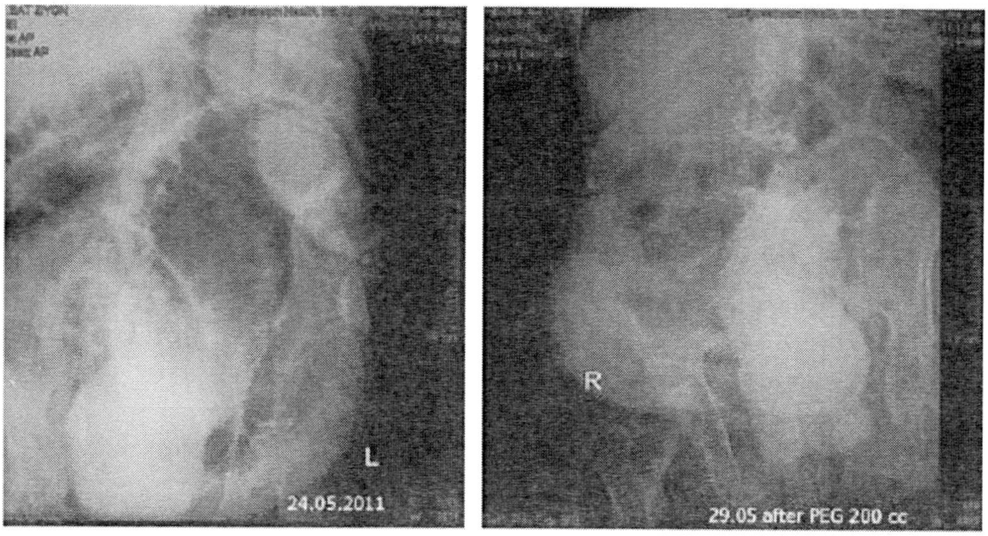


Figure 27. Sequential plain abdominal films surveying purge of the contrast material. There was no elimination of the contrast after one week or on the subsequent week after administration of fleet enema and oral polyethylene glycol.

The patient received 1600 calories/day by tube feeding. She accepted oral intake only when the abdominal distension remitted following decompression via rectal tube. Medications were continued as above. Isotonic fluids were supplied intravenously. As no improvement was observed during the subsequent 10 days and the diagnosis was uncertain the patient was referred for surgical re-evaluation. She underwent a bowel enema with meglumine ioxitalamate (Telebrix) which showed free retrograde passage of the contrast agent: there was neither mechanical obstruction, nor mural pathology or volvulus. The surgeons adopted a palliative approach in view of the patient's advanced age and severe dementia and the patient was returned to our ward. Yet, there was no improvement in her clinical status. The abdomen remained tightly distended with hyperperistalsis and high pitched bowel sounds. The radiocontrast agent she had received by enema was retained in the sigmoid colon in spite of various interventions: fleet enema and rectal tube insertion resulted in decompression of colonic air but not in purging the contrast agent; administration of polyethylene glycol 50 cc and later 200 cc through the gastric tube were of no avail; intravenous neostigmine 1.5 mg caused abdominal cramps and vomiting but purging did not follow (Figure 27). Another surgical consult was requested. The recommendation was unequivocal not to perform cecostomy or other palliative surgery, since results in real life are disappointing and the risks are significant.

During the patient's long hospitalization she suffered repeated episodes of urinary tract infection, which responded to antibiotic treatment. There was no correlation between relapses of sepsis and aggravation of colonic pseudoobstruction. Eventually, with the aid of daily 4-6 hours of colonic decompression via rectal tube the patient's symptoms improved: the abdominal distension diminished, the patient began to eat, and the nasogastric feeding tube could be removed, the bowel sound became normal and the abdominal distension remitted. A later episode of sepsis was not associated with recurrence of the colonic pseudoobstruction. At this time the plain abdominal film showed a dilated sigmoid colon, disappearance of the radiocontrast material, effacement of the haustra and a coffee bean pattern suggesting volvulus of the sigma (Figure 28).

*Acute colonic pseudoobstruction* is caused by a disturbance of the autonomic innervation of the distal colon, which can occur in a variety of clinical settings: severe acute medical illness (stroke, myocardial infarction, peritonitis, sepsis), surgical procedures (orthopedic, cardiovascular, or lung surgery), systemic diseases that affect the neuromuscular component of the gastrointestinal tract (e.g. amyloidosis), and drug effects (phenothiazines, some antiparkinsonian drugs, tricyclic antidepressants, clozapine, anticholinergic agents, opiate analgesics, calcium channel antagonists, clonidine, octreotide).

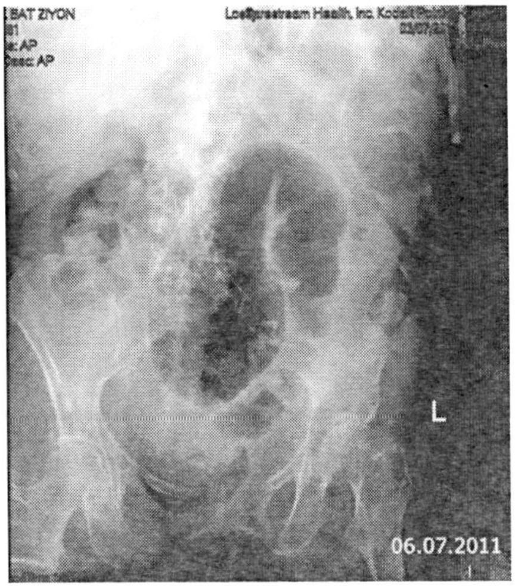


Figure 28. Improvement of radiographical findings one month later, when the clinical symptoms and signs had remitted. Yet, the sigmoid loop remained distended.

*The typical clinical feature* of intestinal pseudoobstruction is severe abdominal distention, with no passage of stool or gas. However, up to 40% of patients with intestinal pseudo-obstruction still pass some gas or even present with diarrhea during the episode. Nausea and vomiting can occur, but in distinction form other entities, nasogastric aspiration provides no relief because pseudo-obstruction affects exclusively the colon. Abdominal distention is usually painless and there is no abdominal tenderness. In fact, the presence of abdominal pain and tenderness suggest colonic perforation or ischemia. Bowel sounds vary from absent to hyperactive and in many cases are high pitched as in mechanical obstruction.

*On plain abdominal film*, the hallmark of intestinal pseudoobstruction is dilatation of the colon. When *air is visible in all colonic segments including the rectosigmoid,* the diagnosis is usually pseudoobstruction. The dilatation preferentially affects the cecum, the ascending and transverse colon, although the left colon including the rectum also may be dilated. The small bowel is involved in some cases. The cecal diameter on abdominal films may have important prognostic significance with implications in management: a cecal 9 cm cut-off is used as a sign of impending perforation in patients with acute colonic pseudo-obstruction. In Vanek and Al-Salti's review, perforation rates for cecal diameters less than 12 cm was 0.7%, with cecal diameter 12 to 14 cm the perforation rate was 7%, and with cecal diameter greater than 14 cm the rate was 23%. Presence of free abdominal air is usually a sign of intestinal perforation. Free air in association with pneumatosis intestinalis, however, may not be associated with perforation and does not necessarily mandates surgical exploration.

*A water-soluble contrast enema* should be performed in all patients in whom the diagnosis is suspected, provided their condition is stable enough. The contrast enema can reliably differentiate between mechanical obstruction and pseudo-obstruction, a differentiation that is essential to guide therapy. Alternatives to contrast enemas are judicious *procto-sigmoidoscopy*, which may provide both the diagnosis and decompression, although not without complications, and *CT of the abdomen*, which has a sensitivity of 96% and specificity of 93%.

*Colonic pseudoobstruction should be differentiated from toxic megacolon*, which is characterized by the combination of colonic distention, colonic inflammation and septic shock. Abdominal upright and plain films may show 'thumb printing' due to submucosal edema and thickening of the colonic wall. Active colitis will be apparent on sigmoidoscopy. The leading cause of toxic megacolon in the elderly is Clostridium difficile infection (it is not necessarily associated with diarrhea). In younger patients, a common cause of toxic megacolon is inflammatory bowel disease.

*Volvulus of the sigmoid colon* is another important differential. Etiologic factors include anatomic variation, chronic constipation, neurologic disease, and megacolon. On plain abdominal film the following are characteristic features of sigmoid volvulus: an inverted U-shaped appearance of distended sigmoid loop, loss of haustra, coffee-bean sign (the midline crease corresponds to the mesenteric root in the greatly distended sigmoid colon). Because volvulus may compromise the circulation of the affected intestinal segment, the bowel may become gangrenous leading to perforation, peritonitis, and sepsis. Immediate detorsion is required to restore blood perfusion to the intestine. Conservative management with rehydration and bowel rest will not release the volvulus and restore the blood flow to the sigmoid and is therefore inappropriate. Endoscopic reduction of the volvulus relieves the obstruction and restores the blood supply to the affected sigmoid. Once sigmoid volvulus is suspected, endoscopic reduction should be performed immediately, before the bowel sustains irreversible ischemic injury. During endoscopy, the clinician can also visualize the colon and observe whether the patient has developed bowel ischemia.

The mortality rate of patients with acute colonic pseudo-obstruction varies from 0 to 32% and is partly determined by comorbidity. Frequent clinical reevaluation, WBC counts and abdominal radiography are the key to timely identify bowel perforation.

*Patients with colonic pseudoobstruction should be kept fasted.* They are often dehydrated as they have lost fluid into the affected bowel. Therefore, *intravenous fluids* are indicated. However, parenteral or enteral nutrition may be necessary in patients with prolonged acute colonic pseudo-obstruction.

*Underlying reversible diseases should be treated,* such as infection or congestive heart failure. Electrolyte imbalances should be corrected, particularly hypomagnesemia, hypocalcemia, and hypokalemia. Acute colonic pseudo-obstruction is often associated with hypokalemia due to secretory diarrhea. Unnecessary medications should be discontinued, especially opiates, sedatives, lactulose, and drugs with anticholinergic side effects.

*Rectal tubes are not useful except* when the sigmoid is involved. In the latter situation (as in our patient) a rectal tube is inserted and attached to gravity drainage. The patient should be placed in a prone position with the hips elevated on a pillow or the knee chest position with the hips held high. These positions should be alternated with right and left lateral decubitus positions each hour.

*Neostigmine*, a parasympathomimetic agent can be administered if after 72 hours of conservative measures the cecal diameter is >9 cm, and there are no contraindications to neostigmine. Intravenous administration of neostigmine 1-2 mg over 3 to 5 minutes may be efficient. The patient is kept supine for at least 60 min after the drug was given with electro-cardiographic and vital sign monitoring. Atropine should be at hand to reverse bradycardia induced by neostigmine. Repeat infusion may be administered after 4 hours if the response is unsatisfactory. Contraindications for neostigmine administration include heart rate less than 60 beats/minute, systolic BP less than 90 mmHg, active bronchospasm, serum creatinine greater than 3 mg/dL, and signs of bowel perforation. After administration of neostigmine the patient promptly passes gas or develops abdominal cramping. However, it has not been shown that such decompression by passage of gas reduces the risk of perforation and mortality.

Enemas have not shown any efficacy except for diatrizoate (Gastrografin) enemas in anecdotal reports. Moreover, enemas may precipitate colonic perforation. Conservative therapy can be continued for 24 to 48 hours provided there is no pain or >12 cm colonic distension. Treatment results in resolution of colonic pseudoobstruction within 2 to 6 days in 83% to 96% of patients. Most patients can be treated in the setting of acute geriatric ward. However, if improvement does not occur within a few days the patient should be referred for *endoscopic decompression*; if there is no response, *percutaneous cecostomy/surgery* may be necessary to decrease cecal distention.

The diagnosis in our patient was uncertain. The suspicion of volvulus of the sigmoid colon was disproved on CT and later on water-soluble contrast enema. There was neither evidence of colonic obstruction nor of toxic megacolon. By exclusion of other causes of colonic distension the patient was managed according to the protocol for colonic pseudoobstruction, with frequent clinical reevaluation, repeated WBC counts, abdominal plain radiographies to detect any possible complication, and consultation with surgeons. Six months later the situation was unchanged. PEG was performed.

Learning Points

- Acute colonic pseudoobstruction is a syndrome of massive dilation of the colon without mechanical obstruction that develops in hospitalized patients with serious underlying medical and surgical conditions.
- The differential diagnosis of a markedly distended colon includes mechanical obstruction, pseudoobstruction and toxic megacolon.
- A water soluble contrast enema should be performed when the diagnosis is suspected.
- The risk of colonic perforation increases when cecal diameter exceeds 12 cm and when the distention has been present for longer than 6 days.
- Management of colonic pseudoobstruction is supportive, with selective use of neostigmine and colonoscopy for decompression.
- Early recognition and management may be important in minimizing complications.

## References

[1] Eisen GM, Baron TH, Dominitz JA, Faigel DO, Goldstein JL, Johanson JF, Mallery JS, Raddawi HM, Vargo JJ, Waring JP, Fanelli RD, Wheeler-Harbaugh J; Standards of Practice Committee of the American Society for Gastrointestinal Endoscopy. Acute colonic pseudoobstruction. *Gastrointest. Endosc.* 2002;56:789-792.

[2] Saunders MD. Acute colonic pseudo-obstruction. *Gatrointestinal Endosc.* 2007;17: 341-360.

## Case 25. Pneumoperitoneum after PEG

In refusing oral intake, the patient described under Case 24 received feeding by nasogastric tube. Her vital signs were normal and routine laboratory tests (CBC, biochemistry panel, prothrombin time and activated partial thromboplastin time) were within the normal range. At this point in time PEG was performed and feeding via the gastrostomy tube was started. By the 11$^{th}$ day after gastrostomy the patient's abdomen became enlarged and tympanic. There was no abdominal tenderness and the peristaltic sounds were unchanged. The patient's body temperature and other vital signs remained normal, the CBC and CRP were unremarkable. A plain abdominal radiography showed free abdominal air (Figure 29). On CT with administration of an oral radiocontrast agent there was neither leakage of gastrographin into the peritoneum nor evidence of damage to a contiguous abdominal structure. The patient was restarted on tube feeding without complications.

*A small amount of free peritoneal air* after PEG is a common and benign finding [1, 2]. It is the air escaped during insufflation of the stomach through the puncture site on the gastric wall into the peritoneal cavity. Pneumoperitoneum may result relative rarely occur by air leakage from the abdominal wall stoma into the peritoneum [3]. In either situation, resolution will occur within a week in most cases. It is often thought that pneumoperitoneum after PEG in the absence of peritonitis has no consequence and should not preclude tube feeding.

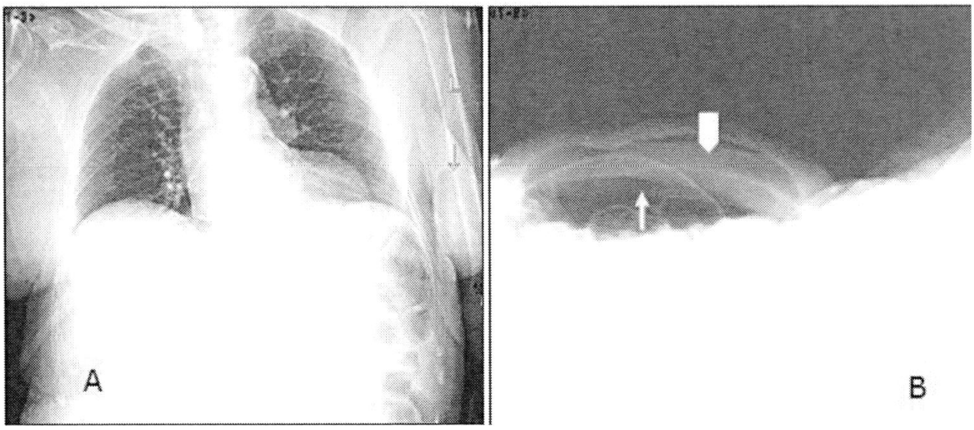


Figure 29. Chest x-ray while the patient was supine is unremarkable (A). Supine cross-table beam examination of the abdomen shows air in the peritoneal space (bold arrow) and air in the dilated sigmoid colon (thin arrow). Rigler's sign is recognized, defined by presence of air on both sides of the intestinal wall, the luminal side and the peritoneal side (B).

However, peritoneal signs and symptoms may not be easily recognized in patients with altered mental status or those who require long-term sedation.

*Incidental perforation of the bowel*, especially the colon, during PEG may also result in pneumoperitoneum [3]. It may be challenging to differentiate the innocent peritoneal free air from pneumoperitoneum resulting from perforation of the colon. In a study of 722 patients who underwent PEG or PEG/J placement, 39 had abdominal free air. Thirty three patients (85%) had no signs of peritonitis and were discharged without surgical intervention. Of the six patients with serious complications related to their procedure, five had clinical signs of peritonitis that helped to guide their management [2]. When clinical features raise concern about a ruptured viscous, contrast radiography through the gastrostomy tube should be obtained to confirm the position of the tube within the stomach and to exclude a leak. Alternatively, a contrast CT scan of the abdomen can disclose damage to an abdominal viscus.

Spontaneous closure of air leakage occurs in most cases of benign pneumoperitoneum after PEG, merely with wound care and proton pump inhibitor treatment. For persistent peristomal leakage, surgical closure and excision of the tract is the traditional treatment. For the same purpose, electrochemical cauterization or clip closure can be performed. Encouraging preliminary results have been reported.

## Learning Points

- Clinical follow-up after PEG is mandatory focused on signs of peritonitis. Abdominal pain, tenderness, rigidity, nausea, vomiting, progressive abdominal distension, arterial hypotension, fever and leukocytosis are ‘red flags’.
- Upon suspicion, a contrast study through the PEG tube or a contrast abdominal CT should be performed to detect possible leakage of gastrographin into the peritoneum or damage to a contiguous abdominal viscus. These investigations guide the subsequent management.

- PEG tube repositioning, electrochemical cauterization, clip closure, or surgical tract closure and excision may be considered.
- If there is no evidence of contrast leakage into the peritoneum, gastrostomy tube feeding can be resumed.
- Serial radiographic imaging is warranted to visualize the resolution of pneumoperitoneum after repositioning the gastrostomy tube.

## References

[1] Wiesen AJ, Sideridis K, Fernandes A, Hines J, Indaram A, Weinstein L, Davidoff S, Bank S. True incidence and clinical significance of pneumoperitoneum after PEG placement: a prospective study. *Gastrointest. Endosc.* 2006; 64:886-889.

[2] Blum CA, Selander C, Ruddy JM, Leon S. The incidence and clinical significance of pneumoperitoneum after percutaneous endoscopic gastrostomy: a review of 722 cases. *Am. Surg.* 2009; 75:39-43.

[3] Milanchi S, Allins A. Early pneumoperitoneum after percutaneous endoscopic gastrostomy in intensive care patients: sign of possible bowel injury. *Am. J. Crit. Care.* 2007;16:132-136.

Chapter V

# Infectious Diseases – Surprises and Mishaps

Diagnosis of common bacterial infections relies on time-honored guidelines. However, surprises are not uncommon and clinicians should be quick in recognizing unusual manifestations of diseases, adverse reactions to treatment and mishaps. In quoting Galen, the physician: '*I call all gods to witness that I have often on further examination seen things I completely missed before*'. Thus, a second evaluation of the patient, his laboratory and imaging data, and a second judgment are justified, worth, and recommended.

## Case 26. Pneumonia Unresponsive to Treatment

An 88-year-old woman was hospitalized with the diagnosis of right lower lobe pneumonia attributed to pulmonary aspiration. Treatment with piperacillin-tazobactam 4.5 g x 3/day was begun. Five days later she was transferred to our ward for subacute care. Remarkable in her medical history were ischemic heart disease, arterial hypertension, colonic diverticulosis, and severe dementia. One month before the present admission she was diagnosed with E. coli urinary tract infection, which remitted on ceftriaxone treatment; an abdominal ultrasound examination at that time did not reveal any abnormality.

The patient was alert, the rectal temperature was 38.2$^0$C, BP 130/72 mmHg, heart rate 76 bpm. Bilateral wet rales and wheezes were perceived over the lower lung fields. Otherwise the examination was unremarkable. The WBC was 12,000/mm$^3$ with 82% polymorphonuclear neutrophils; the CRP was 84 mg/L. Chest radiography showed increased interstitial pulmonary markings. After ten days piperacillin-tazobactam treatment low grade fever persisted (37.6$^0$C-38.2$^0$C) and the WBC, CRP and chest x-rays were basically unchanged. Azithromycin i.v. 500 mg/day was administered for 5 days, however, the fever increased to 39.2$^0$C. A hard and well defined mass with smooth margins became palpable in the patient's left flank. Abdominal CT exposed a large fluid collection surrounding the mid-portion of the descending colon (Figure 30).

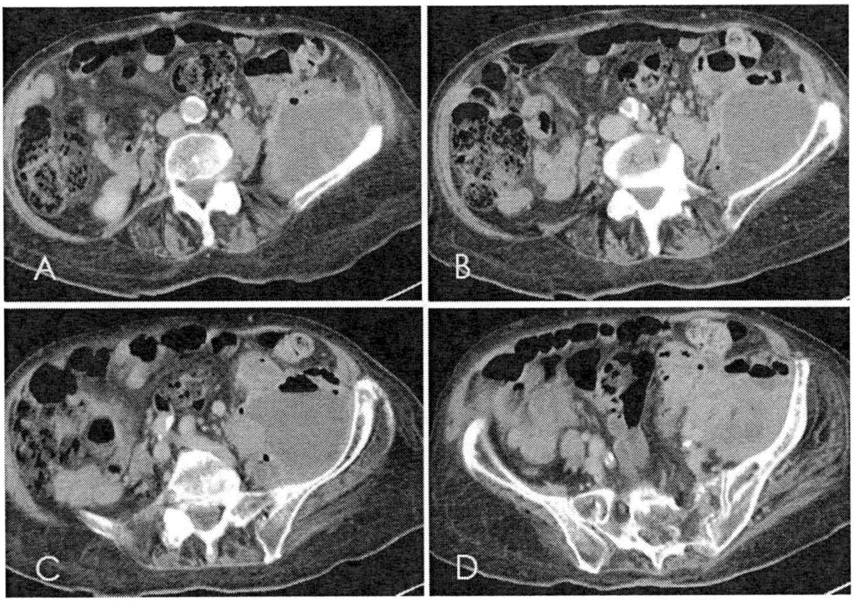


Figure 30. Heterogeneous abscess of low attenuation in the left iliac fossa.

At this point, the cause of sepsis became clear in revealing the paracolic collection, probably an abscess, likely caused by perforation of a colonic diverticle. The patient was referred to surgery. For the beginning external drainage was instituted; the discharge was frankly purulent and grew a mixed aerobic and anaerobic flora.

*The diagnosis of pneumonia* is established when two criteria area met: 1) occurrence of a new infiltrate on chest x-rays, and 2) the 'correct' clinical setting. A clinical suspicion of pneumonia should prompt the ordering of a posteroanterior and lateral chest radiography. Laboratory tests are of little help to advance the diagnosis. Antibiotics should be administered within the first 4 hours and difficulties in obtaining expectorated sputum should not delay drug delivery.

On x-rays, pneumonic infiltrates may be alveolar, interstitial, nodular or mixed, focal or diffuse. Interstitial infiltrates, as seen in this patient, can be found in viral and certain other pneumonias, but also in congestive heart failure, lymphangitic spread of tumor, idiopathic pulmonary fibrosis, collagen vascular diseases, and drug toxicity. Furthermore, the 'interstitial pneumonia pattern' is similar in acute, subacute, poorly resolving acute pneumonia, or chronic interstitial pneumonias. Therefore, review of prior x-rays is mostly important for the interpretation of the current chest x-rays [1].

*For patients who do not respond* to initial empiric antibiotic treatment an aggressive search should be undertaken to detect unusual pathogens, complications of pneumonia (mainly empyema or lung abscess) or an extrapulmonary disorder. Additional diagnostic testing may include sampling of pleural fluid, chest CT, bronchoscopy with collection of respiratory secretions for microbiologic analysis and brush cytology. A paracolic collection was eventually uncovered in our patient. A paracolic collection on the left side is caused by peridiverticulitis, Crohn's disease, or by perforation of a malignant tumor. CT is best suited to the diagnosis and management of these conditions. A paracolic collection on the right side is usually caused by appendicitis, Crohn's disease, perforation of a diverticula or extension of a right subdiaphragmatic abscess. [2].

In the present case, the association of fever with interstitial pulmonary infiltrates pointed to a pulmonary infection. However, the expected improvement did not occur on antibiotic treatment and required to consider other causes of fever. A paracolic abscess was the final diagnosis.

### Learning Points

- The presence of a new pulmonary infiltrate in the appropriate clinical context makes the diagnosis of 'probable pneumonia'.
- Antibiotics should be started quickly.
- The current chest X-rays should be compared with previous radiographies.
- The diagnosis is definitely established only after clinical and radiological resolution of the pulmonary infiltrate – the latter can take several weeks.
- Physicians should be aware of possible pitfalls in the diagnosis.

## References

[1] Mabie M, Wunderink RG. Use and limitations of clinical and radiologic diagnosis of pneumonia. *Semin. Respir. Infect.* 2003;18:72-79.

[2] Touzios JG. Diverticulosis and acute diverticulitis. *Gastroenterol. Clin. North Amer.* 2009; 38: 513-525.

## Case 27. Nephrotoxicity - Vancomycin Implicated by Right or in the Wrong

A 72-year-old man was diagnosed with L1-L2 discitis. He was in poor health for several years, with a history of arterial hypertension, myocardial infarctions, type 2 diabetes mellitus, dyslipidemia and mild renal failure. He suffered numerous episodes of cardiac decompensation. Six months before the present admission he underwent an emergency femoro-popliteal artery bypass operation that complicated by wound infection with methicillin resistant staphylococcus aureus (MRSA). The response to treatment was poor and, eventually, below knee amputation was performed. Subsequently the fever remitted, the WBC and CRP returned to normal. Three weeks later the fever rouse again associated with low back pain. The patient was admitted again to the medical ward. He was cachectic, BP 182/84 mmHg, heart rate 76 bpm, respirations 16 per minute. A grade 3/6 pansystolic murmur was heard over the cardiac apex. There was hepatojugular reflux and grade 1 ankle edema. Laboratory tests were remarkable for CRP 230 mg/L, serum creatinine 1.6 mg/dL, albumin 2.8 g/L. MRSA was recovered in 3 consecutive blood cultures. Gallium scan and CT imaging showed findings consistent with L1-L2 discitis and adjacent vertebral osteomyelitis. Transesophageal echocardiography showed diffusely diminished contractility of the left ventricle, the left ventricular ejection fraction was 30% in the presence of moderate mitral regurgitation; no valvular vegetations were revealed. The estimated creatinine clearance (eCCT) according to the MDRD equation was 45 mL/min/1.73 $m^2$ and according to Cockcroft-Gault equation 30 mL/min/1.73 $m^2$. Treatment with intravenous vancomycin 1 g at 24 hour intervals was administered.

The patient was transferred for subacute care. He continued to receive vancomycin and aspirin 100 mg/day, carvedilol 12.5 mg/day, ramipril 5 mg/day, furosemide 40 mg/day, spironolactone 12.5 mg/day, simvastatin 20 mg/day and insulin. Trough vancomycin levels were measured twice weekly and were found between 5 and 8 μg/mL. Thirty days on vancomycin treatment, the temperature was normal and the CRP had decreased to 18 mg/L. However, the signs of heart failure worsened with generalized edema and pulmonary congestion on x-rays. Results of laboratory tests were unchanged. Furosemide i.v drip 160 mg per day was started. Six days later the serum creatinine had risen to 3 mg/dL and the BUN to 110 mg/dL. There was essentially no change in the patient's BP that remained in the range 124-160/70-82 mmHg. The urinary sediment was unremarkable. The AST, ALT and prothrombin time were within the normal range. The BUN to creatinine ratio was 30:1 at the time of worsened renal status, suggesting renal hypoperfusion. On noting the deterioration in renal function, vancomycin, furosemide and ramipril were discontinued, and treatment with rifampicin was instituted. Gradually, over a period of 10 days the serum creatinine level decreased to 2.6 mg/dL and the BUN to 32 mg/dL. Two months later, the treatment for vertebral osteomyelitis was completed, the heart failure and BP were fairly controlled, but the plasma creatinine was 3 mg/dL.

*Risk factors predisposing to renal hypoperfusion* are well known [1] and were largely present in our patient. These are age >65 years, atherosclerosis, chronic hypertension, chronic kidney disease, sepsis, hypoalbuminemia, and treatment with an ACE inhibitor or ARB. In the context of severe chronic heart failure, the compensatory humoral and neural responses might have been engaged to the maximum with redistribution of blood flow to cerebral and coronary arteries. So, the renal circulation becomes more vulnerable to ischemia. In addition to the latter alterations in renal homeostasis, well known in theory, volume depletion caused by furosemide may have aggravated renal ischemia, and vancomycin possibly has enhanced the predisposition to renal damage.

*Vancomycin is primarily excreted unchanged via the kidneys.* A linear correlation between creatinine clearance and vancomycin levels is recognized, permitting the use of nomograms and formulas to determine the dosing schedule in patients with decreased creatinine clearance. A familiar approach is to administer a fixed loading dose (25 mg/kg) followed by a maintenance dose (19 mg/kg) administered intravenously at a calculated interval

Interval = normal interval x (86 mL/min ÷ [0.689 × creatinine clearance mL/min + 3.66] (where the normal interval is 12 hours)

Creatinine Clearance = [[140 - age(yr)]*weight(kg)]/[72*serum Cr(mg/dL)] (multiply by 0.85 for women)

This schedule should result in an approximate serum peak value of 30 μg/mL and a trough level of 7.5 μg/mL.

*The bactericidal activity of vancomycin* is concentration independent once a concentration of four or five times the MIC for the organism is reached [2].

*Vancomycin serum concentrations should be checked* to optimize therapy and to use as a surrogate marker of effectiveness. A consensus statement from the American Society of Health-System Pharmacists and the Society of Infectious Diseases Pharmacists recommend that vancomycin trough rather than peak levels should be monitored. Trough levels should be checked just before the fourth dose, when steady-state levels are likely to have been achieved. More frequent monitoring may be considered in patients with fluctuating renal function. Trough levels should be higher than 10 mg/L to prevent development of resistance. This aim was not met in our patient. To improve antibiotic penetration trough levels of 15 to 20 mg/L are recommended for pathogens with a vancomycin MIC of 1 mg/L or higher and for complicated infections such as endocarditis, osteomyelitis, meningitis, and hospital-acquired pneumonia. For prolonged courses, it is appropriate to check vancomycin levels weekly in hemodynamically stable patients and more often in those who are not hemodynamically stable or having unstable renal function. Samples for trough concentrations should be obtained within 30 minutes of the next scheduled dose. It was recommended that morbidly obese patients should receive vancomycin loading dose based on their actual total body weight instead of their ideal weight; in order to avoid very high peak values frequent serum level measurements may be worthwhile. In patients with MRSA bacteremia, follow-up blood cultures 2 to 4 days after initial positive cultures and as needed thereafter are recommended to document the clearance of bacteremia.

*Renal function impairment* occurred in our patient under vancomycin treatment. This adverse effect was reported to occur in <1% to 7% of patients; impairment of renal function increased to 14% to 20% when vancomycin was co-administered with an aminoglycoside [1-3]. Occurrence of nephrotoxicity is dose-related; it also is more frequent during prolonged therapy (10 days or longer). Other risk factors associated with aminoglycoside-associated nephrotoxicity include advanced patient age, decreased plasma albumin concentration, poor nutritional status, dehydration, hypercalcemia, rapidly fatal illness, liver or kidney disease, shock, ascites, concurrent and/or sequential systemic or topical use of other potentially nephrotoxic drugs (cisplatin, cephaloridine, kanamycin, amikacin, neomycin, polymixin B, colistin, paromomycin, streptomycin, tobramycin, vancomycin, and viomycin). A retrospective analysis identified the following independent predictors of nephrotoxicity in patients treated with vancomycin: vancomycin serum trough concentrations ≥14 mg/L, duration of vancomycin therapy ≥7 days, and baseline serum creatinine levels ≥1.7 mg/dL. Nephrotoxicity resolved in 81% of cases after treatment with vancomycin was discontinued [3].

In a complex clinical situation such as in the present case, when perfusion of the kidneys was exposed to numerous deleterious influences, it may be their synergistic effect which caused the damage. In fact, it is difficult to distinguish between renal injury induced by an aminoglycoside, sepsis and hypotension, as acknowledged in the literature [4]. In the present case, thorough monitoring of vancomycin serum levels did not prevent the deterioration of renal function.

### Learning Points

- Vancomycin is primarily excreted unchanged via the kidneys. A linear correlation between creatinine clearance and vancomycin levels is recognized.
- Renal function impairment has been reported between zero and 7% of patients on i.v. vancomycin treatment and 14% to 20% when vancomycin is co-administered with another aminoglycoside.
- The occurrence of nephrotoxicity is dose-related and is more frequent when therapy administered for longer than 10 days.
- Other risk factors for vancomycin nephrotoxicity are age greater than 70 years, decreased plasma albumin concentration, poor nutritional status, dehydration, hypercalcemia, rapidly fatal illness, liver or kidney disease, shock, and ascites.
- When numerous deleterious influences might affect the renal perfusion, it is recommended to remove potentially nephrotoxic drugs and to monitor carefully the BP, diuresis, and vancomycin trough levels.
- Vancomycin-induced nephrotoxicity resolves in approximately 80% of cases.

## References

[1] Raveh D, Kopyt M, Hite Y, Rudensky B, Sonnenblick M, Yinnon AM. Risk factors for nephrotoxicity in elderly patients receiving once-daily aminoglycosides. *QJM* 2002;95:291-297.

[2] Leekha S, Terrell CL, Edson RS. General principles of antimicrobial therapy. *Mayo Clin. Proc.* 2011; 86:156-167.

[3] Pritchard L, Baker C, Leggett J, Sehdev P, Brown A, Bayley KB. Increasing vancomycin serum trough concentrations and incidence of nephrotoxicity. *Amer. J. Med.* 2010;123: 1143-1149.

[4] Vance-Bryan K, Rotschafer JC, Gilliland SS, Rodvold KA, Fitzgerald CM, Guay DR. A comparative assessment of vancomycin-associated nephrotoxicity in the young versus the elderly hospitalized patient. *J. Antimicrob. Chemother.* 1994;33: 811-821.

## Case 28. Vancomycin Hypersensitivity Eruption-Treating through

A 66-year-old man was admitted for subacute care after a month-long treatment in the department of internal medicine; the diagnoses were MRSA urinary tract infection, suspected infective endocarditis, and right lower lobe pneumonia. The patient's medical history comprised myocardial infarction, systolic heart failure, ischemic stroke with right hemiplegia, arterial hypertension, and dyslipemia. He was implanted a cardioverter defibrillator. Recent echocardiography revealed an echogenic intraventricular mass adherent to the pacemaker electrode. Blood cultures were negative but have been taken at a time the patient was already receiving ceftriaxone treatment. In the context of MRSA urinary tract infection, the mass lesion attached to the pacemaker electrode was considered potentially to be infected; the diagnosis of possible bacterial endocarditis was proposed. So, antibiotic treatment was started with vancomycin-rifampicin combination for 6 weeks and gentamicin scheduled for 2 weeks and. The patient's usual medications were continued, including simvastatin 20 mg, clopidogrel 20 mg, furosemide 80 mg, spironolactone 12.5 mg, bisoprostol fumarate 1.25 mg, amiodarone 200 mg, doxazocin 1 mg, folic acid 5 mg, and lamotrigene 300 mg/day.

On admission to our ward the patient was in good general state, the rectal temperature was constantly $<37.5^0$ C, BP 110/68, heart rate 80 bpm, and SaO2 in ambient air 92%. The scheduled gentamicin treatment was completed. On the third week of combined vancomycin and rifampicin treatment, an asymptomatic maculopapular eruption was noticed on the dorsum of the left foot and adjacent malleolar area. Two days later the eruption extended along both calves (Figure 31).

There was no interdigital tinea. The patient's temperature remained within the normal range. The WBC was 6100/mm$^3$ with 7% eosinophils. Possible causes of the maculopapular eruption were examined. In considering a drug hypersensitivity reaction, vancomycin and rifampicin were the main candidates since they did not belong to the patient's long-time drug regimen.

*A maculopapular (morbilliform) eruption* as seen in this patient is the most common variant of hypersensitivity drug eruptions. It may be produced by a type IV immunologic reaction or by other mechanisms. Maculopapular eruptions usually begin in dependent body areas and later may generalize. The macules and papules are discrete or coalescing, erythematous, symmetrically distributed. This type of eruption is indistinguishable from a viral exanthema and routine laboratory tests are not helpful in differentiating between the two disorders. The rash clears rapidly following withdrawal of the offending agent, but may fade even if the drug is continued, or may progress to a generalized exfoliative dermatitis [1].

*Vancomycin-induced rash* may occur under various presentations: as leukocytoclastic vasculitis, drug rash with eosinophilia and systemic symptoms (DRES), morbilliform rash, and drug fever associated with a rash [2-4]. The literature review spotted also a few reports of rifampicin-induced exanthema and urticaria.

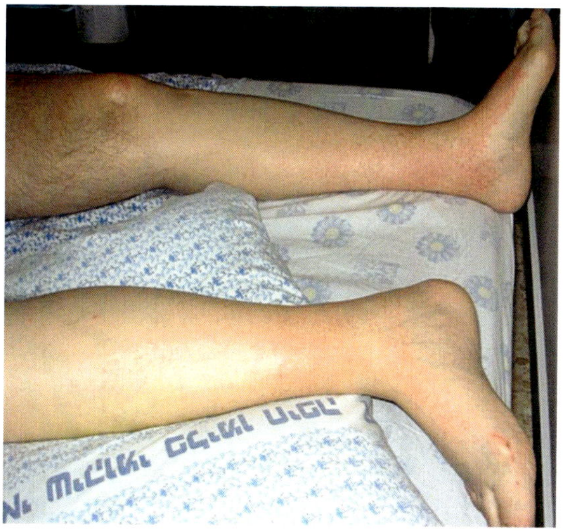

Figure 31. Maculopapular eruption on the dorsum of the feet and calves.

Discontinuation of the responsible medication is essential to the management of a drug eruption. We discontinued rifampicin treatment in being an adjuvant to vancomycin for the treatment of MRSA infections and not considered to be indispensable. On the contrary, treatment with vancomycin or a substitute is essential for the management of MRSA endocarditis. Three alternatives of managing were considered: to replace vancomycin with teicoplanin [5] though sensitivity of the MRSA isolate to teicoplanin had not been tested; vancomycin desensitization [6]; and **'treating through' with vancomycin** [1].

*There are two exceptions to the rule of immediate discontinuation* of the offending medication. First, in a patient with life-threatening enterococcal endocarditis who requires long-term treatment with high-dose penicillin, **'treating through' isolated episodes of urticaria** and generalized pruritus may be necessary. Most such episodes will remit with continuous penicillin therapy. Careful surveillance of hepatic enzymes and renal function is mandatory while continuing administration of the medication that caused the eruption. When treating through such mild type I reaction it is imperative to avoid lapses in treatment because restarting treatment after a lapse may trigger anaphylaxis. Second, a late-occurring macula-papular exanthema with minimal or no pruritus is another setting permitting 'treatment through' if there is a compelling clinical need not to stop the incriminated drug (as illustrated by the present case). Careful monitoring for fever, eosinophilia, proteinuria, arthralgia, lymphadenopathy, and hepatitis is warranted, with prompt cessation of therapy if new signs or symptoms appear.

A treating trough policy was adopted in our patient, based on the clinical setting: the maculopapular pattern of the eruption with limited distribution and no evidence of organ involvement. This is precisely the setting considered appropriate for a trial of 'treating through' the hypersensitivity reaction. Vancomycin administration was continued along with careful clinical monitoring for fever, proteinuria, arthralgia, lymphadenopathy, and laboratory monitoring for eosinophilia and hepatitis. The eruption began to fade after 5 days on continuous vancomycin treatment and without occurrence of clinical or laboratory signs of organ damage. The scheduled six weeks treatment with vancomycin was completed. On discharge from hospital, the patient was advised not to retreat with vancomycin.

*Identification of the causative drug* is in a patient with suspected drug hypersensitivity important, so re-exposure to the culprit drug can be avoided and recurrence of hyper-sensitivity reactions is precluded. Graded challenge and drug provocation is not recom-mended as a routine procedure for the identification of the culprit drug. This test may cause severe relapse and false negative results are possible. More often, tests are performed with alternative drugs to establish a safe substitution. An allergological workup is recommended at least in case of severe hypersensitivity reaction, when the suspected drug cannot easily be omitted or replaced, or when there are uncertainties about cross-reaction of alternative treatment options [7]. However, the predictive value of various tests in less than satisfactory.

*Skin prick or intradermal tests* are easy to perform and may provide help in the identification of the causative drug in both immediate and nonimmediate reactions. Concentrations to be used for prick or intradermal testing have been evaluated especially antibiotics and neuromuscular blocking agents (NMBAs). Patch testing is widely done in Europe but the test procedures and concentrations still need further investigation to be generally recommended. Most researchers recommend performing skin tests 1 to 6 months after the acute event, as effector cells may be exhausted immediately after the reaction. Because the sensitivity of the tests might decrease over time, they should best be performed in the first year after the hypersensitivity reaction. *Specific IgE* for immediate reactions has low sensitivity. The *basophil activation test* is based on flow cytometric quantification of drug-induced CD63 expression or CD203c upregulation. *The lymphocyte transformation test* (LTT) is an in vitro test for the investigation of nonimmediate hypersensitivity reactions or severe IgE-mediated reactions, in which T cells are also involved. The test measures the drug-specific stimulation of cells by assessing proliferation or expression of activation markers. LTT is available only in specialized centers. The specificity of the LTT is >90% but the overall sensitivity is only 30%. This test is performed 1 to 6 months after the acute event. Unfortunately, clinical and laboratory investigations during the florid phase of the hypersensitivity reaction do not provide sufficient support for a reliable diagnosis.

The patients should be informed about their drug allergy. Possible alternatives should be indicated in their 'allergy passport'' [7].

## Learning Points

- Any drug causing a generalized, symmetric, maculopapular rash should be immediately discontinued; the patient should not be treated again with the same drug.
- An exception to this rule is by 'treating through' without discontinuing the causative drug in case of late-occurring, mild maculopapular exanthems with minimal or no pruritus, and when there is a compelling clinical need to continue treatment with the same antibiotic. Careful monitoring for fever, eosinophilia, proteinuria, arthralgia, lymphadenopathy, and hepatitis is warranted, with prompt cessation of therapy if new signs or symptoms appear.
- Also, 'treating through' isolated episodes of urticaria and generalized pruritus may be necessary in patients with life-threatening enterococcal endocarditis, those who require long-term treatment with high-dose penicillin to effect a cure. Most such episodes of drug-induced urticaria are self-limited and will remit with continuous therapy.

# References

[1] Adkinson NF Jr: Middleton's Allergy: Principles and Practice, 7th ed, 2008, Mosby.

[2] Felix-Getzik E, Sylvia LM. Vancomycin-induced leukocytoclastic vasculitis. *Pharmacotherapy* 2009;29:846-851.

[3] Boet S, Noblet C, Haas-Hubscher C, Picard D, Musette P, Dureuil B. Severe vancomycin-induced drug rash with eosinophilia and systemic symptoms syndrome imitating septic shock. *Eur. J. Anesthesiol.* 2009;26:791-793.

[4] Billet SE, Kortuem KR, Gibson LE, El-Azhary R. A morbilliform variant of vancomycin-induced linear IgA bullous dermatosis. *Arch. Dermatol.* 2008 ;144: 774-778.

[5] Hung YP, Lee NY, Chang CM, Lee HC, Wu CJ, Chen PL, Lee CC, Chung CH, Ko WC. Tolerability of teicoplanin in 117 hospitalized adults with previous vancomycin-induced fever, rash, or neutropenia: a retrospective chart review. *Clin. Ther.* 2009;31: 1977-1986.
[6] Kitazawa T, Ota Y, Kada N, Morisawa Y, Yoshida A, Koike K, Kimura S. Successful vancomycin desensitization with a combination of rapid and slow infusion methods. *Intern. Med.* 2006;45:317-321.
[7] Snyder B. Approach to the patient with drug allergy. *Med. Clin. North Am.* 2010;94: 665-670.

## Case 29. Neutropenia Complicating Vancomycin Treatment

A 79-year-old woman with a MRSA-infected hip prosthesis received a course of vancomycin treatment, after removal of the prosthesis. The patient's regular medications were ramipril, hydrochlorothiazide, simvastatin, aspirin and oxycodone. The serum creatinine was 1.2 mg/dL. Vancomycin treatment was administered intravenously 1g at 36 hour intervals and the once measured trough vancomycin level was 2.2 μg/mL (not meeting standards of care). Yet, the clinical response was favorable; after 4 weeks of treatment the temperature was normal and the CRP was 12 mg/L. At this time point, a decline in the WBC was witnessed from 11,200/mm$^3$ with 9,180 neutrophils to 3,400/mm$^3$ with 1,150/mm$^3$ neutrophils and no band forms. The hemoglobin 11g/dL and platelets 230,000/mm$^3$ were essentially unchanged; the CRP was 10.2 mg/L. Common causes of neutropenia could be excluded, mainly infections and a variety of drugs. Thus the possibility was considered that vancomycin was causing the patient's neutropenia. Vancomycin was replaced with rifampin and fusidic acid. Within 3 days the neutrophil count increased to 1,620/mm$^3$ and after one week to 3,100/mm$^3$, the WBC was 6,040/mm$^3$. The subsequent course was uneventful.

*Neutropenia associated with vancomycin treatment* occurs in 1% to 2% of patients. This rate increases with long-term vancomycin administration; in one study 13% of patients treated with vancomycin for a mean 6.2 months developed neutropenia [1]. Neutropenia usually resolves after discontinuation of the drug. In the case described by Mackett et al. neutropenia was noticed on day 17 of vancomycin treatment, it progressed over the next 3 days; after discontinuation of vancomycin a rise in the neutrophil count occurred within 5 days [2]. This is not unlike to the course of neutropenia in the present case. In a patient described by Koo et al. [3], severe leukopenia developed on vancomycin treatment; on discontinuation of vancomycin, the leukocyte and neutrophil counts promptly increased with full recovery after a week. Subsequently, the patient was restarted on a course of vancomycin at a lower dose without recurrence of neutropenia. The latter observation is in disagreement with the common understanding that an immunologic mechanism may be responsible for the reaction. In another study, 12% patients treated with vancomycin developed neutropenia including 4 cases with absolute neutrophil counts $\leq$500 cells/mm$^3$; the mean time of i.v. vancomycin administration to the appearance of neutropenia was 32 days; resolution of vancomycin-induced neutropenia occurred promptly after discontinuation of vancomycin [4]. There was no correlation between total vancomycin doses and serum concentrations with the development of neutropenia. The authors concluded that clinicians should monitor the CBC at least weekly in patients receiving vancomycin therapy for longer than 2 weeks [4].

Learning Points

- Neutropenia may occur on long-term vancomycin treatment.
- CBC should be monitored at least weekly in patients receiving vancomycin therapy for longer than 2 weeks.
- Vancomycin-induced neutropenia may be severe.
- Resolution occurs promptly after discontinuation of vancomycin.

## References

[1] Bernard E, Perbost I, Carles M, Michiels A, Carsenti-Etesse H, Chichmanian RM, Dunais B, Dellamonica P. Efficacy and safety of vancomycin constant-rate infusion in the treatment of chronic gram-positive bone and joint infections. *Clin. Microbiol. Infect.* 1997;3:440-446.

[2] Mackett RL, Guay DR. Vancomycin-induced neutropenia. *Can. Med. Assoc. J.* 1985;132:39-40.

[3] Koo KB, Bachand RL, Chow AW. Vancomycin-induced neutropenia. *Drug Intell. Clin. Pharm.* 1986;20:780-782.

[4] Pai MP. Epidemiology of vancomycin-induced neutropenia in patients receiving home intravenous infusion therapy. *Ann. Pharmacother.* 2006; 40: 224-228.

## Case 30. Spuriously Toxic Vancomycin Levels

A 56-year-old man with sternal osteomyelitis was admitted for vancomycin treatment [1]. The patient's medical history was notable for hypertension, dyslipidemia, diabetes mellitus, and myocardial infarction. In March 2007 he underwent coronary artery bypass surgery. The postoperative course was complicated by sternal wound infection with MRSA. Vancomycin treatment was administered, beginning in March 2007 and terminated in August 2007, after complete closure of the wound. During maintenance treatment, vancomycin 1g once/24 hours achieved therapeutic trough levels of 5 to 10 μg/mL. In September 2007 there was recurrence of the purulent discharge from the sternal wound with MRSA isolates sensitive to vancomycin and rifampicin. Relevant laboratory data at this time were plasma creatinine 0.8 mg/dL and CRP 120 mg/L. Vancomycin was started on September 20$^{th}$ and rifampicin was added. The patient's regular medications, including carvedilol, ramipril, aspirin, simvastatin, and metformin, were continued. On October 12$^{th}$, trough vancomycin was 10.3 μg/mL by using the AxSYM Vancomycin II assay.

Later, the access to superficial veins becoming difficult, a central PermCath catheter was inserted via the axillary vein. According to standard instructions, before use of the line 10 mL of fluid was aspirated and discarded, than blood was sampled as needed. On October 16$^{th}$, the trough vancomycin level in blood sampled via the PermCath was 62 μg/mL; the serum creatinine was 0.8 mg/dL. Vancomycin administration was discontinued. Sixteen hours later, vancomycin trough was 120 µg/mL in blood drawn trough the PermCath. On the same day, repeat sampling produced vancomycin trough level 43.4 µg/mL in blood drawn via the PermCath, while blood collected by puncturing the femoral vein showed vancomycin 10.1 µg/mL. This observation was replicated on October 18$^{th}$. The PermCath was flushed with 50 mL saline and samples were obtained; the vancomycin level was 334 µg/mL in saline retrieved from the central line, 40.4 µg/mL in blood drawn via the central line, and 6 µg/mL in blood drawn from the femoral vein.

Subsequently, vancomycin treatment was reinstituted, 1g once/ 24 hours. After another week of treatment, the trough vancomycin level was 10.2 µg/mL in blood drawn via the femoral vein. After 6 weeks of treatment, the local symptoms of wound infection remitted. Administration of antibiotics was discontinued but the PermCath was kept in place, in anticipating a possible relapse of infection.

In this patient, apparently toxic vancomycin levels were found in blood drawn via the PermCath, but not in samples obtained by venipuncture. Flushing the PermCath with 10 mL or 50 mL of saline did not eliminate the vancomycin from the line, suggesting that spuriously 'toxic' vancomycin levels were the consequence of the antibiotic sticking to the venous catheter. To our surprise, we could not find similar observations in the Medline literature. Indirect evidence, duplicating this observation in vitro, comes from experiments of showing that vancomycin and other antibiotics may adhere to antibiotic-heparin locks for several days [2, 3].

The clinical utility of monitoring vancomycin serum concentration continues to be the subject of much debate. Vancomycin serum concentrations do not predict toxicity, especially when appropriate doses and dosing intervals are used, and clinical data regarding treatment outcomes relative to serum concentrations are sparse. A number of investigators have firmLy taken a position against the routine measurement of vancomycin serum levels [4, 5]. Therapeutic decisions in our patient were not better in that we monitored vancomycin levels, rather we became confused by the results obtained.

### Learning Points

- Vancomycin serum concentrations do not predict toxicity, especially when appropriate doses and dosing intervals are used. A number of investigators have taken a position against routine measurement of vancomycin serum levels.
- Monitoring vancomycin trough serum concentrations might be justified in patients with endocarditis, osteomyelitis, patients receiving other potentially nephrotoxic medications, and with changing renal function.
- Spuriously ‘toxic’ vancomycin levels may arise by drawing blood through venous lines.

## References

[1] Naschitz JE, Gagarin A, Schor RG. Spurious toxic vancomycin levels. *Eur. J. Intern. Med.* 2008;19:e36-37.

[2] Vercaigne LM, Sitar DS, Penner SB, Bernstein K, Wang GQ, Burczynski FJ. Antibiotic-heparin lock: in vitro antibiotic stability combined with heparin in a central venous catheter. *Pharmacotherapy*. 2000;20:394-399.
[3] Haimi-Cohen Y, Husain N, Meenan J, Karayalcin G, Lehrer M, Rubin LG. Vancomycin and ceftazidime bioactivities persist for at least 2 weeks in the lumen in ports: simplifying treatment of port-associated bloodstream infections by using the antibiotic lock technique. *Antimicrob. Agents Chemother*. 2001;45:1565-1567.
[4] American Thoracic Society; Infectious Diseases Society of America. Guidelines for the management of adults with hospital-acquired, ventilator-associated, and healthcare-associated pneumonia. *Am. J. Respir. Crit. Care Med*. 2005;171:388.
[5] Deresinski S. Vancomycin: does it still have a role as an antistaphylococcal agent? *Expert Rev. Anti Infect. Ther*. 2007;5:393-401.

## Case 31. Fever Induced by Ertapenem. The Naranjo Causality Scale

A 91-year-old woman presented with acute onset of fever and delirium. The diagnoses of right lower lobe pneumonia and E. coli bacteriuria were established. The patient's medical history was remarkable for type 2 diabetes mellitus, cholelythiasis and Alzheimer type dementia stage 3. Her regular medication included insulin glargine, doxazocin, atenolol, zuclopethixol, and lactulose, and were unchanged during the preceding month. On admission, the patient was drowsy, the rectal temperature was $38.5^0$C, BP 158/61 mmHg, heart rate 88 bpm, SaO2 92%. Remarkable on physical examination were inspiratory crackles over the right lower lung field. Laboratory studies showed WBC 9700/$mm^3$ with 80% neutrophils and CRP 82 mg/L. Serum levels of bilirubin, ALT, AST and alkaline phosphatase, BUN and creatinine were in the normal range. Chest x-rays showed a homogenous alveolar infiltrate in the right lower lobe. Abdominal ultrasound and CT disclosed a small stone in the not dilated common bile duct. Urine culture grew E. coli >100.000 colony forming units/mL, susceptible to a gamut of commonly used antibiotics. Blood cultures were negative. Treatment with i.v. cefriaxone 1g/day and i.v. azitromycin 250 mg/day was started. After five days of antibiotic treatment, the body temperature fluctuated $37.6^0 – 38.2^0$C. There were no relevant findings on physical examination, bacteriological cultures were negative, and findings on repeat chest x-rays were unchanged. The antibiotic regimen was changed to i.v. ertapenem 1g/day, followed by normalization of the temperature, with the alertness and appetite returning to the usual, and the CRP decreasing to 8.4 mg/L. However, on day 10 of ertapenem treatment the temperature increased to $39.2^0$C. There was neither deterioration in the patient's general state, nor any new finding on physical examination, chest x-rays, and laboratory tests, with CRP 6 mg/L, WBC 8200, and neutrophils 66%. Upon suspicion of drug fever, ertapenem administration was discontinued; 24 hours later the temperature returned to normal and remained so on the following days. Subsequently, there was no recurrence of fever during a period of several weeks. The diagnosis of drug fever induced by ertapenem was posited, supported by the temporality of the association between administration of ertapenem and resurgence of fever, no evidence of an alternative cause of fever, either infectious or non-infectious, and the quick and sustained remission of fever upon discontinuation of ertapenem.

*Drug fever* occurs typically 5 to 10 days after beginning treatment with a particular drug, but it also may occur after the first dose of the drug or late in the course of treatment. Clinicians must not assume that because a patient has been taking a certain medication for a long time it cannot be the cause of fever. Any pattern of fever may be seen in drug fever. Although most patients are surprisingly well while febrile, some are severely sick. Drug fever is usually not accompanied by other signs of drug allergy. However, drug fever may be the first clinical sign of an impending severe drug reaction. Mild normocytic anemia and an elevated erythrocyte sedimentation rate are often accompanying findings, but are not helpful in narrowing the differential diagnosis [1].

Presence of anti-drug antibodies in the patient's serum does not prove a hypersensitivity reaction to the specific drug, since antibodies can also be present in patients without signs of a drug reaction. Also, failure to detect antibodies to the drug does not rule out drug fever since the antibodies may not be directed against the drug itself [1].

Typically, defervescence occurs within 72 to 96 hours after withdrawal of the culprit drug, but delays of five to seven days have also been observed. If the culprit drug is not discontinued the patient may develop a drug rash or other, sometimes severe manifestations of hypersensitivity.

*Discontinuing a recently added drug* may be adequate in considering drug fever. However, removal of the suspected medication should be considered with caution, since the benefits of continued therapy may outweigh the risk of continued fever in some clinical situations. For patients in whom multiple drugs can be the culprits of fever, the discontinuation of all non-essential drugs is recommended. After remission of fever, drugs may be reintroduced cautiously, one at a time, with the most highly suspected drugs avoided if possible. Patient follow-up is mandatory to confirm that the fever subsided spontaneously and only than is the diagnosis of drug fever established. Rechallenge should not be performed solely to confirm the diagnosis of drug fever. If the suspected culprit drug is deemed critical for the patient's management, rechallenge with a single therapeutic dose can be performed very cautiously, with the patient's informed consent [1, 2].

*The Naranjo causality scale* [3] provides a practical means for clinicians to prove causality between a drug treatment and an adverse event, such as fever, suspected to be induced by the drug. The Naranjo questionnaire addresses several characteristics of the association between a drug and a clinical event: temporality, strength, consistency, gradient, specificity, coherence, and results of rechallenge (where applicable). A scoring system permits to compute the total score: >9 is interpreted as definite drug-induced reaction, 5-8 probable drug-induced reaction, 1-4 possible, 0 doubtful drug-induced reaction. In our patient, a score 5 was computed, which is consistent with probable causality between ertapenem treatment and evolving fever.

Antibiotics are the most frequent cause of drug fever and, therefore, it is surprising that we could not find an account of fever induced by ertapenem in the Medline data base [4]. Awareness of this possible adverse event might assist physicians in earlier diagnosis and encourage reports of similar cases. Suspected serious or unusual adverse drug reactions should be reported to the regulator. Indeed, rare adverse reactions cannot be reliably identified before marketing [5].

## Learning Points

- Drug fever may pose diagnostic and therapeutic challenges, in particular when there are few cases reported concerning the particular drug.
- An important clue to the diagnosis is the temporal association between initiation of a drug treatment and onset of symptoms, and waning of symptoms upon discontinuation of the drug.
- Statistical power of probability is important in diagnostic reasoning, but it should not overpower curiosity and recognition of unusual facts.
- The Naranjo causality scale provides a practical means for clinicians to prove causality between a drug treatment and an adverse event

## References

[1] Mackowiak PA, LeMastre CF. Drug fever: a critical appraisal of conventional concepts. An analysis of 51 episodes in the Dallas hospitals and 97 episodes reported in the English literature. *Ann. Intern. Med.* 1987;106:728-733.
[2] Patel RA, Gallagher JC. Drug Fever. *Pharmacotherapy.* 2010;30:57-69. Rubio M, Bousquet PJ, Demoly P. Update in drug allergy: novel drugs with novel reaction patterns. *Curr. Opin. Allergy Clin. Immunol.* 2010;10:457-462.
[3] Naranjo CA, Busto U, Sellers EM, Sandor P, Ruiz I, Roberts EA, Janecek E, Domecq C, Greenblatt DJ. A method for estimating the probability of adverse drug reactions. *Clin. Pharmacol.* 1981;30:239-245.
[4] Naschitz JE. Drug fever induced by ertapenem. *QJM* 2011;104:730-731.
[5] Ferner RE, Beard K. How should we react to adverse drug reactions? *Postgrad. Med. J.* 2011;87:81-82.

# Case 32. Ertapenem-Valproate Interaction

An 84-year-old man was referred from the emergency department with suspected urinary tract infection. Treatment with ceftriaxone 1g/day has been started. The patient's remote history included ischemic stroke with right hemiplegia, aphasia and convulsive spells, carotid stenosis, carotid endarterectomy, gastrointestinal bleeding due to stress ulcer, arterial hypertension, ischemic heart disease, chronic renal failure, benign prostatic hypertrophy, and pulmonary embolism. He received feeding by a gastrostomy tube. The patient's regular medications comprised valsartan 80 mg/day, omeprasol 40 mg/day, and valproate 500 mg/day. During the preceding months plasma valproate levels were regularly within the therapeutic range 50-100 mcg/mL, including a recently measured 65 mcg/mL. On physical examination, the temperature was $37.8^0$C, BP 154/86 mmHg, heart rate 82 bpm, SaO2 in ambient air 92%. The WBC was 6900/$mm^3$ with a normal differential count, serum creatinine 1.7 mg/dL, BUN 61 mg/dL, CRP 13 mg/L; the urine culture did not grow microbiota. A chest x-ray was unremarkable. After 4 days of ceftriaxone treatment the temperature increased to $39,2^0$C, the WBC to 10.200/$mm^3$, and the CRP to 58 mg/L. Blood and urine cultures were negative and another chest x-ray was unchanged. Ceftriaxone was replaced with ertapenem 1g/day for 5 days, and subsequently, in the want of improvement with chloramphenicol.

On routine testing, the valproate plasma level was subtherapeutic - 29.8 mcg/mL. Two days later, while the patient continued to receive the regular dose of the antiepileptic drug through the gastrostomy tube, the valproate plasma level was 3.36 mcg/mL. Therefore the valproate dose was increased to 600 mg/day but another test again showed low plasma valproate: 5.86 mcg/mL. Remarkably, all the samples showing extremely low valproate measurements were taken while the patient was receiving ertapenem. When ertapenem was substituted with chloramphenicol, a repeat measurement three days later detected serum valproate 60.1 mcg/mL. Fortunately the patient did not develop seizures during the period of subtherapeutic valproate blood concentrations. Eventually the fever remitted and the patient could return to the nursing home.

Decreased valproate serum concentration to subtherapeutic levels, sometimes with loss of seizure control, has been noticed in patients during antibacterial treatment with imipenem, meropenem, panipenem, and ertapenem [1-4]. Increasing the dose of valproate did not overcome this interaction, but discontinuation of any of these antibiotics resulted in valproic acid serum level returning to therapeutic levels usually within 2 days; such was the sequence of events in the present case. The mechanism of the interaction between carbapenems and valproic acid has not been elucidated. Product information recommends that carbapenems should not be co-administered with valproate.

### Learning Points

- Clinical judgment is a necessary first step in identification of an adverse drug event. In facing an unexpected event occurring after introduction of a new medication, it is mandatory to consider that it might be an adverse drug effect.
- Decreased valproate serum concentration to subtherapeutic levels has been noted during antibacterial treatment with ertapenem and certain other antibiotics.
- In patients prescribed ertapenem and valproate combination, the valproic acid serum concentration should be carefully monitored to prevent seizure recurrence.
- It possible, concurrent administration of ertapenem and valproate should be avoided.

## References


[1] Liao FF, Huang YB ,Chen CY. Decrease in serum valproic acid levels during treatment with ertapenem. *Am. J. Health Syst. Pharm.* 2010;67:1260-1264.

[2] Lunde JL, Nelson RE, Storandt HF. Acute seizures in a patient receiving divalproex sodium after starting ertapenem therapy. *Pharmacotherapy* 2007;27:1202-1205.

[3] Coves-Orts FJ, Borrás-Blasco J, Navarro-Ruiz A, Murcia-López A, Palacios-Ortega F. Acute seizures due to a probable interaction between valproic acid and meropenem. *Ann. Pharmacother.* 2005;39: 533-537.

[4] Epileptic seizures caused by low valproic acid levels from an interaction with meropenem. *J. Clin. Pharm. Ther.* 2006; 31:393-396.

# Case 33. Discordant Antibiotic Susceptibilities in Laboratory and Clinic

An-88-year-old male, with advanced dementia developed chills and $40^0$C fever. He had suffered from recurrent urinary tract infections and was hospitalized three times during the last year with urinary tract infections. He had an indwelling urinary catheter. At the time of the present admission the WBC was 24.000/mm$^3$, CRP 252 mg/L, and the urinalysis showed pyuria. The chest x-ray was unremarkable. A renal ultrasound examination was unremarkable. The urinary catheter was replaced, urine and blood were sampled for culture, and treatment was started with i.v. ceftriaxone 1g/day. The working diagnosis was urinary tract infection and the choice of empirical antibiotic treatment for the beginning was based on the local sensitivity patterns of common urinary pathogens. The treatment was remarkably successful: within 24 hours the fever remitted, the alertness and appetite returned to usual. After two days on ceftriaxone treatment the WBC and CRP decreased to 10,000/mm$^3$ and 49 mg/L, respectively. At this point, results of bacterial cultures became available. In both, a singe blood and a single urine culture, a MRSA strain was identified susceptible to vancomycin and oxacillin but not to ceftriaxone. Meanwhile the patient had completely recovered on ceftriaxone treatment from the acute illness. Subsequent blood and urine cultures did not grow microbiota. Nasal smears detected MRSA as well and decolonization with intranasal mupirocin was begon.

The excellent clinical response to ceftriaxone in this patient was at odds with the, apparently, lack of susceptibility of the isolates to this antibiotic in the laboratory. Several practical issues came into focus: the choice of empirical antibiotic treatment for the beginning, monitoring the response to treatment, possible error of identification of the staphylococci as MRSA, evaluation and treatment of MRSA blood stream infection, and indication and best approach to patient decontamination.

*Empirical antibiotic treatment for the beginning* is based on clinical judgment, in considering the common pathogens responsible for the disorder in question. It is adequate to start with broad-spectrum antimicrobial agents aiming to cover multiple possible pathogens that are commonly associated with the specific clinical syndrome. In addition, clinicians should consider bacteria known to colonize the patient, as well as the local bacterial resistance patterns for pathogens. The timing of initial therapy is guided by the urgency of the situation. In suspecting a severe bacterial infection, empirical therapy should be initiated immediately after or concurrently with collection of microbiologic specimens.

*Monitoring the clinical response is the most important guide* to establish the efficacy of treatment. It is not uncommon to observe a good clinical response contradicting the apparently poor susceptibility reported by the laboratory (as noticed in the present case) or to see patients failing to respond while laboratory studies suggested that the therapy was adequate.

*Methicillin-resistant Staphylococcus aureus* (MRSA) refers to isolates that are resistant to all currently available beta-lactam antibiotics, including penicillins and cephalosporins. Such a strain was diagnosed in our patient by a battery of laboratory tests: cefoxitin, chromoagar, latex agglutination and fermentation tests. Methicillin resistance is defined in the clinical microbiology laboratory as an oxacillin minimum inhibitory concentration (MIC) $\geq$4 mcg/mL. Isolates resistant to oxacillin are also resistant to all beta-lactam agents including cephalosporins. Methicillin resistance requires the presence of the mecA gene detected by polymerase chain reaction; strains lacking a mecA gene are not methicillin resistant [1].

Health care-associated *MRSA infection* is defined as MRSA infection which occurs >48 hours following admission to hospital or MRSA infection which occurs outside the hospital within 12 months of exposure to healthcare (our patient was hospitalized three times during the last year with urinary tract infections). MRSA isolates were first confined almost exclusively to patients who frequented health care facilities. Other persons at risk for MRSA colonization or infection include those in contact with a person who had a MRSA infection or with a history of illicit drug use. *Health care-associated* MRSA may cause severe, invasive disease, including skin and soft tissue infection, bloodstream infection, and pneumonia. *Health care-associated* MRSA strains tend to be multidrug resistant [2].

In the mid-1990s, MRSA infections began to be detected in the community in persons who did not have contact with the health care system. Molecular typing of isolates from these community-associated cases has shown that they are largely caused by new MRSA strains.

*Vancomycin is the antibiotic of choice* for the treatment of invasive MRSA infections as well as MRSA bacteremia. Alternative agents are teicoplanin, telavacin, daptomycin, linezolid, tigecycline, ceftraroline, to be considered in the setting of adverse effects to vancomycin or infection with a pathogen with inadequate susceptibility to vancomycin. Adjuvant agents to be used in combination with other anti-staphylococcal antibiotics are rifampicin and fucidic acid. The latter should not be administered in monotherapy because resistance may quickly emerge.

*The discrepancy between clinical and laboratory susceptibility* of the isolate in our patient raised questions of major importance: was the result false-positive, by wrongly identifying methicillin-resistant Staphylococcus aureus? Such error may lead to unjustified glycopeptide treatment instead of beta-lactam antibiotics, unjustified decolonization treatments, and isolation of patients and additional constraining infection control measures [3]. For determination of methicillin resistance in S. aureus the gold standard method is mecA detection by PCR assay. However, PCR testing requires a trained staff and special equipment. The latex test is relatively costly, thereby limiting its use. Previously recommended phenotypic MRSA detection methods based on oxacillin disk diffusion or oxacillin screen agar testing may fail to detect MRSA isolates with very heterogeneous subpopulations. Because cefoxitin is a strong inducer of the mecA gene that appears to be less affected than oxacillin by penicillinase-hyperproducing isolates, it is more reliable for MRSA detection and is currently recommended in the CLSI guidelines [1].

Numerous recent studies assessed sensitivities and specificities of familiar laboratory tests for MRSA detection. A comparison of chromogenic media for detection of MRSA showed that BBL-CHROMagar and CHROMagar gave the best overall results for detection of MRSA, irrespective of the sample concentration, investigator, or incubation period. The cumulative average specificity was the highest for BBL-CHROMagar (99%), followed by MRSASelect (98%), CHROMagar (97%), ChromID (89%), and Brilliance MRSA agar (86%). False-positive results were mainly due to methicillin-resistant S. epidermidis [4]. This indicates that staphylococci may be mistakenly identified as MRSA. Another study showed a 12.9% wrongly identified methicillin-resistant Staphylococcus aureus by use of a rapid commercial PCR assay due to presence of staphylococcal cassette chromosome element lacking the mecA gene [3].

In discussing the problem with the laboratory chief of the university hospital, the possibility of wrongly identifying MRSA in the present case was thought to be practically nil.

*Decolonization strategies* are frequently recommended. One such strategy is the use of intranasal mupirocin to reduce nasal carriage of MRSA. However, eradication of nasal colonization appears to be transient, and the use of this agent remains controversial. Moreover, the recent identification of a mupirocin-resistance gene raises serious concern about exposing populations of staphylococci to this agent. Attempts at skin decolonization with chlorhexidine gluconate are commonly suggested, although these approaches have not been rigorously evaluated.

### Learning Points

- A favorable clinical response is the most important testimony for the efficacy of an antibiotic treatment and should lead to reconsideration of conflicting results from the bacteriology laboratory.
- Staphylococci may be mistakenly identified as MRSA.
- In patients with MRSA bacteremia, taking follow-up blood cultures 2 to 4 days after initial positive cultures is recommended, to document clearance of bacteremia.

## References

[1] Clinical and Laboratory Standards Institute. Performance Standards for Antimicrobial Susceptibility Testing: Sixteenth Informational Supplement. M100-S16 Methods for dilution antimicrobial susceptibility tests for bacteria that grow aerobically: Approved Standard. 2006; 26 (3). CLSI, Wayne, Pennsylvania, USA.

[2] Naimi TS, LeDell KH, Como-Sabetti K, et al. Comparison of community- and health care-associated methicillin-resistant Staphylococcus aureus infection. *JAMA* 2003; 290:2976-2984.

[3] Blanc DS, Basset P, Nahimana-Tessemo I, Jaton K, Greub G, Zanetti G. High proportion of wrongly identified methicillin-resistant Staphylococcus aureus carriers by use of a rapid commercial PCR assay due to presence of staphylococcal cassette chromosome element lacking the mecA gene. *J. Clin. Microbiol.* 2011;49:722-724.

[4] Malhotra-Kumar S, Abrahantes JC, Sabiiti W, Lammens C, Vercauteren G, Ieven M, Molenberghs G, Aerts M, Goossens H; MOSAR WP2 Study Team. Evaluation of chromogenic media for detection of methicillin-resistant Staphylococcus aureus. *J. Clin. Microbiol.* 2010;48:1040-1046.

*Chapter VI*

# Venous Thrombosis and Embolism

Diagnosis of venous thromboembolism remains a formidable challenge. Doing our best may not be good enough.

## Case 34. Swollen Calf - A Mishap

An 80-year-old-woman was referred from the emergency department with the diagnosis of recurrent femoral vein thrombosis. Swelling of the left calf was noticed five days before. On Doppler ultrasound examination a thrombus was visualized in the left superficial and the left common femoral veins. The D-dimer test was positive. Similar thrombi have been described on a venous ultrasound examination three years ago; the patient completed a one year course of anticoagulant treatment. Relative to the present event, recurrence of deep vein thrombosis was thought probable, one dose of enoxaparin was administered and warfarin treatment was started in emergency. Her medical history was notable for arterial hypertension, cerebral stroke followed by good functional recovery, stable ischemic heart disease, mild dementia, vitamin B12 deficiency, idiopathic thrombocytopenic purpura in remission, and osteoporosis. The current drug regimen comprised ramipril 2.5 mg, diltiazem 90 mg, doxazocin 4 mg, simvastatin 20 mg, furosemide 40 mg, prednisone 5 mg, chlorpromazine 75 mg, and lorazepam 1 mg/day.

At the time of admission to our ward the patient was alert, BP 132/72 mmHg, heart rate 76 bpm, body temperature 36.2$^{0}$C, respirations 16/min, SaO2 in room air 95%. The left calf was swollen +3 and the distal thigh +1. An ecchymosis 2 x 2 cm in diameter was apparent on the postero-lateral aspect of the left calf. The patient could not recall any trauma. The calf was neither painful nor tender. Among ancillary laboratory findings, the hematocrit was 38.7%, platelets 200,000/mm$^{3}$, PT-INR 1.37, serum creatinine 1.2 mg/dL. Enoxaparin 60 mg x 2/day and warfarin 5 mg was administered; the patient's regular medications and were continued.

On the following morning, 24 hours after beginning anticoagulant treatment, the patient complained of heaviness in the left calf. At that site, a large subcutaneous collection of blood was apparent, covered by a thin layer of skin. The BP was 140/95 mmHg. The tibialis and dorsalis pedis pulses were ample. While examining the patient, the BP dropped to 90/60 mmHg and the heart rate rose to 116 bpm. Obviously, massive subcutaneous bleeding had occurred on anticoagulant treatment. Application of compressive dressing to the calf resulted in erosion of the skin and loss of 250-500 of blood, until bandaging could be completed and the extravasation stopped. The BP had fallen to 70/50 mmHg. The ECG showed sinus rhythm, left bundle branch block, essentially similar to the admission ECG. Fluid resuscitation was started and the patient was rushed to the intensive care unit. The result of the PT- INR in the blood sample taken earlier in the morning was 1.8. Several units of fresh frozen plasma and packed blood cells were administered and the anticoagulant treatment was discontinued. The hematocrit, which upon arrival to the intensive care unit was 22%, was corrected to 31%. The serum creatinine had risen to 3.5 mg/dL.

At this point, revision of the recent venous ultrasound and comparison with ultrasound images recorded 3 years ago invalidated the diagnosis of new venous thrombosis. So, there was no indication for placement of a vena cava filter. On CT of the lower extremities, the left calf hematoma was confined to the subcutaneous layers, in an area 19 cm in length and 11.3 cm in width. The clinical suggestion of compartment syndrome was discarded. Later, debridement of necrotic tissues was performed. Cultures of the exudate from the calf wound grew a mixed flora. Antibiotic treatment was administered. The patient's condition improved slowly. Later, skin grafts were performed to the denuded areas of the calf.

The patient's diagnoses, in retrospect, were 'spontaneous' hematoma in the calf misdiagnosed as deep vein thrombosis, inappropriate anticoagulant treatment causing massive subcutaneous bleeding, shock, acute renal failure and skin necrosis. Mistaking calf hematoma for acute venous thrombosis resulted from a series of omissions. First, by ignoring the faint calf ecchymosis at presentation; this useful hint which might have pointed to the presence of a deeper situated hematoma was disregarded. Second, the confusion between a residual clot and acute thrombosis might have been avoided by comparing the current venous ultrasound with images of the previous examination, which were available having been performed in the same institution. Third, in the diagnostic evaluation of a swollen calf ultrasonography should not be limited to the femoral and popliteal veins but also include imaging the calf's soft tissues, a routine which is useful in the differential diagnosis. Fourth, giving importance to a positive D-dimer test as an argument in favor of actual thrombosis is a mistake, though often met in practice.

*Unilateral swelling of the calf* demands for a differential diagnosis. The following disorders may cause unilateral calf swelling and should not be confounded with venous thrombosis: muscle or soft tissue injury, hematoma, ruptured or dissecting Baker's cyst, cellulitis, superficial phlebitis, postphlebitic syndrome, venous insufficiency, extrinsic compression of a vein by a tumor, S1 radiculopathy even in the absence of radicular pain, and asymmetric peripheral edema resulting from heart failure or liver cirrhosis [1].

*Unrecognized calf hematoma* confused with venous thrombosis is necessarily followed by administration of anticoagulant treatment; this can have serious consequences including bleeding (as observed in our patient) and compartment syndrome. The most common cause of calf hematoma is a partial tear of the medial head of the gastrocnemius muscle; the patient typically reports a sudden onset calf pain that followed to an impulsive dorsiflexion of the ankle. The presence of an ecchymosis around the maleoli is helpful in suggesting calf hematoma in distinction from venous thrombosis. Ultrasound can readily differentiate a hematoma from a Baker's cyst, but is less helpful in diagnosing calf vein thrombosis [2, 3]. After exclusion of deep vein thrombosis, ultrasound, CT or MRI can be used to evaluate the nature of a swollen calf.

*Conservative treatment for calf hematomas* is sufficient when there is no neurological impairment. In a series of 17 patients with calf hematomas, three had simple hematomas, eleven were inflammatory or super-infected hematomas, and three were complicated with ulceration [4]. Needle aspiration after autolysis of the hematoma under CT may be beneficial.

*The D-dimer assay* by ELISA may be useful in the management of suspected deep vein thrombosis. D-dimer is a fibrin degradation product present in the blood after a clot is degraded by fibrinolysis. It is so named because it contains two crosslinked D fragments of fibrinogen. D-dimer is normally undetectable in the blood. While a negative result practically rules out thrombosis, a positive result can indicate a variety of potential etiologies such as inflammation, malignancy, trauma, surgery, liver disease, thrombosis, and advanced age. False negative results can occur if the sample was taken either too early after thrombus formation or if testing is delayed for several days. Additionally, anti-coagulant treatment can render the test negative because it prevents thrombus extension. Consistent with results of prospective studies, deep vein thrombosis can be ruled out in patients who are at low pre-test probability and have a negative D-dimer result (as measured by a sensitive enzyme-linked immunosorbant assay); ultrasonography of the venous system can be safely omitted in such situation. The main use of the D-dimer test, therefore, is to exclude thromboembolic disease in clinical settings where the probability is low. This is not the situation in elderly hospitalized patients; they should not undergo D-dimer testing in the work-up for suspected venous thrombosis.

*Compression ultrasonography* is preferred as the initial test to diagnose venous thrombosis because. It is noninvasive and offers good sensitivity for detecting thrombosis in the popliteal and femoral veins. The limitations of compression venous ultrasound are poor visualization of the iliac and pelvic veins and poor sensitivity in isolated or nonocclusive calf vein thrombosis. An initial negative compression ultrasonography should be repeated after 3 to 5 days if the clinical suspicion of venous thrombosis persists in order to detect the possible propagation of a thrombus from any peripheral vein to a proximal vein [5].

*Differentiation between a new and an old venous clot* may be challenging (1.5). Recurrent symptoms of leg pain and edema can result either from persistent obstruction after an acute venous thrombosis, may be late manifestations of valvular incompetence, or may be signs of recurrent venous thrombosis. Despite early recanalization of a venous clot, compression ultrasound studies remain abnormal after 6 months in 50% of patients and after 1 year in 27% of patients. Thrombus echogenicity and heterogeneity tend to increase with the age of the thrombus, but these characteristics are not consistently useful in differentiating an acute from a chronic clot. Acutely thrombosed veins tend to be dilated whereas the diameter of chronically thrombosed segments is reduced. A free-floating tail if present suggests a new thrombus. In contrast, the presence of venous collaterals and multiple flow channels within the venous lumen are characteristic for chronic thrombosis. A 2-mm or greater increase in compressed thrombus thickness, as compared with previous examinations, has been claimed to have 100% sensitivity and specificity for recurrent proximal venous thrombosis.

*Guidelines provide precise rules for initiation of anticoagulation.* Subcutaneous low-molecular-weight heparin, fondaparinux, or weight-based intravenous unfractionated heparin should be administered for at least 5 days and until the PT-INR is in the therapeutic range (2.0 to 3.0) for 2 consecutive days. Warfarin can be initiated on the first day of therapy. Bed rest is not recommended for deep venous thrombosis unless there is substantial pain and swelling. When pulmonary embolism is diagnosed, inpatient therapy with initial bed rest for 24 to 48 hours is recommended. Anticoagulation should be maintained for 3 to 6 months for venous thromboembolism secondary to transient risk factors and for longer than 12 months for recurrent thromboembolism. While the appropriate duration of anticoagulation for idiopathic or recurrent venous thromboembolism is not definitively known, there is evidence of substantial benefit for extended-duration therapy. Compression stockings should be used routinely to prevent postthrombotic syndrome, beginning within one month of diagnosis of proximal venous thrombosis and continued for a minimum one year after diagnosis.

*Warfarin dosing* can be problematic, since warfarin has a narrow therapeutic index. Effective treatment should be achieved while avoiding the risk of bleeding. Elderly patients require lower dosage than younger patients, although the mechanism for this greater sensitivity to warfarin with aging is not well understood. Elderly patients are also more prone to instability in maintenance of safe anticoagulation with warfarin, because they often have comorbidities, use drugs that interact with warfarin, and respond slower to dose adjustments of warfarin. Algorithms for treatment initiation and close monitoring are recommended. A warfarin induction algorithm was specifically designed for elderly inpatients and is based on the PT-INR measured after three days of 4 mg warfarin taken per day; rules guide the adjustment of warfarin dosages after day 3 according to repeated PT-INR measurements [6, 7]. The latter algorithm slightly differs from the prevalent algorithm with 5 mg warfarin initiation [8]. In having tried both algorithms in elderly inpatients we have not observed an advantage of one over the other. Antibiotic treatment is associated with an increased risk of bleeding among patients receiving warfarin. A case-control study nested within a cohort of 38,762 patients aged 65 years and older who were continuous warfarin users showed that exposure to any antibiotic agent was associated with an increased risk of bleeding: macrolides OR 1.86, quinolones OR 1.69, cotrimoxazole OR 2.70, penicillins OR 1.92, and cephalosporins OR 2.45. Hence, frequent monitoring of the PT-INR is recommended for patients who are concurrently taking warfarin and antibiotics [9].

*Reversal of anticoagulation* may be necessary in case of bleeding, emergent surgery, or elevated PT-INR. Prior to reversing an elevated PT-INR it is required to ensure that the abnormal laboratory value is not artifactual. A blood specimen that is not assayed promptly after blood collection can result in spuriously high PT-INR. To treat minor bleeding or a verified PT-INR that exceeds 9.0 without any bleeding, vitamin K has traditionally been administered parenterally. Vitamin K 10 mg subcutaneously usually reverses the effects of warfarin in 6 to 12 hours. However, this approach makes patients relatively refractory to warfarin for up to 2 weeks, so that reinstitution of warfarin anticoagulation becomes problematic. Merely withholding one or two doses of warfarin and administering 2.5 mg of oral vitamin K is a reliable and safe method for rapidly correcting a PT-INR that exceeds 5.0 in patients who do not have serious concomitant bleeding. Some patients with a PT-INR less than 9.0 simply require interruption of warfarin therapy without administration of fresh frozen plasma or vitamin K, until the PT-INR has returned to the therapeutic range. Normalization of the PT-INR may be delayed in elderly individuals, in patients taking larger warfarin doses, or in those with very high PT-INR values, in patients with poorly compensated heart failure and in patients with active cancer. Life-threatening bleeding due to warfarin overdose has traditionally required immediate treatment with enough cryoprecipitate or fresh frozen plasma to normalize the PT-INR and achieve immediate hemostasis. An improved approach is to use recombinant human factor VIIa concentrate, which provides safe and rapid reversal of warfarin-induced excessive anticoagulation.

*Dabigatran,* a direct thrombin inhibitor*, and rivaroxabane*, a factor Xa inhibitor, are representatives of a new generation of oral anticoagulant medications which do not require laboratory testing [10]. Both drugs are licensed in Europe and Canada for the prevention of venous thromboembolism in patients undergoing elective hip or knee arthroplasty. In October 2010, the U.S. Food and Drug Administration approved high-dose dabigatran (150 mg twice daily) for prevention of stroke and systemic embolism in atrial fibrillation, with reduced dosing available for patients with severe renal impairment (75 mg twice daily). There is no specific antidote for dabigatran, which has a half-life of 12 to 17 hours. *Oral rivaroxaban* (15 mg twice daily for 3 weeks, followed by 20 mg once daily was equally effective for treatment of DVT as compared with subcutaneous enoxaparin followed by a vitamin K antagonist, and was not associated with an increased risk of bleeding [10]. Rivaroxaban is less expensive than low-molecular-weight heparin at therapeutic doses, but costs more than warfarin. Disadvantages of rivaroxaban include bleeding complications that may be catastrophic because there is no antidote.

Selection of patients who could receive dabigatran or rivaroxaban versus warfarin should also consider the availability of an anticoagulation management program for routine monitoring of PT-INR, patient preferences and cost. Dabigatran and rivaroxaban differ in many ways from warfarin, including rapid onset of action, shorter half-life, fewer drug-drug interactions, lack of need for monitoring and no need for titration or dose adjustments. The management of these anticoagulants when transitioning from or back to warfarin, around surgery or in case of major hemorrhage requires knowledge of their pharmacokinetics and mechanism of action. There is a limited evidence base to inform decisions around management of these agents.

### Learning Points

- Unilateral swelling of the calf involves the differential diagnosis between deep vein thrombosis and disorders that may simulate venous thrombosis, e.g. calf hematoma.
- Much of the diagnosis of deep vein thrombosis depends on the expertise of the ultrasonographist.
- The clinician's role is to track symptoms and signs, even if apparently trivial, and to interpret data obtained on imaging in the clinical context.
- Differentiation of a new from an old venous clot may be challenging.
- Administration of anticoagulant treatment in a patient with unrecognized calf hematoma may have devastating bleeding consequences.

## References

[1] Murphy TP, Cronan JJ. Evolution of deep venous thrombosis: a prospective evaluation with US. *Radiology* 1990;177:543-548.

[2] Anouchi YS, Parker RD, Seitz WH. Posterior compartment syndrome of the calf resulting from misdiagnosis of a rupture of the medial head of the gastrocnemius. *J. Trauma* 1987;27:678-680.

[3] Sakakibara Y, Aikawa S, Enomoto Y, Osaka M, Hiramatsu Y, Shigeta O, Terada Y, Atsumi N, Jikuya T, Mitsui T. Lower extremity hematoma as a complication of warfarinization in patients with artificial heart valves. *Jpn. Heart J.* 1999;40:239-345.

[4] Estève E, Armingaud P, Martin L. Cutaneous and subcutaneous hematomas observed in dermatology: 17 cases. *Ann. Dermatol. Venereol.* 2004;131(6-7 Pt 1):555-558.

[5] Prandoni P, Cogo A, Bernardi E, et al: A simple ultrasound approach for detection of recurrent proximal vein thrombosis. *Circulation* 1993; 88(4 Part 1):1730-1735.

[6] Siguret V, Gouin I, Debray M, Perret-Guillaume C, Bnoddaert J, Mahe I, Donval V, Seux M-L, Romain-Pilotaz M, Gisselbrecht M, Verny M, Pautas E. Initiitation of warfarin therapy in elderly medical inpatients: a safe and accurate regimen. *Am. J. Med.* 2005;118:137-142.

[7] Gouin-Thibault I, Levy C, Pautas E, Cambus JP, Drouet L, Mahé I, Bal Dit Sollier C, Horellou MH, Golmard JL, Siguret V. Improving anticoagulation control in hospitalized elderly patients on warfarin. *J. Am. Geriatr. Soc.* 2010;58:242–247.

[8] Kovacs MJ, Rodger M, Anderson DR, Morrow B, Kells G, Kobacs J, Boyle E, Wells PS. Comparison of the 10-mg and 5-mg warfarin initiation nomograms together with low-molecular weight heparin for outpatient treatment of acute venous thromboembolism. *Ann. Intern. Med.* 2003;138:714-719.

[9] Baillargeon J, Holmes HM, Lin Y-L, Raji MA, Sharma G, Kuo Y-F. Concurrent use of warfarin and antibiotics and the risk of bleeding in older adults. *Am. J. Med.* 2012; 125: 183-189.

[10] Bauersachs R, Berkowitz SD, EINSTEIN Investigators.Oral rivaroxaban for symptomatic venous thromboembolism. Oral rivaroxaban is effective for the treatment of symptomatic venous thromboembolism. *N. Engl. J. Med.* 2010;363:2499-2510.

## Case 35. Warfarin Resistance

A 66-year-old man presented to the emergency department following a fall. His medical history was remarkable for duodenal ulcer, gastrointestinal bleeding, chronic hepatitis B, nephrectomy 15 year ago for renal cell carcinoma, vertebral tuberculosis 7 years ago, and cerebellar ataxia attributed to chronic alcoholism. He lived in a shelter in neglect and poor nutrition. He had no personal or family history of venous thromboembolism. He was taking omeprasol 40 mg/day.

The patient was alert and not in acute distress. The body temperature was $36.8^0$C, BP 116/69 mm Hg, pulse 96 bpm, respirations 18 per minute, SaO2 by pulse oxymetry 94% in ambient air. The BMI was 21. The patient's left leg showed considerable swelling extending from the ankle to the upper thigh, and the swollen area was tender. There were no visible venous collaterals. The liver edge was felt 4 to 6 cm below the costal margin. Neurological examination showed ataxia; criteria of Wernicke-Korsakoff syndrome were not met. The patient had normal levels of hemoglobin, WBC, platelets, creatinine, BUN, AST, ALT, lipase, prothrombin time and troponin. A chest x-rays was unremarkable. Venous ultrasonography demonstrated lack of compressibility of the left femoral vein and a clot was visualized extending from the popliteal to the common femoral vein.

The patient was admitted to the department of internal medicine, where treatment was started with enoxaparin 60 mg x 2/day, warfarin 5 mg/day, oral vitamin B1 300 mg/day, and folic acid 5 mg/day; omeprasol was continued 40 mg/day. Three days later he was transferred to our ward for subacute care, being in a clinically stable condition, alert and independent in ADL. His vital signs were within normal limits. He had a great appetite and was encouraged to consume an assorted diet rich in proteins and vitamins. Medications started in the department of medicine were continued.

For the beginning, the response to warfarin was satisfactory with 7.5 mg/day an efficient dose. On the 6$^{th}$ day of treatment the PT-INR was 2.01. Three days later on the same warfarin dose the PT-INR was 1.7; the dose was increased to 10 mg/day. Surprisingly the PT-INR decreased to 1.09 and remained more or less so low for two weeks, though the dosing of warfarin was progressively escalated to 15 mg/day, under enoxaparin coverage. Resistance to warfarin was diagnosed, defined by requirements greater than 70 mg warfarin per week. Obviously, resistance to warfarin was acquired during the current hospitalization.

In an attempt to elucidate the cause of warfarin resistance the following possibilities were considered: laboratory error, non-adherence to medication, food-warfarin interaction, malabsorption, and drug-warfarin interaction. Blood samples for PT assessment were obtained before breakfast, as recommended. Efficiency of the warfarin preparation was confirmed by attesting the responsiveness to warfarin in other patients treated with warfarin provided from the same lot. Competitive antagonism with warfarin by increased dietary vitamin K intake was not thought to play a role, since the patient's diet was strictly controlled with minimal day-to-day variation of food rich in vitamin K. He had no uncontrolled supply of food, alcohol, medications, and had no access to illicit drugs. Furthermore, the medications he was receiving are not listed among drugs known to cause depression of the PT-INR. To eliminate suspicions, the recently started vitamin B1 and folic acid were discontinued, but the PT-INR remained in the range 1.1-1.2. The daily dose of omeprazole was constant along hospitalization.

Warfarin resistance may be due to malabsorption, a possibility which was explored. The patient had one or two pasty stools per day. An iron tolerance test showed no increase in serum iron measured over 2 hours after ingestion of ferum sulphate and was consistent with malabsorption (normal absorption will result in an increase in the serum iron of at least 100 microgram/dL). Tests for antiendomysial IgA, transglutaminsase IgA, and antiphospholipid antibodies were negative. Abdominal CT examination showed a single kidney, an enlarged and slightly irregular liver, but no enlarged lymph nodes or intestinal pathology.

When reaching the 15 mg daily warfarin dose, the INR increased to 2.2 – 2.5. Enoxaparin treatment was terminated. Reinstitution of vitamin B1 and folic acid administration did not affect the PT-INR. With warfarin anticoagulation in the therapeutic range the patient was discharged, recommending strict medical supervision. The cause of the patient's acquired warfarin resistance was obscure.

*Warfarin* is a vitamin K antagonist that inhibits hepatic vitamin K epoxide reductase and thereby interferes with synthesis of clotting factors II (prothrombin), VII, IX and X. Warfarin is rapidly and almost completely absorbed from the gastrointestinal tract. The anticoagulant effect of warfarin is influenced by genetic factors, diet, a variety of drugs, malnutrition, chronic liver disease, alcoholism, antibiotics and the metabolic rate. Patient education is essential to develop a diet with a relatively constant level of vitamin K. Patients taking warfarin should be encouraged to examine nutritional labeling of foods and dietary supplements. Dietary supplements and specialized vitamin and mineral supplements may contain vitamin K and be administered unknowingly. Grapefruit juice does not alter the anticoagulant response to warfarin. Elderly patients taking multiple medications may be subject to unanticipated drug interactions. It is essential to closely monitor the PT-INR when adding or removing any drug from a patient's regimen when he is concurrently taking warfarin.

*The prothrombin time* (PT) used for monitoring warfarin therapy is affected by decreases in the level of coagulation factors II, VII, IX and X. The fasting state is a prerequisite for accurate assessment of the PT. Plasma turbidity can interfere with the optical system of the instrument used for measurement of the PT and cause artifactual results, as it occurs in lipemic plasma, and hemolyzed or icteric specimens. When the hematocrit is high, the relative volume of plasma to anticoagulant is proportionately reduced resulting in an artifactual prolongation of the PT. Alerting the laboratory about a high hematocrit and adjusting the volume of anticoagulant in the collection tube for patients with hematocrits >55% yields more reliable results. Blood samples for PT assessment should be obtained in the morning, allowing time in the afternoon to obtain the results and indicate the next dose. Warfarin should be administered in the early afternoon if PT-INR monitoring is done the following morning. PT-INR testing is best done 15 hours or more following administration of the drug allowing for sufficient time for the warfarin effect to be demonstrated.

*The target PT-INR* is set 2.0 to 3.0 for most indications except patients with mechanical heart valves where a target PT-INR 2.5 to 3.5 is recommended. Because warfarin has a narrow therapeutic window, frequent coagulation monitoring is essential to ensure that a therapeutic anticoagulant response is obtained. Elderly patients are at high risk of over-anticoagulation when treated with warfarin, especially during treatment induction. For this reason, a dosing initiation and maintenance nomogram has been specifically designed for elderly patients [1]. Even patients with stable warfarin dose requirements should have their PT-INR determined every 2 to 4 weeks. More frequent monitoring is necessary when new medications are introduced because many drugs enhance or reduce the anticoagulant effects of warfarin. A stable PT-INR is more commonly obtained in anticoagulation clinics staffed by pharmacists and nurses than with individual physician regulation of the PT-INR; in addition, bleeding complications are reduced. Monitoring warfarin therapy can be problematic in patients with antiphospholipid antibody.

*Genotypes* of the cytochrome p450 isoform CYP2C9 and the vitamin K epoxide reductase complex subunit 1VKORC1 shape the warfarin dose requirements. The *2 (R144C) and *3 allele (I359L) variants of CYP2C9 cause reductions in enzymatic activity by 30% and 80%, respectively, and increase the bleeding risk. Ten VKORC1 single nucleotide polymorphisms and 5 inferred haplotypes determine low-, intermediate-, and high-dose requirements. Scolars have proposed that these genotypes together with clinical characteristics could predict one half of interindividual dose variability. However, an algorithm guided by pharmacogenetic and clinical criteria did not improve the rate of out-of-range PT-INRs [2].

*Warfarin resistance* is defined by requirements greater than 70 mg warfarin/week to maintain the PT-INR in the target therapeutic range [3]. Hereditary warfarin resistance is rare. In patients with persistent sub-therapeutic PT-INR levels, non-adherence, laboratory errors and drug-warfarin or food-warfarin interactions should be excluded:

1) Serious comorbid diseases leading to poor oral intake and malnutrition can cause an increase in the activity of warfarin because of a decline in vitamin K intake, vitamin K stores, and in hepatic synthesis of clotting factors.
2) Broad-spectrum antibiotics can alter the production of vitamin K by the gastrointestinal flora, particularly in patients with poor nutrition and limited vitamin K stores.
3) Chronic alcohol use can increase the clearance of warfarin, but the presence of concomitant liver disease can potentiate the action of warfarin. Significant wine use in patients taking warfarin apparently has little effect on the PT-INR.
4) The metabolic rate has an impact upon warfarin metabolism: there is increased catabolism of coagulation factors with fever or hyperthyroidism.
5) Drug interactions that alter the pharmacokinetics of warfarin may affect warfarin's absorption (e.g., cholestyramine), plasma-binding (the presence of excessively albumin-bound drugs causes an increase in free serum warfarin and therefore an increase in antithrombotic activity), and metabolism either by 2C9 enzyme induction which increases warfarin clearance and thereby reduces its antithrombotic activity (e.g. phenytoin, rifampin), or enzyme inhibition (e.g. amiodarone, cimetidine, sulfamethoxazole, metronidazole) which increases its antithrombotic effect and the PT-INR.
6) Studies with omeprazole and lansoprazole in healthy volunteers have indicated changes in warfarin bioavailability, but there is no clear evidence on the effect on clotting [4]. The continuous co-prescription of omeprazole with warfarin does not affect steady-state anticoagulation, but their intermittent use could explain some of the fluctuations in PT. True warfarin resistance can rarely be ascribed solely to omeprazole-warfarin interaction.
7) Competitive antagonism by increased dietary vitamin K intake impedes warfarin's anticoagulant activity.
8) Interactions of warfarin with herbal medications are increasingly recognized. An interaction with ginkgo was described and attributed to an inhibition of CYP2C9, but a controlled trial failed to demonstrate this interaction. Hyperforin found in St. John's wart may induce the CYP2C9 microsomal enzymes and reduce the anticoagulant effect of warfarin. Ginseng has also been found to inhibit warfarin action.
9) An interaction between dietary supplements of omega-3-polyunsaturated fatty acids contained in fish oils (2 gram per day or more) with warfarin causes an increased PT-INR. A registry of anticoagulant interactions with food supplements is available at http://www.clotcare.com
10) Alterations in the vitamin K control loop and receptor may cause warfarin resistance, an uncommon condition.
11) Elderly individuals taking multiple medications may be subject to unanticipated interactions. Because of the numerous potential drug interactions it is essential to closely monitor the PT-INR when adding or eliminating a medication from a patient's drug regimen while taking warfarin.
12) Warfarin resistance may be due to malabsorption [6].
13) Hereditary warfarin resistance is rare, with four previous cases confirmed.

*An algorithm* has been proposed for evaluation of suspected warfarin resistance [3]. First, if the patient's PT-INR is less than 2.0 while taking more than 15 mg warfarin per day, possible noncompliance with treatment should be addressed. Second, the patient's medications and diet should be reviewed for potential interference with warfarin. Next, the possibility of malabsorption should be pursued. In the following, clotting assays of factors II, VII, IX, and X may be the more precise way to assess the pharmacodynamics of warfarin, although there is no strong evidence to support their routinely use. Factor II and factor X activity <40% of normal suggest therapeutic dose of warfarin and unreliable PT-INR (e.g. lupus anticoagulant); in this situation it may be useful to check warfarin plasma level to confirm the diagnosis. Factor II and factor X activity >40% of normal are consistent with pharmacokinetic or pharmacodynamic resistance to warfarin or noncompliance. The latter can be excluded by measuring the warfarin plasma level. The therapeutic total plasma warfarin level is between 0.5 μg/mL and 3.0 μg/mL, though the range may vary among laboratories and patient populations.

In the patient here described, a normal response to warfarin was observed at the beginning, but later warfarin resistance emerged. Hence, hereditary warfarin resistance was not a consideration. There was no evidence of confounding factors which could interfere with PT measurement in the laboratory. Malabsorption was a reasonable consideration. Results of an iron tolerance test were consistent with malabsorption. The patient was malnourished. It is well known that severe starvation may compromise the normal functioning of the gastrointestinal tract and can lead to an incomplete tolerance to enteral re-feeding. Was malabsorption exacerbated by re-feeding? It is speculative but unproven that incomplete tolerance to enteral re-feeding might have aggravated malabsorption and, as a result, warfarin absorption was disturbed. Measurement of warfarin plasma levels could clarify this possibility but was not available when the patient was in our care several years ago.

Acquired warfarin resistance, induced by partial intolerance to re-feeding or by another obscure cause, may be transient. Therefore, the steady-state anticoagulation achieved in hospital may be transitory. Therefore, the need for dose readjustments is predicted and the need for close monitoring the PT is stressed. A preferable alternative to warfarin in this patient could be the novel oral anticoagulants. However, dabigatran and rivaroxabane were not in clinical use at the time the patient was in our care.

## Learning Points

- Warfarin resistance is defined by requirements greater than 70 mg warfarin per week to maintain the PT-INR in the target therapeutic range.
- Assessment for suspected warfarin resistance includes evaluation for laboratory error, non-adherence to treatment, food-warfarin interaction, malabsorption, drug-warfarin interaction, and hereditary warfarin resistance.
- In managing warfarin resistance, increasing the daily dose of warfarin or choice of another oral anticoagulant (e.g. dabigatran, rivaroxaban) are valuable options.

## References


[1] Gouin-Thibault I, Levy C, Pautas E, Cambus JP, Drouet L, Mahé I, Bal Dit Sollier C, Horellou MH, Golmard JL, Siguret V. Improving anticoagulation control in hospitalized elderly patients on warfarin. *J. Am. Geriatr. Soc.* 2010;58:242–247.

[2] Anderson JL, Horne BD, Stevans SM, Grove AS, Barton S, Nicholas ZP, Kahn SF, May HT, Samuelson KM, Muhlestein JB, Carlquist JF; Couma-Gen Investigators. Randomized trial of genotype-guided versus standard warfarin dosing in patients initiating oral anticoagulation. *Circulation* 2007;116:2563-2570.

[3] Osinbowale O, Malki MA, Schade A, Bartholomew J. An algorithm for managing warfarin resistance. *Cleve Clin. J. Med.* 2009;76:724-730.

[4] Unge P, Svedberg LE, Nordgren A, et al. A study of the interaction of omeprazole and warfarin in anticoagulated patients. *Br. J. Clin. Pharmacol.* 1992;34:509–512.

[5] Sutfin T, Balmer K, Bostrom H, Eriksson S, Hoglund P, Paulsen O. Stereoselective interaction of omeprazole with warfarin in healthy men. *Therapeut. Drug Monitor.* 1989;11:176–184.

[6] Sobieraj DM, Wang F, Kirton OC. Warfarin resistance after total gastrectomy and Roux-en-Y esophagojejunostomy. *Pharmacotherapy.* 2008;28:1537-1541.

[7] Pushpakom SP, Gambhir N, Latif A, Hadfield KD, Campbell S, Newman WG. Exacerbation of Hereditary Warfarin Resistance by Azathioprine. *Clin. Appl. Thromb. Hemost.* 2011;17:293-296.


## Case 36. Venous Thromboembolism Long Term Management

An 85-year old community-dwelling man was admitted to hospital with intestinal obstruction. Adenocarcinoma of the sigmoid colon was diagnosed and a Hartman procedure was performed, whereby the rectosigmoid colon was resected and a right sided colostomy was established. He had suffered two months earlier from shortness of breath, diagnosed on CT as pulmonary embolism, and treated with enoxaparin and subsequently with warfarin. The patient's medical history was remarkable for arterial hypertension, stable ischemic heart disease, mild renal failure, and prostatectomy for benign prostatic hypertrophy. He had suffered an ischemic stroke one year before the present admission. He experienced numerous falls during the preceding several months. His medications included enoxaparin, warfarin (treatment restarted), famotidine, lercanidipine, hydrochlorothiazide, and haloperidol.

On admission to our ward for subacute care the temperature was 36.8°C, BP 143/70 mmHg, heart rate 76 beats/minute, respiratory rate 20 breaths/minute, and oxygen saturation 94% in breathing ambient air. The patient was intermittently confused, having paranoid delusions. Muscle wasting was prominent, the body weight was 57 kg, and the BMI 17. The surgical wound, stoma and findings on abdominal examination were unremarkable. Laboratory studies showed hemoglobin 11.7 g/dL, mean corpuscular volume 97 fL, and serum creatinine 1.5 mg/dL. Serum electrolytes, blood glucose, transaminases, arterial blood gases and urinalysis were within the normal range. The PT-INR was 1.37.

The discussion at this point will focus on issues related to anticoagulant treatment. The problems during hospitalization were, however, not limited to reinstitution of anticoagulant treatment, but also involved the management of delirium, urinary tract infection, severe orthostatic hypotension, unsteady balance and gait. The latter will be discussed under the heading 'Falls, cerebrovascular disease, orthostatic hypotension and anticoagulant treatment' (Case 54).

*For initiation of anticoagulation,* guidelines provide precise rules: subcutaneous low-molecular-weight heparin (LMWH), fondaparinux or weight-based intravenous unfractionated heparin is started with concomitant initiation of warfarin treatment. LMWH or equivalents should be administered for at least five days until the PT-INR is in the therapeutic range (2.0 to 3.0) for two consecutive days [1, 2]. Because warfarin's antithrombotic effect depends on the clearance of prothrombin which may take up to five days, LMWH, heparin, or fondaparinux is administered concurrently with warfarin for at least five days to prevent thrombus propagation. This practice also protects against development of a hypercoagulable state because of the precipitous reduction of protein C during the first 36 hours of the warfarin treatment.

After anticoagulation has been started in patients with venous thromboembolism (VTE), three issues need to be addressed: the length of therapy, a basic workup for malignancy in patients with idiopathic VTE, and measures to prevent development of the postthrombotic syndrome [3].

*The length of anticoagulant treatment* should be tailored to the patient's specific circumstances. The risk of recurrent VTE is related to clinical risk factors. If surgery was the risk factor, patients with VTE treated for approximately 6 months had a 0% at 2 years rate of recurrence. The risk was 9% if the risk factor was nonsurgical and 19% if there were no detectable risk factors [4]. The American College of Chest Physicians recommends three months of anticoagulation for VTE caused by a reversible risk factor and indefinite treatment for idiopathic VTE in patients without risk factors for bleeding and who can get anticoagulation monitoring [5]. The high rate of recurrence of idiopathic VTE (4% to 27% when anticoagulation is limited to 3 months) suggests that a longer duration of treatment is reasonable [6]. However, increasing the length of therapy from 3 to 12 months delays but does not prevent recurrence, the risk of which begins to accumulate once anticoagulation is stopped [6]. There are two promising strategies to identify subgroups of patients with idiopathic VTE who are at highest risk of recurrence and who would most benefit from prolonged anticoagulation: d-dimer testing and evaluation for residual vein thrombosis.

*VTE can be the first manifestation of cancer,* as probably it was in the present case. Patients with cancer have a higher risk of developing VTE than the non-cancer population due to secretion of cancer related procoagulants and the increased activation of coagulation factors (tissue factor, thrombin anti-thrombin complex and factor VIIa). The prevalence of clinically apparent VTE in cancer patients is up to 15%, yet as the cancer progresses so does the prothrombotic tendency. Studies in patients with advanced cancer have shown an incidence of asymptomatic VTE in up to 52% of patients. This figure is similar to postmortem studies which showed evidence of pulmonary emboli in 50% of cancer patients [7]. A systematic review of 34 studies [8] found that, in patients with idiopathic VTE, cancer was diagnosed within 1 month in 6.1%, within 6 months in 8.6%, and within 1 year in 10.0%. Since cancer is a well-known risk factor for VTE, it seems logical to screen for cancer in patients with VTE of unknown cause. However studies were disappointing. Extensive screening of 1383 patients with deep venous thrombosis would have resulted in beneficial earlier cancer diagnosis in only two patients [9]. In another study, the detection rate for prevalent cancers was 5% with limited screening and 7% with extensive screening soon after the diagnosis of idiopathic VTE [10].

*Which work-up is appropriate for which patients?* To make an informed decision one needs to understand the utility of extensive cancer screening. Solitary idiopathic lower limb thrombosis merits a 'hunt for cancer' only if there are abnormalities on physical examination, blood count, erythrocyte sedimentation rate or chest X-ray film [9, 11]. It is considered appropriate medical practice to discuss with the patient and proxies whether to engage into extensive investigations in search of an occult neoplasia possibly underlying to the VTE. So they can balance the benefits and risks of the medical work-up versus the lack of proven survival benefit and cost-effectiveness.

*VTE recurrence is three times more likely in patients with cancer* than in primary VTE, with a cumulative rate of recurrence at one year of 21% vs. 7% [12]. Cancer patients are also twice as likely to suffer major bleeding complications while on anticoagulation [12]. Current thinking suggests that VTE should be treated until the cancer is resolved. However, this hypothesis has not been adequately tested, and consequently, the American College of Chest Physicians gives it only a level 1C recommendation [3].

*The management of cancer-associated VTE differs* from management of VTE of other etiologies. LMWH has proven advantages over warfarin in cancer patients with respect to VTE recurrence, drug–drug interactions and safety. However, in considering long term anticoagulation, there will still come a time when the continuation of LMWH offers no symptomatic benefit or improvement in quality of life [7]. Clinical judgment and discussion with the patient is the cornerstone of management in the palliative stage.

*Prevention of the postthrombotic syndrome* should begin soon after starting anticoagulant therapy. Damage to the venous valves produces chronic venous insufficiency with subsequent leg pain, venous dilation, edema, pigmentation, skin changes, and venous ulcers, i.e. the post-thrombotic syndrome. For patients with symptomatic proximal venous thrombosis, evidence supports the use of knee-high graduated compression stockings exerting a pressure of 30 to 40 mmHg at the ankle. Guidelines recommend use of compression stockings started within one month of proximal deep vein thrombosis, and continued for a minimum of one year after diagnosis [13]. A systematic review of three randomized trials concluded that elastic compression stockings reduce the risk of postthrombotic syndrome from 43% to 20% and the risk of severe postthrombotic syndrome from 15% to 7% [14]. Use of compression stockings is contraindicated in patients with evidence of severe occlusive arterial disease.

*If elective surgery is scheduled* in a patient receiving, warfarin administration should be timely discontinued and substituted with intravenous standard heparin or low molecular weight heparin. This approach was associated with very low rates of thromboembolism in major surgery (surprisingly, the rates of thromboembolism were also low if warfarin was discontinued without adding heparin).

*Minor invasive procedures* can be performed safely in patients who are receiving anticoagulation at therapeutic levels. There is no need to decrease the level of anticoagulation before placement of pacemakers and defibrillators, intramuscular injection of influenza vaccine, coronary angiography, arthocenthesis and joint injection (shoulder, knee, hip). This approach simplifies the periprocedural management of anticoagulation and may lead to improved outcomes and reduced health care costs [15].

The patient described in this report made his choice in favor of warfarin anticoagulation, in not willing to accept parenteral treatment for a prolonged period of time (enoxaparin was recommended). On oncology consultation palliation alone was offered in considering the patient's poor metabolic state and comorbidities that affect his prognosis.

### Learning Points

- VTE can be the first manifestation of cancer.
- However, there is lack of proven survival benefit or cost-effectiveness in engaging into extensive investigations in search of an occult neoplasia possibly underlying to the VTE.
- Long-term anticoagulation with LMWH in cancer-associated VTE is preferred over warfarin, taking in account the advantages with respect of recurrent thrombosis, drug–drug interactions and safety.
- In patients with cancer-associated VTE it is recommendation to administer LMWH therapy for at least 6 months.

## References

[1] Gouin-Thibault I, Levy C, Pautas E, Cambus JP, Drouet L, Mahé I, Bal Dit Sollier C, Horellou MH, Golmard JL, Siguret V. Improving anticoagulation control in hospitalized elderly patients on warfarin. *J. Am. Geriatr. Soc.* 2010;58:242–247.

[2] Anderson JL, Horne BD, Stevans SM, Grove AS, Barton S, Nicholas ZP, Kahn SF, May HT, Samuelson KM, Muhlestein JB, Carlquist JF; Couma-Gen Investigators. Randomized trial of genotype-guided versus standard warfarin dosing in patients initiating oral anticoagulation. *Circulation* 2007;116:2563-2570.

[3] Katz S, Quershi W, Lavender RC. Venous thromboembolism: what to do after anticoagulation is started. *Cleeveland Clin. J. Med.* 2011;78:609-618.

[4] Baglin T, Luddington R, Brown K, Baglin C. Incidence of recurrent venous thromboembolism in relation to clinical and thrombophilic risk factors: prospective cohort study. *Lancet* 2003; 362:523–526.

[5] Kearon C, Kahn SR, Agnelli G, Goldhaber S, Raskob GE, Comerota AJ; American College of Chest Physicians. Antithrombotic therapy for venous thromboembolic disease: American College of Chest Physicians Evidence-Based Clinical Practice Guidelines (8th Edition). *Chest* 2008;133(suppl 6):454S–545S.

[6] Agnelli G, Prandoni P, Becattini C, et al; Warfarin Optimal Duration Italian Trial Investigators. Extended oral anticoagulant therapy after a first episode of pulmonary embolism. *Ann. Intern. Med.* 2003; 139:19–25.

[7] Nobel S. The challenges of managing cancer related venous thromboembolism in the palliative care setting. *Postgrad. Med. J.* 2007;83:671-674.

[8] Carrier M, Le Gal G, Wells PS, Fergusson D, Ramsay T, Rodger MA. Systematic review: the Trousseau syndrome revisited: should we screen extensively for cancer in patients with venous thromboembolism? *Ann. Intern. Med.* 2008; 149:323–333.

[9] Nordstrom M, Lindblad B, Anderson H, Bergquist D, Kjellstrom T. Deep venous thrombosis and occult malignancy: an epidemiological study. *Br. Med. J.* 1994;308: 891-894.

[10] Blom JW, Doggen CJ, Osanto S, Rosendaal FR. Malignancies, prothrombotic mutations, and the risk of venous thrombosis. *JAMA* 2005; 293:715–722.

[11] Buller H, Ten Cate JW. Primary venous thromboembolism and cancer screening. *New Engl. J. Med.* 1998;338:1221-1222.

[12] Prandoni P, Lensing AW, Piccioli A, et al. Recurrent venous thromboembolism and bleeding complications during anticoagulant treatment in patients with cancer and venous thrombosis. *Blood* 2002; 100:3484–3488.

[13] Kahn SR, Partsch H, Vedantham S, Prandoni P, Kearon C; Subcommittee on Control of Anticoagulation of the Scientific and Standardization Committee of the International Society on Thrombosis and Haemostasis. Definition of post-thrombotic syndrome of the leg for use in clinical investigations: a recommendation for standardization. *J. Thromb. Haemost.* 2009;7:879–883.

[14] Kolbach DN, Sandbrink MW, Hamulyak K, Neumann HA, Prins MH. Non-pharmaceutical measures for prevention of post-thrombotic syndrome. *Cochrane Database Syst. Rev.* 2004; CD004174.

[15] Ahmed I, Gerner E. Safety of arthrocenthesis and joint injection in patients receiving anticoagulation at therapeutic levels. *Am. J. Med.* 2012;125:265-269.

*Chapter VII*

# Hypertensive Spells – Dealing with Uncertainty

Treatment of chronic stable hypertension is properly settled in clinical guidelines. Yet, treatment of unstable hypertension may be challenging. Work-up of possible etiologies should be the rule, but too often in practice a 'try and see' type of management is applied.

## Case 37. Pseudopheochromocytoma

A 72-year-old woman, by profession a physician, was seen on emergency during a hypertensive spell. The patient complained of attacks of palpitations, dizziness, headache, diaphoresis and tremor, associated with BP surges that exceeded 200/110 mmHg. She reported having six similar episodes over eight months. During the same time period she began suffering from panic attacks, which she considered to be secondary to the hypertensive spells. She was diagnosed with arterial hypertension and diabetes mellitus for well longer than 10 years. She was a nonsmoker and nondrinker. Her current medications were aspirin 100 mg/day, amlodipine 10 mg/day, ramipril 5 mg/day, spironolactone 12.5 mg/day, hydrochlorothiazide 12.5 mg/day, simvastatin 20 mg/day and metformin 2550 mg/day.

On physical examination the patient appeared calm, the BP was 166/92 mmHg, heart rate 82 bpm, temperature 36.5$^0$C, respiratory rate 20 per minute, oxygen saturation by pulse oxymetry 98% on ambient air, BMI 29. There was corneal arcus and a grade II goiter; otherwise the physical examination was unremarkable. The hemoglobin was 15.1 g/dL, serum creatinine 1.3 mg/dL, potassium 4.8 mmol/L, glucose 133 mg/dL. Other routine laboratory tests were normal. The ECG showed sinus rhythm with left ventricular strain. Chest x-rays and recent mammography, gynecologic examination, transvaginal and abdominal ultrasound examinations were unremarkable. Funduscopy showed stage II hypertensive retinopathy. The diagnosis of hypertensive bouts on the background of chronic arterial hypertension was entertained, i.e. the differential diagnosis of adrenergic spells.

*Pheochromocytoma crisis* is the prototype of adrenergic spells [1]. Pheochromocytoma crises are characterized by episodic symptoms that typically include palpitations, tremor, headache and diaphoresis. The spells tend to be stereotypical for each person, but the type of spell may greatly differ among patients. Peripheral vasoconstriction during the spell results in cold hands and feet and facial pallor. An increased sense of body heat and sweating occurs toward the end of the spell. Spells may be either spontaneous or precipitated by postural change, anxiety, medications (e.g. metoclopramide, anesthetic agents), exercise, and maneuvers that increase intraabdominal pressure (e.g. change in position, lifting, defecation, exercise, and trauma). Spells can occur several times per day or as infrequently as once monthly. The typical duration of a pheochromocytoma spell is 15 to 20 minutes, but it may be much shorter or may last for several hours. Nearly all patients have increased urinary excretion of the catecholamine metabolites vanilmandelic acid and metanephrines as well as free catecholamines. Measurement of total metanephrine excretion/24 hours is the most useful diagnostic test for pheochromocytoma, but false-positive results can occur (especially when the patient is treated with labetalol or buspirone). Sampling blood for catecholamines yields more frequent false positive results. In case of high clinical suspicion of pheochromocytoma and a more than 2-fold increase of urinary catecholamines or metanephrine, imaging should be ordered to locate the suspected adrenal mass. Abdominal CT or 123 MIBG scan serve for this purpose. On the contrary, with low clinical suspicion and normal 24-hour urinary catecholamines or metanephrine other causes of adrenergic spells should be investigated. Indeed, most patients having typical adrenergic spells do not have a pheochromocytoma and among patients suspected to have pheochromocytoma the diagnosis is rarely confirmed [1].

*Adrenergic spells other than pheochromocytoma* may occur in the following settings: essential hypertension, panic attacks, sympathomimetic ingestion, withdrawal of clonidine ('rebound hypertension'), baroreflex failure, familial dysautonomia, crack cocaine ingestion, serotonin syndrome, neuroleptic malignant syndrome, spinal cord injury, amyotrophic lateral sclerosis, diencephalic epilepsy, orthostatic hypotension, autonomic neuropathy, cerebrovascular insufficiency, thyrotoxicosis, insulinoma, hypoglycemia, mast cell disease, treatment with monoamine oxidase inhibitor with concomitant ingestion of tyramine or a nasal decongestionant, cerebral infarction, and renovascular disease. The most commonly encountered sympathetic crises in adults, less so perhaps in geriatrics, are induced by recreational use of cocaine, amphetamine or phencyclidine.

In all clinical situations characterized by sympathetic overstimulation, use of beta-adrenergic antagonists should be avoided because beta-receptor antagonism results in unopposed alpha-adrenergic activity; the latter may result in BP surge and/or coronary constriction. High BP is managed in these situations with nicardipine, fenoldopam or verapamil in combination with a benzodiazepine. In being a combined alpha- and beta-adrenergic antagonist, labetalol has been considered the ideal agent for the treatment of sympathetic overstimulation, but studies do not support its use in this clinical setting.

*The serotonin syndrome* is a result of excessive serotonergic activity in the central and peripheral nervous system. At risk are patients taking one or more medications that increase serotonin levels such as SSRIs, monoamine oxidase inhibitors or tricyclic antidepressants. The serotonin syndrome can present with mental status changes (anxiety, restlessness, disorientation), autonomic hyperactivity (tachycardia, hypertension, hyperthermia, diaphoresis, diarrhea), and/or neuromuscular abnormalities (hyperreflexia, myoclonus, ocular clonus, spontaneous or inducible clonus, tremor, bilateral Babinski sign, muscle rigidity). Prompt removal of the offending drug is mandatory along with administration of intravenous fluids and cardiovascular monitoring. Most cases of serotonin syndrome are self-limiting.

*The parkinsonism-hyperpyrexia syndrome* is a rare but potentially fatal complication met in patients with Parkinson's disease, most commonly following reduction of the dose or cessation of antiparkinsonian medications. Clinically it resembles neuroleptic malignant syndrome with rigidity, pyrexia, reduced level of consciousness and autonomic failure indicated by labile hypertension, less often hypotension, and tachycardia. Management consists of dopaminergic drug replacement, supportive measures and treatment of complications.

*Baroreflex failure* is characterized by marked and frequent fluctuations in BP, with alternating high and low readings. Baroreflexes normally buffer BP fluctuations; this function is impaired in baroreflex failure usually consequent to neck irradiation or surgery. Orthostatic tests typically are normal.

*The dysautonomic 'hyper-hypo syndrome'* is characterized by co-existent supine hypertension and orthostatic hypotension. It is often seen in patients with diabetes mellitus or Parkinson's disease (see Case 39).

*Panic disorder* is characterized by episodes of fear or panic, and is commonly associated with physical symptoms such as chest pain, headache, palpitations, flushing, and dizziness, along with some degree of BP elevation. Panic disorder is present in as many as 40 percent of patients evaluated for suspected pheochromocytoma compared with 5 percent of control patients with hypertension.

*Anxiety syndrome* is a common cause of adrenergic hypertensive spells. Nevertheless, patients usually insist that episodes are unrelated to emotional distress. With careful interviewing the diagnosis can be made and the adrenergic spells can be attributed to emotions that patients were not aware of. With treatment based on this understanding, further paroxysms were eliminated in the majority of cases in a study by Mann SJ: alpha-blockade plus beta-blockade was used, combined when necessary with an antidepressant agent, with or without an anxiolytic agent.

*Atherosclerotic renal artery stenosis* can manifest with hypertensive spells. Manifold manifestations of atherosclerotic renal artery stenosis have been described: renovascular hypertension, ischemic nephropathy, flash pulmonary edema, refractory heart failure, and unstable angina. Percutaneous vascular intervention to the management of renal artery stenosis has met much uncertainty and confusion. There are conditions for which most experts agree that renal stents are useful, such are bilateral 90% renal artery stenosis and flash pulmonary edema. There are conditions for which it is agreed that renal stents are not useful: this is the case of less than 50% renal artery stenosis without a translesional pressure gradient. There are borderline conditions for which there is uncertainty regarding the efficacy of percutaneous renal intervention [2].

*Acute management of hypertensive spells* may require an oral or an i.v. agent. If the BP elevation is not extreme, oral agents such as clonidine can be administered acutely. An anxiolytic agent, e.g. alprazolam alone or in combination with an antihypertensive agent can bring quick relief of symptoms and high BP. Intravenous labetalol, beginning with a bolus of 20 mg initially, followed by 40 to 80 mg every 10 minutes to a maximum dose of 200 to 300 mg is usually very effective [3].

*Concerning BP variability,* recent studies have shown that visit-to-visit variability in BP and episodic hypertension are powerful risk factors for stroke. The benefits of certain blood-pressure-lowering drugs are attributable partly to their effect of reducing variability in BP [4]. This insight needs to be integrated in medical practice.

Our patient described denied an emotional background to her symptoms and hypertensive bouts, but her spouse readily supported this possibility. Indeed, treatment with escitalopram in the past had resulted in some improvement; the patient unwilling to accept to have psychological troubles had discontinued the drug. On further evaluation, a postural test and postprandial BP monitoring showed normal results, the thyrotropin level and urinary 24 hour catecholamines and metanephrine were normal. Escitalopram treatment was resumed and the dose was gradually increased. In reaching a 15 mg daily dose the symptoms subsided and an acceptable BP control was reported; this was attested on 24 hours ambulatory BP monitoring. On three and six months follow-up visits the patient reported that no further spells had occurred.

### *Learning Points*

- Symptomatic paroxysmal hypertension should raise a suspicion of pheochromocytoma. However, an adrenal tumor is rarely found in patients in whom it is considered.
- Adrenergic spells other than pheochromocytoma may occur in a variety of disorders. More frequent among these are labile essential hypertension, autonomic neuropathy, anxiety syndromes, and panic attacks.
- Anxiety syndrome is a common cause of adrenergic hypertensive spells, though patients usually insist that episodes are unrelated to emotional distress.
- An anxiolytic agent can bring quick relief.

## References

[1] Mann SJ. Severe paroxysmal hypertension (pseudopheochromocytoma). *Curr. Hypertens. Rep.* 2008; 10:12.
[2] White CG. The need for randomized trials to prove the safety and efficacy of parachutes, bulletproof vests, and percutaneous renal intervention. *Mayo Clin. Proc.* 2011;86:603-606.
[3] Rodriguez MA, Kumar SK, De Caro M. Hypertensive crisis. *Cardiol. Rev.* 2010;18: 102-107.
[4] Rothwell PM, Algra A, Amarenco P. Medical treatment in acute and long-term secondary prevention after ischaemic attack and stroke. *Lancet* 2011;377:1681-1692.

## Case 38. Orthostatic Hypotension Associated with Supine Hypertension

A 76-year-old man was referred to our institution with a history of recurrent falls. Dementia with Lewy bodies has been diagnosed five month previously, based on progressive cognitive decline, visual hallucinations, extra pyramidal signs, sleep disturbance and repeated falls. CT showed mild cerebral atrophy.

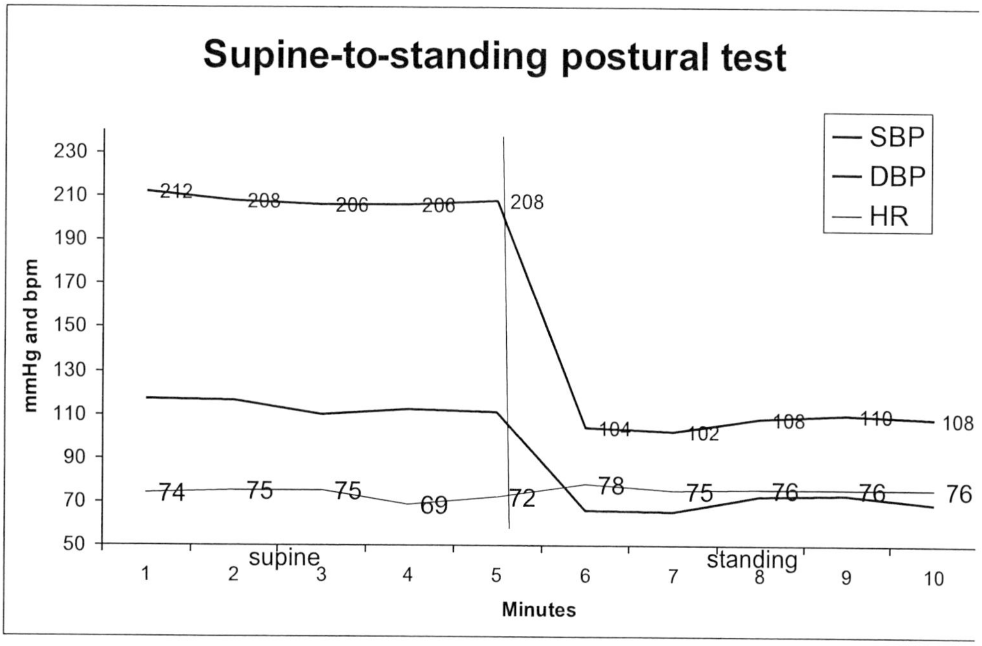


Figure 32. Supine hypertension with severe orthostatic hypotension.

His medical history was remarkable for arterial hypertension, coronary artery disease, and mild fasting hyperglycemia. He was a nonsmoker and nondrinker. Ramipril and hydrochlorothiazide were recently discontinued because of severe orthostatic hypotension. The patient's current medications were aspirin 100 mg/day, simvastatin 20 mg/day, and midodrine 5 mg x 2/day. Yet, the BP was poorly controlled. The supine BP on admission was 208/116 mmHg and the seated BP was 102/65 mmHg.

There was resting tremor, muscle rigidity and parkinsonian gait. Results of routine laboratory tests, ECG and chest x-rays were unremarkable. The main problem at this point was how to treat supine hypertension associated with orthostatic hypotension (Figure 32).

The commonly used management for this syndrome was instituted. During day-time, increased fluid intake, compression bandages to the calves and thighs, oral midodrine 7.5 mg x 3/day and later 10 mg x 3/day were prescribed (the first dose is taken 20 minutes before standing up in the morning and the last dose at 4 p.m.), and emphasis was given to avoid recumbence during day-time. Over night the bandages were removed and a nitroglycerine 10 mg transdermal patch was applied. The improvement of BP control was remarkable, with the patient able to stand. On a 10 minute supine-5 minute standing postural test the systolic blood pressure was in the range 112-130 mmHg and the diastolic blood pressure was 60 to 74 mmHg. In the seated position, the postprandial blood pressure was recorded at 10 minute intervals for 2 hours: the blood pressure was in the range 116-127/62-78 mmHg, while the patient was free of symptoms. The supine BP at 10 p.m. was 150/88 mmHg and at 7 a.m. 148/80 mmHg. These results were considered largely satisfactory.

*The 'hyper-hypo syndrome'* is characterized by co-existent supine hypertension and orthostatic hypotension. It is usually due to autonomic failure and is often met in patients with diabetes mellitus or Parkinson's disease. Autonomic failure by other causes is rarely met in acute geriatric care (e.g. Guillain-Barre syndrome, Shy-Draeger syndrome). More than 50%

of primary autonomic failure patients have high BP when supine, with values reaching 230/140 mm Hg and carrying the risks of stroke, cerebral hemorrhage, papiledema, and heart failure. The mechanisms of the paradoxical hypertension in the setting of a generalized sympathetic failure involve hypersensitivity of postsynaptic β-adrenoreceptors, nocturnal fluid retention and baroreflex failure. Orthostatic hypotension in patients with autonomic failure is due to interruption of the homeostatic reflex arch which is responsible to correct the effective hypovolemia occurring upon assuming the upright posture, when blood is pooling in the lower body areas. Orthostatic hypotension can be asymptomatic or associated with symptoms of cerebral hypoperfusion; there is relief of symptoms when the patient lies flat. Severely affected patients are unable to stand or sit but for few seconds before symptoms of cerebral hypoperfusion oblige them to assume the supine position. The management entails treatment of orthostatic hypotension when the patient is upright and treatment of hypertension when the patient is supine.

*The definition of orthostatic hypotension* was updated in a 2011 consensus statement [1]. Accordingly, orthostatic hypotension is a sustained reduction of systolic BP of at least 20 mmHg or diastolic BP of at least 10 mmHg within 3 minutes of standing or head-up tilt to at least $60^0$ on a tilt table. In patients with supine hypertension, a reduction in systolic BP of 30 mmHg may be a more appropriate criterion for orthostatic hypotension because the magnitude of the orthostatic BP fall is dependent on the baseline BP [1]. Many patients with neurogenic orthostatic hypotension have supine hypertension. Some of these patients have BP falls on standing that fulfill criteria for orthostatic hypotension although the BP remains above the normal range. The clinical significance of this phenomenon is unknown. Some patients have symptomatic orthostatic hypotension that occurs beyond 3 minutes of standing. The latter is diagnosed by extending the duration of standing or head-up tilt beyond 3 minutes. The clinical significance of 'delayed orthostatic hypotension' is unknown [1].

*Epidemiologic studies* show an increased prevalence of orthostatic hypotension in the elderly. Among community dwelling individuals older than 65 years of age the prevalence of orthostatic hypotension is about 20%; in those older than 75 years the prevalence may be as high as 30%. In frail elderly individuals living in nursing homes, the prevalence of orthostatic hypotension may be up to 50%. The orthostatic BP drop is more common and more severe in the morning. Beside orthostatic hypotension, elderly subjects and patients with autonomic failure are susceptible to postprandial hypotension. Postprandial hypotension is induced or aggravated by large meals, by meals high in carbohydrate, and by alcohol intake.

*Characteristic symptoms* of orthostatic hypotension are lightheadedness, dizziness, presyncope and syncope. Loss of consciousness is usually of gradual onset but may occur suddenly. Some patients have general complaints such as weakness, fatigue, cognitive slowing, leg buckling, visual blurring, headache, neck pain, orthostatic dyspnea or chest pain. Orthostatic hypotension may be asymptomatic [2]. Orthostatic hypotension per se is rarely hazardous, but complications are related to the risks associated with falls. The treatment therefore is symptomatic and a stepwise approach is recommended based on the severity of the symptoms. On the contrary, supine hypertension may complicate with stroke, cerebral edema, heart failure, and coronary events, and is associated with increased mortality [3].

*The goal of management of the 'hyper-hypo syndrome'* is to raise the patient's standing BP without also raising his supine BP, and specifically to reduce orthostatic symptoms, increase the time the patient can stand, and improve the ability to perform daily activities. No specific treatment is currently available that achieves all these goals [2].

First, aggravating conditions such as anemia, hypovolemia, heart failure, deconditioning should be treated and alleviated if possible. Erythropoietin treatment for anemia may be beneficial in the appropriate clinical context. If the patient is taking any drug that may cause orthostatic hypotension it should be either discontinued, the dose reduced, or substituted. Especially antiparkinsonian medications, nitrates, antidepressants, diuretics, prostate medications, and antihypertensive medications are suspect. The patient should avoid dehydration, alcohol ingestion, carbohydrate-heavy meals, quickly standing up after prolonged sitting or recumbence, prolonged motionless standing, vigorous or isometric exercise, heat exposure, and straining during micturition or defecation.

In order to avoid orthostatic deconditioning, adequate orthostatic stress should be maintained during the day, i.e. upright activity. Mild physical exercise improves orthostatic tolerance by reducing venous pooling and increasing plasma volume. Training in a supine or sitting position, such as swimming or recumbent biking, is recommended.

Elastic compression to reduce venous capacitance is a key factor in the treatment of orthostatic hypotension. Abdominal compression by using an elastic binder is the preferred means [2]. Compression of the legs is not as beneficial as compression of the abdomen because the venous capacitance of the calves and thighs is relatively small compared with that of the splanchnic mesenteric bed. Moreover, compression garments and stockings that are strong enough to produce a measurable effect on orthostatic hypotension are cumbersome to put on and uncomfortable to wear. Advantages of the abdominal binder include the immediate effect which can be easily assessed. The binder or compression garments should be tight enough to exert gentle pressure. They should be put on before rising from bed and taken off when lying supine thereby avoiding enhancement of supine hypertension.

Boluses of water drinking (500 mL of cold water) help to expand the plasma volume and elicit within a few minutes a significant pressor effect. This can be used when prolonged standing is expected. It is recommended that patients drink daily 1.25 to 2.5 L of fluids. Salt intake should be 10 to 20 g per day. However, caution is needed in patients who have severe supine hypertension, heart failure or edema. Some patients are very sensitive to sodium supplementation and can fine-tune their orthostatic control with salt alone. Patients need to maintain a high-potassium diet, as the high sodium intake combined with fludrocortisone promotes potassium loss. Fruits and vegetables have high potassium content.

Vasopressor drugs are a mainstay of therapy for orthostatic hypotension. Midodrine is effective and safe when used for treating neurogenic orthostatic hypotension. A common starting dose is 5 mg three times a day; most patients respond best to 10 mg three times a day. As midodrin's duration of action is 2 to 4 hours, the drug should be taken before getting up in the morning, before lunch, and in the mid afternoon. To avoid nocturnal supine hypertension, midodrine should not be taken after the mid afternoon. The main side effects of midodrine are supine hypertension, scalp paresthesias, and pilomotor reactions. Midodrine is ineffective when the plasma volume is reduced [2].

Fludrocortisone is a synthetic mineralocorticoid that has a pressor effect by the ability to expand the plasma volume and to increase the alpha-adrenoceptor sensitivity. Fludrocortisone is helpful when the plasma volume fails to adequately increase with salt supplementation. The usual dose is 0.1 to 0.2 mg/day, but may be increased to 0.4 to 0.6 mg/day in patients with refractory orthostatic hypotension. Administration of fludrocortisone is contraindicated in the presence of congestive heart failure and in chronic renal failure. The potential adverse effects are severe hypokalemia and excessive supine hypertension. Frequent monitoring of serum potassium, a diet high in potassium, and regular checks of supine BP are advised, especially at higher doses when added to midodrine. Elderly patients may poorly tolerate midodrine.

Yohimbine 5.4 mg may be worth a trial when orthostatic hypotension is difficult to control; pyridostigmine, contrary to early claims, was shown to be ineffective for treatment of orthostatic hypotension [4].

*For treatment of supine hypertension* the patient should not take pressor agents before bedtime and fluid intake at bedtime should be avoided. A snack before bedtime is recommended and minimal alcohol consumption before going to bed is permitted. Compressive binders, stockings and bandages should be removed before going to bed. The head of the bed should be raised by 15–30 cm. Pharmacologic measures employed while the patient is supine are transdermal nitroglycerin (a 10 mg patch when going to bed and to be removed before standing up) or clonidine 0.1 mg early in the evening. Preference is given to transdermal nitroglycerin because of its versatility.

*Education* is probably the single most important factor in the proper control of the 'hyper-hypo syndrome' [2]. Patients should be taught the mechanisms that maintain postural normotension and how to recognize the onset of orthostatic symptoms. They should be taught nonpharmacologic approaches to deal with orthostatic symptoms. They should be aware that other drugs they start may worsen symptoms of the 'hyper-hypo syndrome' [2].

### Learning Points

- Orthostatic hypotension associated with supine hypertension entails the double threat of orthostatic syncope and hypertensive complications.
- The treatment is demanding and the patients' and caregiver's understanding and compliance are essential for success.

## References

[1] Freeman R, Wieling W, Axelrod FB, Benditt DG, Benarroch E, Biaggioni I, Cheshire WP, Chelimsky T, Cortelli P, Gibbons CH, Goldstein DS, Hainsworth R, Hilz MJ, Jacob G, Kaufmann H, Jordan J, Lipsitz LA, Levine BD, Low PA, Mathias C, Raj SR, Robertson D, Sandroni P, Schatz I, Schondorff R, Stewart JM, van Dijk JG. Consensus statement on the definition of orthostatic hypotension, neurally mediated syncope and the postural tachycardia syndrome. *Clin. Auton. Res.* 2011; 21:69-72.

[2] Figueroa JJ, Basford JR, Low PA. Preventing and treating orthostatic hypotension: As easy as A, B, C. *Cleveland Clinic Journal of Medicine* 2010;77:298-306.

[3] Biaggioni I, Robertson RM. Hypertension in orthostatic hypotension and autonomic dysfunction. *Cardiology Clinics* 2002;20:291-301.

[4] Shibao C, Okamoto LE, Gamboa A, Yu C, Diedrich A, Raj SR, Robertson D, Biaggioni I. Comparative efficacy of yohimbine against pyridostigmine for the treatment of orthostatic hypotension in autonomic failure. *Hypertension* 2010;56:847-851.

# Case 39. Orthostatic Hypertension

An 87-year-old man was referred to our ward with a history of hypertensive spells which occurring in a stereotypical fashion during the preceding two months. According to the description of staff members from the nursing home where he was living, the symptoms occurred 30 to 120 minutes after being seated in a geriatric chair, featuring pallor, more prominent muscle rigidity than usual, tachycardia up to 110 bpm, BP surge as high as 210/130 mmHg, and profuse sweats, and an apparent pause of urine output for several hours (the patient had a permanent urinary catheter). The event ended soon when the patient was brought back to bed, the BP returning to usual levels of 130/70 mmHg and subsequent polyuria (about 500 cc within an hour). The blood sugar measured at the height of a spell was 118 mg/dL and the body temperature was normal. These hypertensive spells were not linked to intake of food. The patient's medical history was notable for stroke, vascular dementia with parkinsonism, an enlarged and firm prostate, and prostate specific antigen 42 ng/mL (normal < 4 ng/mL). Further investigation of suspected prostatic carcinoma was declined by the patient's apotropos. The patient's medications were memantine 20 mg/day and doxazocin 4 mg/day. Doxazocin has been discontinued, than oxycontin was administered for a few days; neither influenced the occurrence of the hypertensive spells. On physical examination, the patient's temperature was $36.7^0$C, BP 130/60 mmHg, heart rate 62 beats/min, respirations 18/minute, and oxygen saturation 94% while breathing room air. The prostate was enlarged and felt hard. Laboratory studies showed normal CBC, liver-function tests, erythrocyte sedimentation rate, CRP, lactic dehydrogenase, uric acid, calcium and thyrotropin.

The BP was measured in supine and in erect position with the aim to reproduce the hypertensive spell and symptoms described. For this purpose a variant of a passive postural test was performed adapted to the patient's special physical condition. A geriatric chair was shifted in supine position with the patient lying on his back for 15 minutes, than the configuration of the chair was adjusted to sitting for 10 minutes. The BP and heart rate were monitored. The supine BP was about 130/70 mmHg and the heart rate 73 bpm with minimal variation. The sitting BP gradually increased to 160/76 while the heart rate decreased to 64 bpm. During both phases of the postural test, the oral temperature was $36.4^0$C and the ECG showed sinus rhythm. The patient's typical symptoms, told to occur regularly together with the BP surges, were not reproduced during the test. These data were interpreted as orthostatic hypertension with adequate baroreflex heart rate response.

On a different occasion the test was repeated after the patient was given his regular meal; postprandial BP measurements were taken at 10 minute intervals for 2 hours. The results were essentially similar with those recorded on the short orthostatic test. A 24-hour urine collection for catecholamines showed normal epinephrine, norepinephrine, dopamine and metanephrine levels; the collection included a four hours period of continuous sitting on a chair. In summarizing these findings, the diagnosis of orthostatic hypertension was proposed.

*Orthostatic hypertension* is defined as a rise in systolic BP upon assuming an upright posture. There is no generally agreed definition of orthostatic hypertension and the diagnostic criteria adopted by different study groups vary: increase in the systolic BP upon assuming upright posture by ≥10 mmHg or by ≥5 mmHg in other studies [1]. The prevalence of orthostatic hypertension and its association with morbidity and subsequent mortality was examined prospectively in 3741 Japanese-American men aged 71-93 years. The prevalence of postural hypertension in this cohort was 39%; there were no significant correlations with morbidity and subsequent mortality [2]. The mechanism responsible for orthostatic hypertension is unknown. Some of the more severely affected patients have baroreflex failure, mastocytosis, hyperadrenergic postural tachycardia syndrome or pheochromocytoma. Postural change may trigger hypertensive spells in patients with pheochromocytoma (see discussion in Case 38). Impairment of cerebellar autonomic modulation or dysfunction of the baroreflex circuit may result in orthostatic hypertension. A comparable phenomenon was described in a patient with cerebellar hematoma and acute hydrocephalus who had a vermian and partial right cerebellar hemisphere resection. Neurosurgery was followed by incident orthostatic hypertension: on standing the patient's systolic BP rose by 60 mmHg with a fivefold increase in plasma noradrenalin level. After a period of eight weeks the postural BP regulation improved and orthostatic hypertension diminished [3].

In the current case the main diagnostic considerations were adverse effects of medications (but he was receiving only memantine which has not been shown to cause adrenergic hyperactivity), pheochromocytoma (yet, urinary catecholamines were in the normal range), and an obscure neurological disturbance of BP homeostasis. A therapeutic trial with tamsulosin 5 mg/day, that may be useful in the treatment of sympathetic hyperactivity [4], was of no avail in this patient. Eventually the diagnosis was labeled idiopathic postural hypertension.

### Learning Points

- Orthostatic hypertension is defined as a rise in systolic BP upon assuming upright posture by $\geq$10 mmHg.
- Orthostatic hypertension is common in elderly persons and often no underlying cause can be found.
- Orthostatic hypertension may occasionally be a manifestation of pheochromocytoma, as postural change may sometimes triggers an adrenergic crisis.

## References

[1] Fessel J, Robertson D. Orthostatic hypertension: when pressor reflexes overcompensate. *Nat. Clin. Pract. Nephrol.* 2006;2:424-431.

[2] Alagiakrishnan K, Masaki K, Schatz I, Curb JD, Blanchette P. Postural hypertension in elderly men - the Honolulu Heart Program. *Hawaii Med. J.* 2000;59:48-50.

[3] Idiaquez J, Fadic R, Mathias CJ. Transient orthostatic hypertension after partial cerebellar resection. *Clin. Auton. Res.* 2011;21:57-59.

[4] Ohno T, Shimizu T, Kato S, Hayashi H, Hirai S. Effect of tamsulosin hydrochloride on sympathetic hyperactivity in amyotrophic lateral sclerosis. *Auton. Neurosci.* 2001;88: 94-98.

# Case 40. Unstable BP

A 52-year-old woman with advanced-stage amyotrophic lateral sclerosis suffered for several years of weakness of the muscles, impaired speech, dysphagia, dyspnea at rest and sleep apnea. Noninvasive ventilation with bi-level positive airway pressure was administered first; eventually the patent became ventilator dependent. Nutrition was provided via a gastrostomy tube. She received riluzole 50 mg x 2/day. Supine BP oscillations became worrying: swings of the systolic BP ranged between 78 and 220 mmHg and those of the diastolic BP between 40 and 120 mmHg. Urinary catecholamines and metanephrine were on the upper normal levels. The BP fluctuations could not be ascribed to the only medication the patient was receiving, to inefficient ventilation or to pulmonary aspirations. A trial of tamsulosin treatment 0.4 mg/day did not curb the BP fluctuations.

*Amyotrophic lateral sclerosis* is a neurodegenerative disease of the systemic motor neurons. Involvement of the limbic system, particularly the central and basolateral nuclei of the amygdala and the hypothalamus might be responsible for the fluctuations both in emotional behavior and in autonomic regulation. Respirator-dependent patients with amyotrophic lateral sclerosis may have marked BP fluctuation followed by circulatory collapse or sudden death. High plasma norepinephrine concentrations in some cases indicate sympathetic hyperactivity [1]. A study showed that tamsulosin, a selective long-acting alpha-1 adrenergic blocker, which usually is used for the treatment of benign prostatic hypertrophy, may be helpful in preventing sympathetic hyperactivity and hypertensive spells in patients with amyotrophic lateral sclerosis [2]. This was not the case in this patient.

## Learning Point

- BP fluctuations in patients with advanced amyotrophic lateral sclerosis may be refractory to treatment.

# References

[1] Shimizu T, Hayashi H, Kato S, Hayashi M, Tanabe H, Oda M. Circulatory collapse and sudden death in respirator-dependent amyotrophic lateral sclerosis. *J. Neurol. Sci.* 1994; 124:45-55.

[2] Ohno T, Shimizu T, Kato S, Hayashi H, Hirai S. Effect of tamsulosin hydrochloride on sympathetic hyperactivity in amyotrophic lateral sclerosis. *Auton. Neurosci.* 2001; 88:94-98.

# Cases 41,42 and 43. Flush Hypertension during Infusion of Saline

Salt-sensitivity is present in approximately half the population with essential hypertension [1]. Weinberger's saline infusion test is widely accepted to diagnose salt-sensitivity; this test compares the BP measured after infusing two liters of isotonic saline over 4 hours with the BP measured during a salt-restricted diet and administration of three 40-mg oral doses of furosemide. A 10 mmHg or greater difference in mean BP between the salt-loaded and salt-depleted phases of the test is named salt sensitivity [2]. In the three patients to be described infusion of isotonic saline induced a surge of BP far in excess to the mild hypertensive effect required to diagnose salt-sensitive hypertension. Such episodes are not well described in the literature.

*Case 41.* A 96-year-old-woman was referred with the diagnosis of left lower lobe pneumonia. Amoxicillin/clavulanate i.v. 1g x 3/day was started. Notable in the patient's medical history were multi-infarct dementia, dysphagia, grade I arterial hypertension, vitamin B12 deficiency and iron deficiency. Her regular medications were simvastatin 20 mg, furosemide 40 mg, vitamin B12 and ferum sulfate 160 mg/day. The patient's BP readings on the day of admission were 185/90, 139/77, 145/65 mmHg, the heart rate 72 bpm, temperature 38.6$^0$C. The serum creatinine was 0.7 mg/dL, WBC 12,300/mm$^3$, polymorphonuclear leukocytes 79%. Two days later, the temperature returned to normal but the abdomen became distended with no passage of stool or gas and high pitched bowel sounds suggesting intestinal obstruction or pseudoobstruction. On plain abdominal x-rays the colon was distended, air was visible in all colonic segments including the rectosigmoid, and the maximum cecal diameter was 7 cm. The BP was 138/70 mmHg. Serum levels of sodium, potassium, calcium and thyrotropin were within the normal range. On surgical consultation a diagnosis of colonic pseudoobstruction was posited and conservative management was recommended. The patient was kept fasted and i.v. saline was started. Four hours later she became tachypneic and the BP increased to 220/107 mmHg. Relief was achieved by administration of furosemide and clonidine. Repeated episodes of intestinal pseudoobstruction followed. During another episode of intestinal pseudoobstruction one liter of normal saline was started slowly, keeping in mind the recent incident. Nonetheless, the patient became dyspneic with the BP 214/111 mmHg, heart rate 72 bpm, and auscultatory findings consistent with pulmonary edema. The saline infusion was discontinued and furosemide, nitroglycerin and clonidine were administered, followed briefly by hemodynamic stabilization. Subsequently, the administration of saline was avoided; for hydration i.v. glucose 5% was administered.

Throughout 12 days of hospitalization the patient received enteral and, repeatedly, parenteral hydration. Only infusion of saline was associated with hypertensive spells, on challenge and, by necessity, on rechallenge. The BP remained in the range 110-138/72-80 mmHg when receiving large quantities of fluids other than saline.

*Case 42.* An 81-old-woman was referred with the diagnosis of right lower lobe pneumonia. Empirical treatment with ceftriaxone and azithromycin was started. Remarkable in her medical history were fairly controlled arterial hypertension, diabetes mellitus type 2, left bundle branch block and chronic renal failure. The patient's regular medications comprised insulin mixtard, simvastatin 20 mg/day and clonidine 0.150 mg x 2/day. On admission to our ward the patient's temperature was 37.0$^0$C, supine BP 177/70 mmHg, heart rate 60 bpm, oxygen saturation on room air 98%. The chest x-rays showed an alveolar infiltrate with air bronchogram in the right lower lung field. The serum creatinine was 3.5 mg/dL and BUN 84 mg/dL. Acute oliguric renal failure was diagnosed and infusion of isotonic saline 12 gtts/minute was started. Four hours later the patient became tachypneic, the BP had increased to 230/130 mmHg, and wet rales were perceived over the lower lung fields. The ECG was unchanged. To this time the patient had received 180 mL of saline. The infusion was discontinued. With 40% oxygen administered by face mask, morphine 10 mg, sublingual clonidine 0.150 mg and 80 mg furosemide i.v. it took about 30 minutes to observe improvement: the BP decreased to 190/98 mmHg and soon 154/76 mmHg, and the rales withdraw to the lung bases. During her hospital stay, the patient's median BP was 134/50 mmHg with furosemide 120 mg/day added and all other medications continued. A control chest x-rays showed no pulmonary congestion. Ahead of discharge to the nursing home the serum creatinine was 3.7 mg/dL and the BUN 91 mg/dL.

A severe and unexpected rise of the BP had occurred during infusion of merely a small volume of isotonic saline; predisposing factors were chronic systolic hypertension and renal failure.

*Case 43.*A 63-year-old usually healthy, normotensive women underwent elective lumpectomy for carcinoma of the beast. Her preoperative BP was 120/68 mmHg. As part of the postoperative care she received infusion with 1000 mL of isotonic saline. She made a swift recovery and was in good mood. Unexpectedly, 24 hours after surgery her BP was 193/110 mmHg and remained elevated for 24 hours. Routine biochemistry and urinalysis were unremarkable. Infusion of saline was discontinued. No antihypertensive medication or sedative was administered. Urinary catecholamines were normal. The patient remained under close observation for another day and had all BP measurements within the normal range. On 24-hours ambulatory monitoring and during outpatient follow-up the BP remained within the normal range.

This case illustrates an unexpected upsurge of the BP after saline infusion in a normotensive subject; the BP returned to normal after discontinuation of saline infusion. Although hospitalization might be responsible for stress-hypertension, an argument can be made against this possibility. Indeed, normal BP values were recorded in the hospital before surgery and the BP returned to normal while she was still in the hospital. The rise and fall in BP in this patient is not in line with a psychogenic vasopressor reaction.

*Studies with intravenous saline loading* have shown adaptive responses in healthy adult volunteers: intravenous infusion of 20 to 30 mL/kg of normal saline over 30 minutes (1500 - 2000mL) yielded an increased pulmonary capillary blood volume by 12%, increased the cardiac output, concomitant increase of the systolic BP by merely 7 mmHg without significant change in diastolic BP [3]. In contrast to the former, altered adaptive mechanisms might be operative in salt-sensitive hypertension.

*A variety of etiologic factors* are involved in salt-sensitive hypertension. Older age, black race, and female sex are associated with an increased frequency of salt sensitivity [4]. Salt sensitive hypertension may be acquired as a consequence of microvascular and tubulointerstitial renal injury; this is mediated in part by lymphocytes and macrophages infiltrating the tubulointerstitium, which produce angiotensin II and stimulate oxidative stress [5]. Salt sensitive hypertension may be genetically determined. The rare, Mendelian, juvenile forms of hypertension involve excessive activation of the epithelial Na+ channel (ENaC), i.e. the final common pathway for reabsorption of sodium in the distal nephron. Mutations in the kinases WNK1 and WNK4 have been identified to be responsible for some forms of Gordon's syndrome. The ADD1, ACE, WNK1 and NEDD4L variants [6] and a polymorphism of the PRKG1 gene [7] modulate, at different targets, the acute BP response to salt load. The mechanisms of hypertension driven by sodium retention include volume-mediated effects, volume-independent direct effects of sodium such as production of ouabain-like steroids, angiotensin-mediated central effects of sodium, increased sympathetic nervous system activity, increase in the production of nuclear factor kappa B, and increased expression of the angiotensin 1 receptor in renal tissues [4].

*The pathophysiology of the incidents observed* in the portrayed three patients is obscure. The medical background of the three patients was remarkably different: normal BP, chronic arterial hypertension without renal failure, and chronic arterial hypertension with renal failure. Yet, the three patients had in common a transient and severe BP surge during infusion of relatively low volumes of saline. The patient describes in Case 41 had repeated hypertensive spells upon administration of i.v. saline, but tolerated salt free solutions administered i.v. Hence, flush hypertension in this patient appeared to be independent of volume overload. The excessive BP surge during infusion of saline in the three patients contrasts with the generally mild hypertensive response elicited by large volumes of saline, which is typical for salt-sensitive hypertension [2].

The extreme BP reactivity in the three patients might stand for an extreme variant of salt sensitive hypertension or could be a different syndrome, which has not received emphasis in the literature. Temporality of the association, illustrated by the parallel time course of saline infusion and BP surge, might be an argument supporting the idea of causality. That saline infusion was responsible for flare hypertension in Case 41 is attested by replication of the reaction on rechallenge, improvement on dechallenge, and no placebo response on hydration with i.v. glucose. The clinical implication of these incidents is important.

Transient severe hypertension occurring during saline infusion is not well described in the literature and deserves to be purposely studied. Assessment of the genetic polymorphism in this context may be instructing.

## Learning Points

- Normotensive adults may unexpectedly develop flush hypertension under infusion of moderate volumes of normal saline. If such was the case, an alert should be added to the patient's diagnoses.
- Hypertensive adults, with or without renal failure, may be excessively sensitive to intravenous saline infusion.
- When saline is administered for treatment of dehydration, sepsis or worsening renal failure the BP should be checked repeatedly as long as the infusion is administered and preferably over the subsequent 24 hours.
- Salt free isotonic solutions might be tolerated by these patients.

# References


[1] Appel LJ, Brands MW, Daniels SR, Karanja N, Elmer PJ, Sacks FM. Dietary approaches to prevent and treat hypertension: a scientific statement from the American Heart Association. *Hypertension* 2006;47:296-308.

[2] Weinberger MH, Fineberg NS. Sodium and volume sensitivity of BP: age and pressure change over time. *Hypertension* 1991;18:67-71.

[3] Prisk KG, Olfert MI, Arai TJ, Wagner PD, Hopkins SR. Rapid intravenous infusion of 20 mL/kg saline does not impair resting pulmonary gas exchange in the healthy human lung. *J. Appl. Physiol.* 2010;108:53–59.

[4] Rodriguez-Iturbe B, Romero F, Johnson RJ. Pathophysiology of salt-dependent hypertension. *Am. J. Kidney Dis.* 2007;50:655-672.

[5] Rodríguez-Iturbe B, Quiroz Y, Herrera-Acosta J, Johnson RJ, Pons HA. The role of immune cells infiltrating the kidney in the pathogenesis of salt-sensitive hypertension. *J. Hypertens. Suppl.* 2002;20:S9-S14.

[6] Beeks E, Kessels AG, Kroon AA, van der Klauw MM, de Leeuw PW. Genetic predisposition to salt-sensitivity: a systematic review. *J. Hypertens.* 2004;22: 1243-1249.

[7] Citterio L, Simonini M, Zagato L, Salvi E, Delli Carpini S, Lanzani C, Messaggio E, Casamassima N, Frau F, D'Avila F, Cusi D, Barlassina C, Manunta P. Genes involved in vasoconstriction and vasodilation system affect salt-sensitive hypertension. *PLoS One.* 2011;6:e19620.

*Chapter VIII*

# Hyponatremia

Hyponatremia is common among hospitalized patients. Its management is well established. In certain situations, however, hyponatremia management may be demanding. The importance of diagnosing the cause of hyponatremia and treating hyponatremia has been convincingly demonstrated. Even mild, chronic, so-called 'asymptomatic' hyponatremia (serum natrium 125-130 mEq/L) is associated with poorer performance on attention tests, unstable posture, gait disturbance, falls and bone fractures; severe hyponatremia is associated with additional morbidity.

## Case 44. Treatment of Severe Hyponatremia in Patients with Heart Failure

An 80-year-old community dwelling woman was treated in emergency for cardiogenic pulmonary edema. The ECG showed atrial fibrillation, the heart rate was 122 bpm. The serum sodium was 126 mEqu/L, potassium 3.1 mEq/L, glucose 190 mg/dL, and troponin I <0.2 ng/mL. Her medical history was remarkable for arterial hypertension, obesity, episodes of paroxysmal atrial fibrillation, and glaucoma. She was a lifelong nondrinker and nonsmoker. Her recent medications were enalapril 40 mg/day, hydrochlorothiazide 25 mg/day, simvastatin 20 mg/day, aspirin 100 mg/day, doxazosin 4 mg/day, amiodarone 200 mg/day, omeprazole 20 mg/day, and latanoprost and dorzolamide eye drops. Her state stabilized and furosemide treatment she had received for a few days was discontinued. The patient was transferred to subacute care. On admission the patient was drowsy but arousable. The oral temperature was 37.3$^0$C, BP 128/65 mmHg, the pulse was irregular, heart rate 82 bpm, SaO2 92% by pulse oxymetry on room air, BMI 30. There was a grade 2 pansystolic murmur perceivable at the cardiac apex; respiratory sounds and neurological examination were unremarkable. Interrogation of the patient's family members revealed that her mental status has acutely changed. Usually she was well oriented and calm, but from the time of arrival to hospital she became confused, with episodes of hallucinations and delusions. During the 'lucid intervals' she was easily distractible. There was hyponatremia while the urinary osmolarity was 384 mOsm (Table 1). The CBC, serum creatinine, potassium, TSH and cardiac biomarkers were normal.

**Table 1. Course of hyponatremia and delirium**

Pulm. edema Delirium

| | ER | | | ER | AGC | | | | | | AGC |
|---|---|---|---|---|---|---|---|---|---|---|---|
| Date | 1Feb | 2 | 2 | 3 | 3 | 4 | 4 | 5 | 6 | 7 | 9 Feb |
| sNa | **126** | **119** | **126** | **119** | **119** | **120** | **117** | **126** | **135** | **138** | **144** |
| sK | 3.1 | 2.8 | 3.1 | 3.0 | 3.0 | 2.8 | 3.3 | 3.4 | 3.7 | 3.5 | 3.9 |
| sOsm | | | | | | 252 | | | | | |
| uOsm | | | | | | 365 | | | | | |
| i v NaCl 0.9% (cc) | | | | | 1000 | 1000 | | | | | |
| Nacl 3% (cc) | | | | | | | 300 | 300 | | | |
| Fusid | ++ | | | | | | | | | | |

Water restriction

ER = emergency department, AGC = acute geriatric care, sNa = serum sodium, sK = serum potassium, sOsm = serum osmolarity, uOsm = urine osmolarity, Fusid = furosemide.

Treatment of heart failure, delirium and hyponatremia were the main concerns at this time point. Delirium occurring in the context of hyponatremia is considered to be a complication of hyponatremia if other causes can be excluded. Hyponatremia causing delirium is a medical emergency; quick intervention is recommended to increase the serum natrium by 8 to 10 mEq/L. On the other hand, because the patient just had recovered from pulmonary edema, an imprudent sodium load exposes the patient to another episode of pulmonary edema. One more concern was to distinguish hyponatremia secondary by inappropriate antidiuretic hormone secretion (SIADH) from diuretic-induced hyponatremia.

*Delirium* affects about 30% of older patients admitted to hospital. Delirium in elderly persons is often the presenting symptom, sometimes the only symptom, of a serious underlying disease such as sepsis, heart failure, or an acute coronary event. Patients who develop delirium have high mortality, high rates of institutionalization and complications, and have increased lengths of hospital stay compared to non-delirious patients [1]. Hence, delirium may perform as a barometer of the patients' overall health state.

Four cardinal features of delirium (confusional state) serve for the diagnosis: 1) acute onset and fluctuating course of a change in the mental status from the patient's baseline; 2) inattention illustrated by the patient's difficulty in focusing attention; 3) disorganized thinking, exemplified by incoherent or irrelevant conversation or unpredictable switching from one subject to another; 4) altered level of consciousness, that means a level of consciousness which is other than alert, maybe hyperalert, lethargic, drowsy but easily aroused, or difficult to arouse. Illusions, hallucinations and delusions may occur. Diagnosis of delirium requires the presence of features 1 and 2, supplemented by either feature 3 or 4. The confusional state often worsens with the coming of night, a phenomenon called 'sun downing'. Patients may display 'lucid intervals', especially in the morning, wherein their consciousness appears clear. Such lucid intervals during morning rounds may mislead clinicians. Delirium may be precipitated by sepsis, medications, failure of a major organ system, hypoxemia, hypercarbia, hyponatremia, etc.

*Hyponatremia is defined* as a serum sodium concentration less than 135 mEq/L, although the adverse clinical effects are rarely seen until the serum sodium is less than 130 mEq/L. Hyponatremia is characterized by low effective serum osmolarity. Hyponatremia occurs in 15% to 30% of both acutely and chronically hospitalized patients. Most cases are mild and asymptomatic, but acute and severe hyponatremia can cause important morbidity: lethargy, delirium, seizures, coma and death [2]. On the other hand, over-rapid correction of chronic hyponatremia can lead to severe neurological injury due to osmotic demyelination (see Case 46).

Hyponatremia is usually caused by excessive water retention and infrequently by excessive sodium excretion by the kidneys.

*Advanced renal failure* may be the cause of impaired renal water excretion.

*Increased secretion of arginine vasopressin* (AVP) may depend on physiological triggers - increased serum osmolarity as well as hypovolemia. A 2% increase in extracellular fluid osmolarity produced by solutes such as sodium chloride (but not urea) shrinks the osmoreceptor cells and in this manner stimulates the release of AVP from storage sites in the posterior pituitary gland. When osmolarity falls below a genetically determined osmotic threshold, plasma AVP levels become undetectable and renal excretion of solute-free water results, preventing further decrease in plasma osmolarity. Failure to suppress AVP secretion below the normal osmotic threshold results in water retention and hyponatremia, conditioned by sufficient intake of hypotonic fluids. In a different way, a reduction of 8-10% from the normal body volume of water will result in AVP secretion, initiated by pressure receptors located in the atria, pulmonary arteries and veins that convey their input to the hypothalamus. In most physiological situations, there is synergy between the effects of increased osmolarity and decreased effective plasma volume to stimulate release of vasopressin. So, with dehydration osmolarity increases jointly with the decrease of the effective intravascular volume and each stimulate the release of AVP. Under pathologic conditions, AVP secretion may occur in the absence of hyperosmolarity and reduced effective arterial volume; this is the syndrome of inappropriate antidiuretic hormone secretion (SIADH). The opposite occurs with excess of water load, which results in decreased osmolarity and increased effective intravascular volume, and both inhibit AVP secretion.

*Primary polydipsia* can produce hyponatremia because the gastrointestinal tract is able to absorb water faster than the kidney can excrete.

*Hyponatremia can also be the consequence of a negative sodium balance.* Impairment of one or more of the tubular sodium reabsorptive mechanisms can generate a sodium deficit. This occurs in specific renal and endocrine disorders, or in response to diuretic medications.

Obtaining a drug history is useful in the evaluation of patients with hyponatremia: thiazide diuretics (by increase natriuresis) and SSRIs (by stimulating secretion AVP) are among the most common causes of hyponatremia in the elderly.

*Genuine or false hyponatremia?* The initial step in the diagnostic work-up is to distinguish genuine hyponatremia from a false laboratory result. Spurious hyponatremia (pseudohyponatremia) is a laboratory miscalculation which may be the result of in vitro hemolysis, hyperlipidemia, hyperproteinemia, hyperglycemia, or mannitol which has been administered to the patient. The effective extracellular osmolarity is not reduced in pseudohyponatremia, in distinction from true hyponatremia which always is associated with decreased serum osmolarity.

*Estimation of the extracellular fluid volume is the second step* in evaluation of hyponatremia. Hyponatremia is commonly classified into euvolemic, hypervolemic, and hypovolemic types. The diagnosis of the extracellular fluid status is an estimate, based on the clinician's impression. Patients with orthostatic hypotension, tachycardia, dry mucus membranes and decreased skin turgor are considered hypovolemic (though it is understood that the specificity of any of these signs is poor in elderly subjects). Increased BUN, serum creatinine, BUN/creatinine ratio, and uric acid level indicate volume depletion; however, these findings are neither sensitive nor specific markers of hypovolemia. Patients without clinical and laboratory signs of volume depletion are considered to be euvolemic unless they are edematous, indicating excessive extracellular fluid volume.

*Measurement of the spot urinary sodium concentration* is the third step in the diagnostic work-up. Three situations are distinguished with this simple test: 1) Patients with euvolemic hyponatremia having a spot urinary sodium ≥30 mmol/L the diagnosis of SIADH should be considered, with a few differentials. The expected augmented sodium reabsorption, meant to correct the low sodium serum concentration, is offset by euvolemia. 2) In patients with hypovolemic hyponatremia the spot urinary sodium should be <30 mmol/L because tubular sodium reabsorption is enhanced through sensing hypovolemia, a mechanism engaged to correct hypovolemia. 3) When patients with hypovolemic hyponatremia have spot urinary sodium ≥30 mmol/L, renal salt wasting is suspected.

*In subjects taking a diuretic,* however, the spot urinary sodium and fractional excretion of sodium are of limited diagnostic utility because the diuretic inhibits the tubular sodium reabsorption. Other markers are required for classifying these cases: the uric acid may be such an indicator. Uric acid is excreted predominantly by the kidneys, with urate transport confined exclusively to the proximal tubule. Therefore, urate excretion is not directly affected by furosemide. On this basis, measurement of the fractional excretion of uric acid might differentiate the SIADH from other causes of hyponatremia regardless of the use of loop diuretics.

FEua = Uua:Pua/ Ucr:Pcr

(where FEua is fractional excretion of uric acid; Uua uric acid concentration in the urine, Pua uric acid concentration in the plasma; Ucr is creatinine concentration in the urine; Pcr is creatinine concentration in the plasma).

In one study [3], fractional excretion of uric acid >12% was consistent with SIADH (sensitivity 86% and specificity 100%) while fractional excretion of uric acid < 8% excluded SIADH (sensitivity and negative predictive value 100%). There are limitations to this principle, since other factors may also augment fractional excretion of uric acid; such are thiazide diuretics, losartan and probenecid.

*A trial of isotonic saline infusion* can be helpful in establishing the diagnosis of extracellular volume depletion. After infusion of 0.5 to 1 liter of isotonic saline patients with hypovolemic hyponatremia will begin to correct their hyponatremia without developing signs of volume overload. On the contrary, the serum natrium will decrease or remain unchanged in patients with the SIADH since the infused water is retained while the infused sodium is excreted in the urine.

*The syndrome of inappropriate antidiuretic hormone secretion (SIADH)* is the prototype of euvolemic hyponatremia. The secretion of arginine vasopressin in this situation is considered inappropriate because it occurs in the absence of a reduced effective arterial volume or hyperosmolarity. Common causes of SIADH are tumors, pulmonary diseases, central nervous system disorders, drugs that stimulate arginine vasopressin release or potentiate arginine vasopressin's antidiuretic effects, AIDS; the cause of SIADH remains unknown in a large proportion of cases. The criteria necessary to diagnose SIADH are: 1) plasma osmolarity <275 mOsm/L (thereby excluding pseudohyponatremia), 2) urine osmolarity >100 mOsm/L with normal renal function, 3) clinical euvolemia, 4) urinary sodium >30 mEq/L (>20 mEq/L according to other experts), 5) exclusion of other causes of euvolemic hypoosmolarity (hypothyroidism, Addison's disease, pituitary ACTH insufficiency, and diuretic use). Hypouricemia is often present, but does not serve as a diagnostic condition. The hope that measurement of plasma vasopressin levels might become the definitive test for diagnosis of SIADH has not been met.

*Diuretic induced hyponatremia* is very common in the elderly. Treatment with diuretics may cause or aggravate hyponatremia. Thiazide drugs are the predominant cause. In a literature review, 73% of cases of diuretic-induced hyponatremia were caused by thiazides alone, 20% were caused by thiazides in combination with antikaliuretic agents, and 8% were caused by furosemide. Furosemide-induced hyponatremia tends to occur after many months of treatment or when an intercurrent illness develops, whereas thiazide-induced hyponatremia frequently occurs within a few days or weeks after initiation of therapy. A high urinary sodium level is expected to be present if diuretic use is ongoing [4, 5]. Even modest levels of hyponatremia in patients with congestive heart failure are associated with increased mortality. Hospital admission for heart failure and hyponatremia is associated with a 60-fold increase in morbidity/mortality.

*The treatment of hyponatremia is determined by three factors* [6]. First, the severity of symptoms: the presence or absence of lethargy, delirium, seizure, or coma. Second, the rapidity of onset: hyponatremia onset within 48 hours versus hyponatremia with onset more than 48 hours before beginning treatment. Third, the patient's volume status. Symptomatic hyponatremia is a medical emergency, particularly if associated with hypoxia. A quick raise in serum natrium by 8 to 10 mEq/L within 4 to 6 hours is recommended by infusion of hypertonic saline.

*The rate of correction of hyponatremia should* take in consideration the patient's susceptibility to develop osmotic demyelination by quick correction. Water moves freely between the intracellular and extracellular compartments. Hence, when the serum sodium concentration is low water enters cells and the cells swell with water. Swelling is most hazardous in the brain: when hyponatremia develops over a few hours exceeding the brain's ability to adapt, cerebral edema results. Thus, patients with acute hyponatremia (<48 hours duration) may present with severe neurological symptoms and eventually brain herniation; administration of hypertonic saline intending to quickly increase in the serum sodium concentration by 2 to 4 mmol/L effectively reduces brain swelling. The situation differs in lasting hyponatremia: given due time brain cells extrude organic solutes from the cytoplasm allowing intracellular osmolarity to equalize with plasma osmolarity without swelling of the neurons. When hyponatremia develops over ≥48 hours, brain swelling is minimized. This explains why patients with chronic hyponatremia have moderate neurological symptoms or no symptoms at all. However, the adaptation which permits neuronal survival in chronic hyponatremia also makes the brain vulnerable to injury from too rapid correction of the hyponatremia, which may exceed the brain's capacity to recapture the lost organic osmolytes. Because water moves freely between the intracellular and extracellular compartments, too fast increase in the serum sodium concentration results in an osmotic shift of water out of neurons. Large water egress from the brain can result in neurological damage, i.e. the osmotic demyelination syndrome or 'central pontine myelinolysis'. The osmotic demyelination syndrome can usually be avoided by limiting correction of chronic hyponatremia to <10 mmol/L (maximum 12 mmol/L in 24 hours and <18 mmol/L in 48 hours).

*Correction of acute symptomatic hyponatremia in SIADH* is best accomplished with hypertonic (3%) saline given via continuous infusion, because patients with euvolemic hypo-osmolarity such as SIADH will not improve on administration of isotonic saline. An initial infusion rate can be estimated by multiplying the patient's body weight in kilograms by the desired rate of increase in serum natrium in mmol/L/hour (e.g. in a patient weighing 70 kg an infusion of 3% NaCl at 70 mL/hour will increase the serum natrium by approximately 1 mmol/L per hour; infusing 35 mL/hour will increase the serum natrium by approximately 0.5 mmol/L per hour). Intravenous furosemide 20 to 40 mg should be used to treat volume overload, or prevent volume overload in patients with heart failure. Infusion with hypertonic saline should be terminated when one of three endpoints is reached: 1) the patient's symptoms are abolished; 2) a safe serum natrium level is achieved (generally ≥120 mmol/L); 3) a total magnitude of correction of 18 mmol/L is accomplished. It follows from these recommendations that serum natrium levels must be frequently monitored during the acute phase of treatment, preferably every 2 hours but at least every 4 hours, in order to adjust therapy. Subsequently, the treatment follows the principles adopted for mild-to-moderate hyponatremia in SIADH (see below). The use of vasopressin receptor antagonists might become a mainstay of treatment for euvolemic hyponatremia. Today, insufficient data are available from clinical trials to know if sufficiently rapid and safe correction of acute and severe hyponatremia can be achieved by vasopressin receptor antagonists and without the use of hypertonic saline [7].

*For mild-to-moderate hyponatremia in SIADH, fluid restriction represents the treatment of choice.* Generally, fluids should be limited to 500 mL/day below the average daily urine volume. All fluids, not only water, must be included in the restriction. Sodium intake should not be restricted. Efforts should be made to overcome thirst, e.g. by substituting hard candy or ice chips for drinking fluids. Several days of restriction are usually necessary before a significant increase in plasma osmolarity occurs. Drugs known to be associated with SIADH should be discontinued or changed. Failure of hyponatremia to correct under fluid restriction past several days of confirmed negative fluid balance should prompt reconsideration of other possible causes of hyponatremia, including clinically unapparent hypovolemia.

*In patients with diuretic-induced hyponatremia* the diuretics should be immediately discontinued, the hypovolemia corrected and hypokalemia or hypomagnesemia, if present, should be treated. Serum sodium should be closely monitored to avoid overcorrection. Some authors recommend for this reason not to use hypertonic saline for treatment of diuretic-induced hyponatremia [8].

In the patient under discussion, the working diagnosis SIADH was supported by the following: the patient appeared to be euvolemic; she presented elevated urinary sodium and osmolarity that persisted several days past discontinuation of diuretics; hyponatremia was aggravated by infusion of isotonic saline; the serum thyrotropin was normal. Only after hypertonic saline was administered and the patient was on fluid restriction could hyponatremia be corrected (Table 1). Hence, hyponatremia was attributed to SIADH, possibly enhanced by diuretics. Correction of hyponatremia was achieved safely without recurrence of pulmonary congestion. The delirium remitted and the patient returned to the community in good condition.

N.B., treatment with isotonic saline in a patient with SIADH is contrary to the routine that is compulsory in our department.

## Learning Points

- Symptomatic hyponatremia is a medical emergency.
- Euvolemic hyponatremia, with urinary sodium >30 mEq/L and exclusion of other potential causes of euvolemic hypoosmolarity is consistent with SIADH.
- Administration of isotonic saline may aggravate hyponatremia in patients with SIADH, but correct the hyponatremia in hypovolemic patients.
- Symptomatic hyponatremia should be treated with hypertonic saline under frequent monitoring of the serum sodium concentration.

# References

[1] Inouye SI. Delirium in older Persons. *N. Engl. J. Med.* 2006;354:1157-1165.

[2] Wald R, Jaber BL, Price LL, Upadhyay A, Madias NE. Impact of hospital-associated hyponatremia on selected outcomes. *Arch. Intern. Med.* 2010;170:294-302.

[3] Fenske W, Störk S, Koschker A-C, Blechschmidt A, Lorenz D, Wortmann S, Allolio B. Value of fractional uric acid excretion in differential diagnosis of hyponatremic patients on diuretics. *J. Clin. Endocrino. Metab.* 2008; 93:2991-2997.

[4] Felker MG, Lee KL, Bull DA, Redfield MM, Stevenson LW, Goldsmith SR, LeWinter MM, Deswal A, Rouleau JL, Ofili EO, Anstrom KJ, Hernandez AF, McNulty SE, Velazquez EJ, Kfoury AG, Chen HH, Givertz MM, Semigran MJ, Bart BA, Mascette AM, Braunwald E, O'Connor CM, for the NHLBI Heart Failure Clinical Rcscarch Network. Diuretic strategies in patients with acute decompensated heart failure. *N. Engl. J. Med.* 2011; 364:797-805.

[5] De Vecchis R, Ciccarelli A, Pucciarelli A. Unloading therapy by intravenous diuretic in chronic heart failure: a double-edged weapon? *J. Cardiovasc. Med.* (Hagerstown). 2010;11:571-574.

[6] Verbalis JG, Goldsmith SR, Greenberg A, Schrier RW, Sterns RH. Hyponatremia treatment guidelines 2007: Expert Panel Recommendations. *Amer. J. Med.* 2007;120, (11 Suppl 1):S1-21.

[7] Jaber BL, Almarzouqi L, Borgi L, Seabra VF, Balk EM, Madias NE. Short-term efficacy and safety of vasopressin receptor antagonists for treatment of hyponatremia. *Amer. J. Med.* 2011;124, 977.e1-977.e9.

[8] Vaidya C, Ho W, Fred BJ. Management of hyponatremia: providing treatment and avoiding harm. *Cleveland J. Med.* 2010;77:715-726.

# Case 45. Renal Salt Wasting

An 83-year-old woman was transferred from the department of internal medicine, where she has been admitted for severe, yet asymptomatic hyponatremia. Remarkable in her medical history were arterial hypertension, dyslipemia, and frequent falls. The patient has been repeatedly diagnosed in the past five years with hyponatremia in the range 115-133 mEq/L. Hyponatremia has also been diagnosed in her father 'for as long as medical records existed'. Six months before the present episode the patient had been admitted to the medical ward with symptomatic hyponatremia. CT showed several small cerebral infarctions and an empty sella turcica. The serum thyrotropin level, cortisol at baseline and cortisol after ACTH stimulation were within the normal range. On a second admission for hyponatremia the serum sodium was 114 mEq/L, urinary osmolarity 279 mOsm, urinary sodium 44 mEq/L, serum creatinine 1.7 mg/dL, BUN 43 mg/dL, and uric acid 8 mg/dL. The patient's medications at that time were enalapril, spironolactone, simvastatin, and micropirin. Infusion of saline 0.9% resulted in progressive attenuation of hyponatremia to 116, 117, 125, 131 mEq/L. On abdominal ultrasound examination the kidneys' sizes were 8.6 and 9.7 cm, respectively. Spironolactone and enalapril were discontinued. On discharge from hospital the renal failure had remitted, the serum creatinine was 0.8 mg/dL and the BUN was 23 mg/dL. On a third, the latest, hospital admission for severe yet asymptomatic hyponatremia the serum sodium was 116 mEq/L, serum potassium 4.5 mEq/L, uric acid 1.4 mg/dL, urinary sodium 52 mEq/L. The patient received a 5 days course of isotonic saline infusion and the hyponatremia improved progressively as can be seen on day-to-day serum sodium measurements: 116,118,117,122,124 mEq/L. Cerebral CT showed old parietal and basal ganglia infarctions and periventricular lucency. Subsequently, the patient was referred for subacute care to our department.

She was alert and appeared to be euvolemic. The BP was 130/84 and the heart rate 74 bpm. A bedside postural test 15 minutes supine to 5 minutes standing showed normal BP and heart rate reactivity. A regimen of water restriction was instituted but hyponatremia did not get better. The hyponatremia improved subsequently on intravenous infusion of saline 0.9% and was effectively controlled by eating a salt enriched diet. Before discharge, the serum sodium concentration was consistently 134 mEq/L or higher, the serum potassium 4.35 mg/dL, uric acid 8.9 mg/dL, creatinine 0.8 mg/dL, and BUN 16 mg/dL. At this point in time a 24 hour urine collection contained 95 mEq/L sodium (equivalent with 12 g salt/day), potassium 26 mEq/L, and uric acid 532 mg/L. The diagnosis of hyponatremia went past the common causes.

*A diagnosis of SIADH was discarded* since hyponatremia did not improve by water restriction but corrected on isotonic saline administration (see discussion relating to Case 44).

*The reset osmostat* [1] is associated with hyponatremia. The reset osmostat is characterized by a lower than usual osmotic threshold for secretion of antidiuretic hormone, but the secretion ceases when the serum osmolarity is greatly reduced. Thus, in the presence of mild hyponatremia the urine spot sodium is <30 mmol/L while during severe hyponatremia the urine spot sodium is >30 mmol/L. In our patient there was urine spot sodium is >30 mmol/L equally in the presence of mild hyponatremia and during severe hyponatremia - this opposes to the diagnosis of reset osmostat, but is a feature common to SIADH and to several salt wasting syndrome.

*Cerebral salt wasting* is characterized by inappropriately increased natriuresis and the resulting volume contraction appearing in the context of a cerebral pathology, e.g. head injury, brain tumor, intracranial surgery, stroke, intracerebral hemorrhage, or meningitis [2]. While the cerebral salt wasting syndrome mimics the SIADH, it can be differentiated from the latter by three distinguishing features: the total body fluid is decreased in the salt wasting syndrome, the BUN and natriuretic peptides are increased, and there is a negative sodium balance [2]. The importance of making the distinction between salt wasting syndrome and SIADH is in their different treatment. SIADH is usually treated with water restriction whereas patients with salt wasting syndrome require fluid and salt supplementation with sometimes addition of the mineralocorticoid fludrocortisone. Fludrocortisone acts directly on the renal tubule to reduce sodium excretion. Computing the sodium balance prior to treatment of hyponatremia is important for the diagnosis, although difficult to perform. The sodium intake should take count of the oral and intravenous routes and the sodium excretion be measured by multiplying urinary sodium concentration with the daily urine volume.

The cerebral salt wasting syndrome resolves spontaneously in 2-4 weeks. In the present patient, hyponatremia and salt wasting spanned a period of years; this makes a case against cerebral salt wasting syndrome.

*Renal salt wasting* is characterized by urine spot sodium >30 mmol/L in the presence of hypovolemic hyponatremia and a negative sodium balance. Measurement of the 24-hour natrium excretion is essential for the diagnosis. The urine spot sodium is >30 mmol/L both in the presence of severe and mild hyponatremia, in distinction from reset osmostat where in the presence of mild hyponatremia the urine spot sodium is <30 mmol/L. Cortisol deficiency, hypoaldosteronism and pseudohypoaldosteronism are among the causes of renal salt wasting [3]. Tubular injury of various causes may be responsible for pseudohypoaldosteronism, i.e. the diminished response to aldosterone. So, pseudohypoaldosteronism with renal salt wasting has been described in association with obstructive uropathy, urinary tract infection, tubulointerstitial nephritis, lupus nephropathy, amyloidosis, multiple myeloma, and renal transplantation. Also drugs that impair renin or aldosterone synthesis or cause mineralocorticoid resistance can induce renal salt wasting (e.g. beta-adrenergic antagonists, heparin, ACE inhibitors, spironolactone, amiloride, triamterene, and cyclosporine).

In conclusion, the findings in the present patient were inconsistent with SIADH, reset osmostat, and cerebral salt wasting syndrome. Renal salt wasting syndrome was diagnosed and effectively treated with a salt enriched diet. The etiology or renal salt wasting, including the possibility of a hereditary disorder, was not further investigated. An elaborate work-up (plasma ANP and BNP, renin, aldosterone, genetics, and chromosomal studies of Na and K channels) was not considered necessary for the patient's management and was not implemented [4].

## Learning Points

- Symptomatic hyponatremia is a medical emergency, asymptomatic hyponatremia is not.
- Taking a spot urine sample should be part of the routine workup of hyponatremia; in doing so first the treatment is not delayed.

- Urinary spot sodium >30 mmol/L is consistent with salt wasting by various mechanisms: SIADH, defective osmostat, cerebral salt wasting, or renal salt wasting.
- After infusion of 0.5 to 1 liter of 0.9% saline, patients with hypovolemic hyponatremia will begin to correct their hyponatremia without developing signs of volume overload. Conversely, in patients with SIADH the serum natrium will remain unchanged or decrease.
- Measurement of the 24-hour sodium excretion is essential in approaching the diagnosis of salt losing syndromes.

## References

[1] Kahn T. Reset osmostat and salt and water retention in the course of severe hyponatremia. *Medicine* (Baltimore) 2003;82:170-176.

[2] Cerdà-Esteve M, Cuadrado-Godia E, Chillaron JJ, Pont-Sunyer C, Cucurella G, Fernández M, Goday A, Cano-Pérez JF, Rodríguez-Campello A, Roquer J. Cerebral salt wasting syndrome: review. *Eur. J. Intern. Med.* 2008;19:249-254.

[3] Zennaro MC, Borensztein P, Soubrier F, Armanini D, Corvol P. The enigma of pseudohypoaldosteronism. *Steroids* 1994;59:96-99.

[4] Wiebke Fenske, Maier SK, Blechschmidt A, Allolio B, Störk S. Utility and limitations of the traditional diagnostic approach to hyponatremia: a diagnostic study. *Am. J. Med.* 2010;123:652-657.

# Case 46. Osmotic Demyelination Syndrome?

An 82 year-old woman suffered an accidental fall with contusion of the chest. She was until recently living independently; now she was admitted to a nursing home, to be comforted. Her medical history was remarkable for arterial hypertension, retinal vein thrombosis and polymyalgia rheumatica, the latter diagnosed five years ago. Two years before the present event she had an episode of hyponatremia. The patient's current medications included cilazapril 5 mg/day, amlodipine 5 mg/day, prednisone 5 mg/day, omeprazole 20 mg/day, and warfarin. Lately she complained of fatigue. Laboratory tests taken in the nursing home revealed serum sodium 115 mEq/L. The patient denied having diarrhea, vomiting, and the use of diuretics or laxatives. She was treated in the nursing home with i.v. hypertonic saline. The other day the serum sodium was 128 mEq/L, but the patient developed delirium, disturbed balance and gait, and urinary retention with leukocyturia. The body temperature remained normal. A urinary catheter was inserted and treatment with ciprofloxacine 1 g/day was started empirically. The daily dose of prednisone was increased to 15 mg and she was brought to the emergency department. The serum sodium 127 mEq/L, potassium 3.2 mEq/L, plasma osmolarity 270 mOsm/L, urine osmolarity 273 mOsm/L, urinary sodium 83 mEqu/L, and PT-INR 2.2. Findings on chest x-rays and cerebral CT were unremarkable. The patient was referred to our ward.

On admission she was alert, oriented, the body temperature was 36.4$^0$C, BP 131/72 mmHg, heart rate 90 bpm, respirations 16/minute, SaO2 92%, diuresis 800 mL/24 hours.

Neurological examination revealed ataxia. Family members were surprised by the dramatic change that occurred in the patient's behavior after correction of hyponatremia: 'she never was such a nuisance', 'forgiveness for her behaving'. Laboratory tests were remarkable for hemoglobin 11.6 g/dL, MCV 78 fl, WBC 11,500/mm3, sodium 128 mEqu/l. The thyrotropin and FT4 were within the normal range. Chest x-rays and ECG were unremarkable. The patient's temperature remained normal on the following days, the pre-treatment urine culture was negative, so antibiotic treatment was stopped and the patient was weaned from the urinary catheter. The daily dose of prednisone was tapered to 7.5 mg.

On water restriction the serum sodium concentration increased within two days to 134 mEq/L and remained at similar values on follow-up. The serum potassium was 4.5 mEq/L. Physical therapy for reconditioning was initiated. Nurses and physicians reported the patient's disagreeable assertiveness persisted, and according also to family members the patient's recent behavioral changes had not improved. Neurologic and psychiatric consultations were unrewarding. The MMSE was 30/30. The patient was discharged to the nursing home, with scheduled cerebral MRI, lung CT, and ACTH testing. Afterwards it turned out the patient was unwilling to submit to diagnostic tests. Four months later the patient was free of complaints and had returned to live alone in her apartment. The behavioral disturbances had disappeared.

The cause of the patient's transient behavioral disorder was intriguing. In recognizing the proximity between the hurried correction of hyponatremia and subsequent behavioral change the possibility of causality was considered. It is well known that too fast correction of hyponatremia results in an osmotic shift of water out of the brain to the extravascular space; large water egress from the brain can cause neurological damage, i.e. central pontine myelinolysis also known as osmotic demyelization syndrome. Was the patient's behavioral disorder a manifestation of osmotic demyelization?

*Osmotic demyelization* is a serious complication caused by rapid correction of severe hyponatremia or fluctuating serum osmolarity due to hyperglycemia or hyperammonemia. It is characterized by a loss of oligodendrocytes and myelin in the central basis of the pons, basal ganglia and cerebellum with relatively preserved neurons. Due to the specific vulnerability of the pons to rapid changes in electrolyte balance this region is affected first. The risk for development of osmotic demyelization is associated with the severity and chronicity of hyponatremia and the correction rate of hyponatremia. Osmotic demyelization rarely occurs if the serum sodium was greater than 120 and hyponatremia was acute in onset. Occurrence of osmotic demyelization can usually be avoided by limiting correction of chronic hyponatremia to <10 to 12 mmol/L in 24 hours and <18 mmol/L in 48 hours.

Severe demyelization syndrome can lead to permanent brain damage, coma, or death. Gross neurological symptoms, such as spastic quadriparesis, pseudobulbar palsy, dysarthria, loss of pain sensations, may occur. Behavioral manifestations can arise, either coexisting with neurological deficits, or as the predominant disturbance, or sometimes as the sole manifestation of osmotic demyelization.

*Neuropsychological deficits* reported in central pontine myelinolysis span the domain of attention and concentration: high distractibility, difficulty in mental tracking, slow visual scanning, and impaired sustained attention. Memory functions were impaired in some patients. Visualmotor and fine motor speeds were slow. Behavioral manifestations may be the most prominent clinical feature of the milder variant of demyelization syndrome and probably remain undiagnosed or are labeled 'hysterical'. During the forthcoming several months the symptoms usually improve or remit completely [1-4].

*The diagnosis* of osmotic demyelization can be suspected clinically on the basis of 1) inappropriate brisk correction of hyponatremia and 2) progressive neurological deficits resulting in a 'locked-in' syndrome. The definite diagnosis is provided on CT or MRI. Radiological abnormalities are not necessarily confined to the pons and may occur in the basal ganglia and the internal capsule. Whereas the presence of positive MRI findings strongly supports the diagnosis, MRI often fails to demonstrate the characteristic demyelinative lesions because scans are usually negative until 3 to 4 weeks after the onset of neurological symptoms. Though MRI is helpful in diagnosing demyelization, the extent of pontine signal abnormality should not be considered a prognostic indicator. Patients with extensive pontine lesions can have a complete recovery [5].

*The Naranjo causality scale* [6] provides a practical means for clinicians to prove causality between a drug treatment and an adverse event. The Naranjo questionnaire addresses several characteristics of the association between a treatment and a clinical event: temporality, strength, consistency, gradient, specificity, coherence, and results of rechallenge (where applicable). A scoring system permits to compute the total score: >9 is interpreted as definite drug-induced reaction, 5-8 probable drug-induced reaction, 1-4 possible, and 0 doubtful drug-induced reaction. Relevant to the case of our patient are following features: there exist conclusive reports of this reaction (1 point), the adverse event occurred after the specific treatment was administered (2 points), the adverse reaction did improve after the treatment was discontinued (1 point), there was no alternate cause other than the treatment which could have caused the reaction (2 points). A score of 6 points in our patient supports 'probable causality'. So, the patient's behavioral disturbance that appeared a few days after the precipitous correction of severe hyponatremia could be attributed to treatment with hypertonic saline. A definite diagnosis could not be established because the patient worried to undergo cerebral MRI.

### Learning Points

- Precipitous correction of severe hyponatremia may be dangerous, in sometimes causing osmotic demyelination (pontine and extrapontine myelinolysis).
- The osmotic demyelination syndrome can usually be avoided by limiting correction of chronic hyponatremia to 10-12 mmol/L in 24 hours and 18 mmol/L in 48 hours.
- Serum sodium levels must be frequently monitored during the acute phase of correction of hyponatremia, preferably every two hours but at least every four hours.

## References

[1] Vermetten E, Rutten SJ, Boon PJ, Hofman PA, Leentjens AF. Neuropsychiatric and neuropsychological manifestations of central pontine myelinolysis. *Gen. Hosp. Psychiatry.* 1999;21:296-302.

[2] Lee TM, Cheung CC, Lau EY, Mak A, Li LS. Cognitive and emotional dysfunction after central pontine myelinolysis. *Behav. Neurol.* 2003;14:103-107.

[3] Bridgeford D, Arciniegas DB, Batkis M, Sandberg E, Beresford TP. Methylphenidate treatment of neuropsychiatric symptoms of central and extrapontine myelinolysis. *J. Stud. Alcohol.* 2000;61:657-660.

[4] Silbert PL, Knezevic WV, Peake HI, Khangure M. Behavioural changes due to pontine and extrapontine myelinolysis. *Med. J. Aust.* 1992;157:487-488.

[5] Graff-Radford J, Fugate JE, Kaufmann TJ, Mandrekar JN, Rabinstein AA. Clinical and radiologic correlations of central pontine myelinolysis syndrome. *Mayo Clin. Proc.* 2011;86:1063-1067.

[6] Naranjo CA, Busto U, Sellers EM, Sandor P, Ruiz I, Roberts EA, Janecek E, Domecq C, Greenblatt DJ. A method for estimating the probability of adverse drug reactions. *Clin. Pharmacol.* 1981;30:239-245.

*Chapter IX*

# Miscellaneous

The following will reveal that the aphorism 'practice makes perfect' is merely wishful thinking and a nice saying.

## Case 47. Acute Onset Parkinsonism

A 73-year-old man, living in the community alone and in neglect, was brought to the emergency room after a fall. His medical history was remarkable for depressive disorder, alcoholism, and repeated falls. The MMSE scored 28 on recent cognitive assessment. Cerebral CT one year before the present event showed a callus of the calvarium without mention of other abnormalities. He was prescribed aspirin 100 mg, propranolol 80 mg, citalopram 20 mg, and prysoline 250 mg/day, but admitted taking none. On examination in the emergency department the vital signs were found to be normal. There was a tremor of both hands at rest and during exertion, increased muscle tonus, cogwheel sign, bradykinesia, stiff face, freezing of gait, and a positive pull test. No focal neurological deficit was found. Treatment with Dopicar (L-dopa in combination with carbidopa) ¼ tb x 3/day was initiated. A cerebral CT was not ordered. The patient was referred to the Acute Care for Elderly Unit for supervised treatment with Dopicar.

On admission, the BP was 146/55 mmHg, heart rate 71 bpm, temperature 37.1$^{0}$C, SaO2 by pulse oxymetry on room air 95%. There were prominent extrapyramidal signs, as described above. The patient insisted that the tremor had begun three weeks ago. The BP and heart rate reactivity were found to be normal on supine-to-standing postural and on post-prandial monitoring. Routine laboratory tests, chest x-rays and the ECG were unremarkable. On the following days the patient developed bizarre behaviors that were suspected to be adverse effects of Dopicar. Our neurologist consultant recommended to discontinue Dopicar and the drug was replaced with rasagiline 0.5 mg/day. Evaluation for secondary causes of parkinsonism was initiated, beginning with cerebral CT.

The CT examination performed on urgency showed bilateral large subdural hematomas (Figure 33), and the patient was referred to neurosurgery. The subsequent course was complicated by urosepsis, shock and the patient died in deep coma.

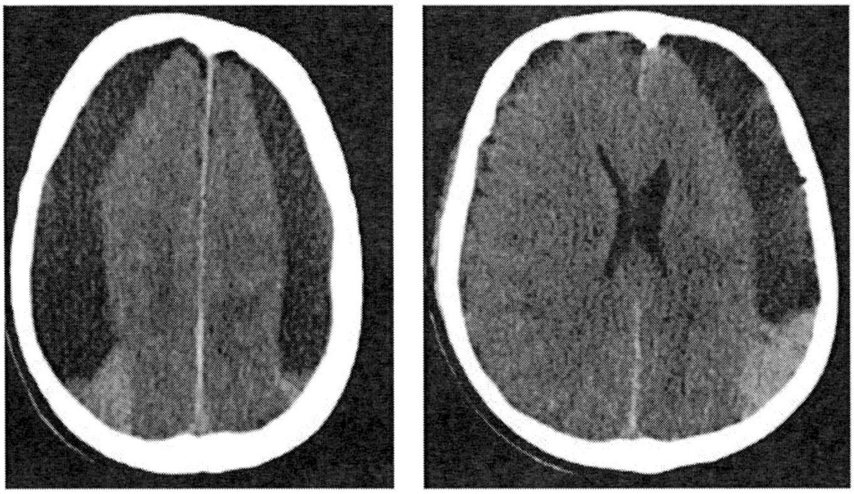

Figure 33. The noncontrasted computed tomography scan shows bilateral crescentic areas in the parietal regions between the brain and the skull, with bright high-density sediments below and lower fluid densities above.

*The parkinsonian syndrome* (parkinsonism) is defined by bradykinesia associated with at least one of the following signs: muscular rigidity, 4–6 Hz rest tremor, and postural instability that is not caused by primary visual, vestibular, cerebellar, or proprioceptive dysfunction [1].

*Bradykinesia* may be apparent as soon as the patient enters the consulting room, or when undressing to be examined. The facial expression can be immobile and rigid, and the ability to express emotions is slow. The speech might also be slow. Bradykinesia may be unapparent, but can be readily exposed by rapid repetitive tapping of the index finger on the thumb for about 20 sec on each hand, followed by sequential touching of each finger on the thumb. Bradykinesia in the leg is assessed by fast foot tapping and asking the patient to walk. Bradykinesia is confirmed with the demonstration of slowness and a progressive reduction of speed and amplitude on sequential motor tasks.

*Tremor* is a rhythmic oscillation of a body part. The presence of a regular cycle of motion differentiates tremor from other dynamic movement disorders such as chorea (manifesting as an irregular activity that sometimes seems to flow from one area to another) and from tics (showing repeated brief but more complex stereotyped movements that are under some voluntary control).

Pill rolling tremor of the hands (4–6 cycles/sec) may be only evident when the hand is truly at rest, such as when the patient is asked to do fine finger movements with the other hand or to walk. The tremor improves with purposeful movement. Parkinsonian tremor usually starts asymmetrically. Although the presence of rest tremor is helpful for the diagnosis of Parkinson's disease, a similar tremor can occur in some cases of dystonic and atypical tremor syndromes. Tremor of the hands is aggravated by emotional situations. Older patients may have tremor of the jaw, chin, lips, and tongue.

Clues to the differential diagnosis of tremor have been proposed: tremor at rest is characteristic for Parkinson’s disease, tremor which appears by stretching out the pronated arms (positional tremor) is characteristic for essential tremor or is induced by drugs, tremor that worsens with movement, e.g. when the patient is asked to perform finger–nose coordination testing, characterizes cerebellar tremor. The diagnosis of essential tremor is supported by the presence of an associated head tremor or voice tremor, a family history of tremor in more than one first-degree relative, normal olfaction, and an improvement of symptoms with small amounts of alcohol. Among commonly prescribed drugs, the following can induce tremor: β receptor agonists, theophylline, antidepressants, lithium, thyroxine and amiodarone, as well as lifestyle drugs such as caffeine, alcohol, marijuana, cocaine and amphetamines. Sodium valproate often causes a tremor that resembles essential tremor, but can also produce a resting tremor.

*Rigidity* of the cogwheel type is the expression of increased muscle tone that persists throughout the range of passive movement of a joint. Rigidity is usually asymmetric at onset.

*Postural instability* is assessed with the 'pull test'. The examiner stands behind the patient and briskly gives a quick backward pull on the patient's shoulders. On the first attempt, it is advisable to use only mild to moderate force when pulling. If the patient recovers well, then a stronger pull is used. The patient may require a practice with a mild pull to appreciate what is expected of him or her. The examiner needs to be prepared to catch the patient should he or she not recover balance. The retropulsion test is positive when the patient is falling straight back. This is not usually severe early on in Parkinson's disease; if falls and postural reflexes are much impaired early in the course of the disease then other diagnoses should be considered.

*Parkinson's disease* is the prototype of parkinsonism [1]. Parkinson's disease commonly presents with impairment of dexterity or a slight dragging of one foot. Fatigue and stiffness are common complaints. A change in the patient's writing can be present for several years before diagnosis, with a tendency to slope usually in an upward direction and for the writing to get progressively smaller and more cramped after a line or two. The onset is gradual and the earliest signs might be unnoticed or misinterpreted, ascribed to old age or rheumatism. A delay of 2–3 years from the first symptoms to diagnosis is not unusual. The characteristic stiff face, hangdog appearance, flexion of one arm with lack of swing, the monotonous speech, and an extreme slowing down are late signs of Parkinson's disease.

*The diagnosis of Parkinson's disease* evolves in three steps [2]:

- Step 1 – comprises diagnosis of the parkinsonian syndrome, that requires the presence of bradykinesia and at least one of the following signs to be met: muscular rigidity, 4–6 Hz rest tremor, and postural instability (not caused by primary visual, vestibular, cerebellar, or proprioceptive dysfunction).
- Step 2 - comprises exclusion criteria: a history of repeated strokes with stepwise progression of parkinsonian features, history of repeated head injury, history of definite encephalitis, oculogyric crises, neuroleptic treatment at onset of symptoms, more than one affected relative, sustained remission, strictly unilateral features after 3 years, supranuclear gaze palsy, cerebellar signs, early severe autonomic involvement, early severe dementia, Babinski sign, presence of a cerebral tumor or communicating hydrocephalus on CT scan, negative response to large doses of L-dopa (if malabsorption is excluded), MPTP exposure (a neurotoxin that causes permanent extrapyramidal by destroying neurons in the substantia nigra).
- Step 3 – provides supportive prospective criteria, among them three or more are required for the diagnosis of definite Parkinson's disease: unilateral onset, rest tremor present, progressive disorder, persistent asymmetry, excellent response to L-dopa

(most patients with Parkinson's disease have a sustained benefit from L-dopa), severe L-dopa-induced chorea, L-dopa response for 5 years or longer, clinical course 10 years or longer, hyposmia, and visual hallucinations.

In most cases, the diagnosis of Parkinson's disease can be made on clinical grounds. Neurology consultation is recommended on initial diagnosis.

*'Red flags'* which should raise the possibility of an alternative diagnosis are falls within the first 2 years of the disease (as in the propositus), an accelerated course (as in the propositus), fainting, urinary incontinence, disturbed swallowing, amnesia, and delirium.

*Parkinson's plus syndromes* comprises some signs of Parkinson's disease with added symptoms, such as inappropriate eye movement control, autonomic dysfunction, muscle weakness and atrophy, profound memory difficulties and behavioral disturbances. Parkinson's plus syndromes include dementia with Lewy bodies, progressive supranuclear palsy, multiple system atrophy, corticobasal degeneration, parkinsonism in late Alzheimer's dementia, and Parkinson's disease with amyotrophic lateral sclerosis. With Parkinson's plus syndromes, the response to L-dopa is usually poor or absent. In patients suspected to have Parkinson's disease who fail to respond to therapeutic doses of L-dopa (at least 600 mg/day administered for 12 weeks), cerebral MRI scanning is needed to exclude rare secondary causes (e.g. supratentorial tumors, normal pressure hydrocephalus, extensive subcortical vascular pathology).

*Secondary parkinsonism* may occur in brain neoplasms, drug effects, post-encephalitis, AIDS, hypothyroidism, Wilsons's disease, normal pressure hydrocephalus, head trauma, toxins. Drug-induced parkinsonism includes dopamine antagonists such as prochlorperazine for giddiness, metoclopramide for dyspepsia, chlorpromazine for bipolar depression, calcium-channel blockers, and sodium valproate used to control epilepsy or migraine – any of these medications can cause reversible parkinsonism. Herbal remedies such as the western Pacific sedative kava kava or the Indian snake root Rauwolfia serpentina can also cause parkinsonism.

*Acute or subacute onset parkinsonism is due to a secondary cause,* except for the rare form of the dominantly inherited rapid-onset dystonia-parkinsonism linked to chromosome 19. A variety of etiologies are related to acute-onset parkinsonism: medications, infections, toxins, metabolic disturbances and various structural lesions. The possibility of secondary parkinsonism was raised in our patient. Eventually, bilateral subdural hematoma was diagnosed on cerebral CT.

*Subdural hematoma* is bleeding into the subdural space caused by rupture of any bridging vein between the brain and venous sinuses, especially where stretched by underlying cerebral atrophy. Nearly all cases are caused by trauma, although the trauma may be trivial [3]. Coagulation abnormalities and especially anticoagulant therapy in the elderly are significant risk factors. A subdural hematoma typically expands over most of the cerebral convexity; spread to the contralateral hemisphere is limited by the falx cerebri. Because subdural hematomas often are associated with damage to the underlying brain tissue, contusions and swelling of the ipsilateral cerebral hemisphere are common. Subdural hematomas may be acute, subacute, or chronic.

*Acute subdural hematomas* are symptomatic within 24 hours after trauma. Patients with acute subdural hematoma often have a decreased level of consciousness; 12 to 38% of patients will have a lucid period at some point in their presentation. The overall mortality of patients who have an acute subdural hematoma and require surgical intervention is between

40% and 60%. Current consensus guidelines recommend that acute subdural hematoma with a thickness greater than 10 mm or a midline shift of more than 5 mm on CT should be evacuated surgically.

A *subacute* subdural hematoma becomes symptomatic between 24 hours and 2 weeks after injury. Patients complain of headache, altered mental status, muscle weakness, or frank paralysis. On CT the hematoma may appear hypodense or isodense. Most patients with subacute subdural hematoma require surgical evacuation of the lesion.

A *chronic subdural hematoma* becomes symptomatic 2 weeks after trauma or longer. The signs and symptoms may be subtle or nonspecific, but many patients demonstrate unilateral weakness or hemiparesis. Most patients have an altered level of consciousness. In 20% of cases, chronic subdural hematomas are bilateral (as in the present case). A chronic subdural hematoma may have initially been small and asymptomatic, but expand and became symptomatic due to recurrent hemorrhage. On CT scan, a chronic subdural hematoma may appear isodense or hypodense to brain parenchyma; blood of various ages is seen as a mixed-density lesion (as in the present case). Indirect evidence of the lesion includes a midline shift, effacement of the ipsilateral cortical sulci, and ventricular compression. Symptomatic chronic subdural hematomas require surgical evacuation. Most patients have a favorable outcome after surgery. Overall, the mortality from surgically drained chronic subdural hematomas approaches 4%, with decreased survival in the old.

*Subdural hematoma presenting as subacute parkinsonism* has been reported infrequently [4-6]. Parkinsonism was attributed to the mass effect produced by the subdural hematoma. Evacuation of the hematoma may result in the disappearance of parkinsonian symptoms without the need for antiparkinsonian medication.

## Learning Points

- Acute/subacute parkinsonism is a syndrome not to be confused with Parkinson's disease and deserves evaluation for its cause.
- Acute/subacute parkinsonism is acknowledged as a "red flag" situation that requires quick intervention.
- Cerebral CT may reveal an anatomic lesion and determine subsequent management.
- Early diagnosis of subdural hematoma and neurosurgical treatment may preserve neurological functions and save life.
- The clinical symptoms of subdural hematoma may occur with delay after the causal event.

# References

[1] Lees AJ, Hardy J, Revesz T. Parkinson's disease. *Lancet* 2009;373:2055-2066.

[2] Litvan I, Bhatia KP, Burn DJ, Goetz CG, Lang AE, McKeith I, Quinn N, Sethi KD. Shults C, Wenning GK. Movement Disorders Society Scientific Issues Committee Report SIC Task Force Appraisal of Clinical Diagnostic Criteria for Parkinsonian Disorders. *Movement Disorders* 2003;18: 467-486.

[3] Greenberg M: Handbook of Neurosurgery. 5th ed. New York, Thieme, 2001.
[4] Bostantjopoulou S, Katsarou Z, Michael M, Petridis A. Reversible parkinsonism due to chronic bilateral subdural hematomas. *J. Clin. Neurosci.* 2009;16:458-460.
[5] Krul JM, Wokke JH. Bilateral subdural hematoma presenting as subacute parkinsonism. *Clin. Neurol. Neurosurg.* 1987;89:107-109.
[6] Giray S, Sarica FB, Sen O, Kizilkilic O. Parkinsonian syndrome associated with subacute subdural haematoma and its effective surgical treatment: a case report. *Neuro Neurochir. Pol.* 2009;43:289-292.

# Case 48. Low Back Pain

A 71-year-old hypertensive man presented with low back pain of eight months duration. The pain was of moderate intensity, unaffected by motion, and was not relieved by bed-rest. He noted 4 kg loss of weight during the preceding months. Laboratory examination revealed normocytic anemia and CRP 86 mg/dL. Plain radiographs showed degenerative changes of the lumbar spine. The latter were considered 'red flags' and, therefore, thoracic and abdominal CT was performed. The CT showed, in addition to degenerative changes of the lumbar spine, severe atherosclerotic changes along the thoracic and abdominal aorta; there was heavy thickening of the wall of the abdominal aorta exhibiting a periaortic rind and an irregularly narrowed lumen (Figure 34). These findings were consistent with localized abdominal periaortitis.

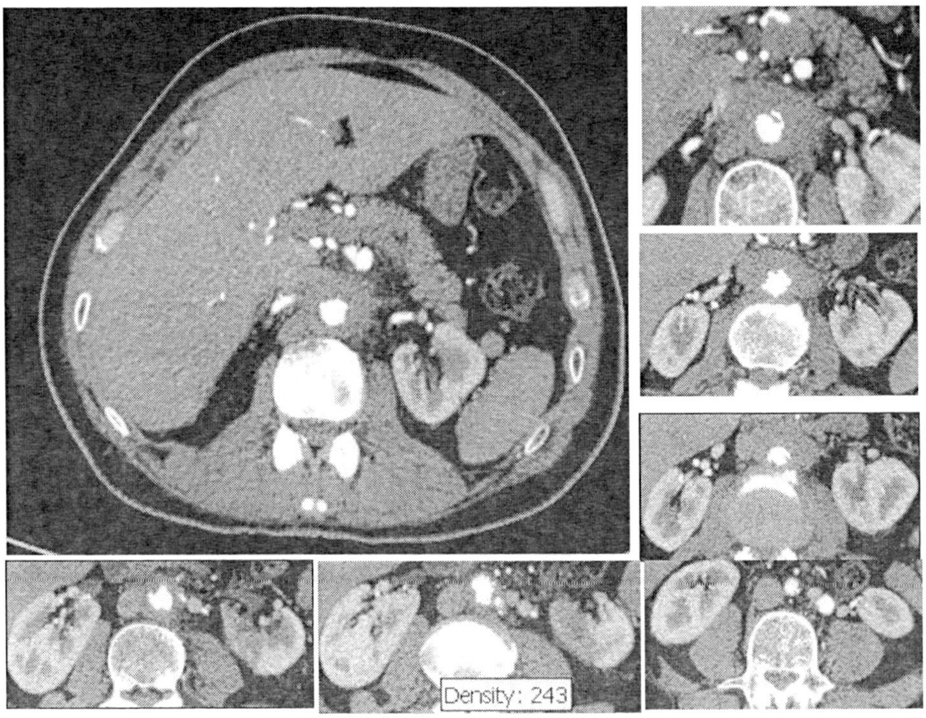


Figure 34. CT angiography with the aid of 64-row MDCT. Axial image at the level of the renal arteries shows narrowing of the aortic lumen, aortic wall thickening and a periaortic rind.

*Low back pain* is not a clinical entity but a symptom, with different stages of impairment, disability, and chronicity [1]. Many people have episodes of low back pain, but most incidents are self-limiting and the pain diminishes within days or weeks. Specific spinal disorders such as vertebral fractures, tumors, infections, inflammatory diseases, symptomatic disc herniation or spinal stenosis occur in only a few patients with acute low back pain. Measures of function such as range of motion and back strength are weakly associated with outcomes.

*Chronic low back* pain, lasting longer than 3 months, accounts for about 10% of cases but is one of the greatest health problems in industrialized societies. After a brief diagnostic triage, including a scrutiny for 'red flags' and a limited neurological and musculoskeletal examination, about 85% patients can be classified as having non-specific low back pain. The following features are 'red flags', indicating possible serious spinal pathology: low back associated with thoracic pain, fever, unexplained weight loss, urinary retention or incontinence, bowel dysfunction, history of carcinoma, ill health, progressive neurological deficit either motor or sensory, saddle anesthesia, disturbed gait, pain unrelieved by rest, osteoporosis, significant trauma related to age, and onset after age 55. No routine imaging is recommended in the absence of any of the mentioned alarm signals. Diagnostic imaging should be reserved to patient in whom a systemic disease is suspected or for patients who are candidates for surgery. Patients diagnosed with non-specific low back pain should be informed, reassured and advised to continue their regular daily activities. Analgesia is prescribed, with first choice paracetamol and second choice non-steroidal anti-inflammatory drugs. Paracetamol is in general preferred because its better side-effect profile, while side effects of NSAID on the gastrointestinal tract, the water and mineral metabolism, and atherothrombosis are common. Safety considerations are particularly important in the elderly, when age associated decline in cardiac and renal function and presence of co-morbidities may augment the risks related to antalgic treatment.

'Red flags' were present in the patient described in this vignette, including weight loss, normocytic anemia, no pain relief by bed-rest, and increased CRP. Therefore a thoracic and abdominal CT examination was performed. Unexpectedly, periaortitis was revealed.

*Periaortitis* [2] includes a variety of conditions belonging to a spectrum of retroperitoneal inflammation: idiopathic retroperitoneal fibrosis, perianeurysmal retroperitoneal fibrosis, inflammatory abdominal aortic aneurysms, and isolated periaortitis (typified by the present case). Periaortitis may be the expression of a local immune response to antigens in atherosclerotic plaques or may be a manifestation of a systemic disease. Some cases of inflammatory abdominal aortic aneurysm represent a manifestation of the IgG4-related systemic disease [3]. The latter, a recently recognized entity, is characterized by high serum IgG4 concentrations, inflammatory-sclerosing infiltrates containing numerous IgG4-positive plasmacytes, and involvement of multiple organs (autoimmune pancreatitis, aortitis and periaortitis, Sjogren's syndrome, pleurisy, pulmonary infiltrates, as well as biliary, periorbital, renal, meningeal, mammary, prostatic, thyroid, pericardial and skin inflammation). The histopathological features bear similarities across organs, regardless of the site of disease.

There are no specific laboratory tests for chronic periaortitis. The CRP and ESR are increased, but are not reliable markers for monitoring disease activity. Imaging has a major role in the diagnosis and should be performed in patients with unexplained back, flank, or abdominal pain. Although ultrasound is useful for detecting urinary tract obstruction or aortic aneurysms, it is limited in defining the extent of retroperitoneal fibrosis or in distinguishing between inflammatory and non-inflammatory aortic aneurysms. Contrast enhanced MRI and CT permit more detailed imaging of chronic periaortitis. Steroid therapy alone or with added immune suppressive medications (cyclophosphamide, azathioprine, cyclosporine A, or mycophenolate mofetil) results in resolution of abdominal pain and systemic symptoms. Average length of therapy in one study was 41 months.

Our patient was referred to the rheumatology clinic for management and long-term follow-up of periaortitis. Prednisone and methotrexate treatment was administered and there was a gradual improvement of symptoms over several weeks. Repeated CTs showed slow but consistent regression of the periaortic pseudotumor. There was no evidence of involvement of other organ systems and the test for IgG4 was negative.

### Learning Points

- Low back pain is a symptom with different degrees of impairment, disability, and chronicity.
- Possible indicators of serious pathology ('red flags') are low back pain with associated thoracic pain, fever, unexplained weight loss, urinary retention or incontinence, bowel dysfunction, history of carcinoma, progressive neurological deficit, saddle anesthesia, disturbed gait, pain unrelieved by rest, and osteoporosis.
- After a brief diagnostic triage and pursuit of 'red flags', if none is found no imaging is recommended.
- Diagnostic imaging should be reserved to patient in whom a systemic disease is suspected as well as for patients who are candidates for surgery.
- Imaging should not be limited to the spine.

## References

[1] Balagué F, Mannion AF, Pullise F, Cedraski C. Clinical update; low back pain. *Lancet* 2007;369:726-728.

[2] Mitnick H, Jacobowitz G, Krinsky G, Eberle M, Rosenzweig B, Willis D, Rockman C, Riles T. Periaortitis: Gadolinium-enhanced magnetic resonance imaging and response to therapy in four patients. *Ann. Vas. Surg.* 2004;18:100-107.

[3] Leise MD, Jakobson KM, Chaari ST. 75-Year-old man with abdominal pain and weight loss. *Mayo Clin. Proc.* 2008;83:1161-1164.

## Case 49. End-stage Heart Failure

A 73-year-old man, suffering from severe chronic congestive heart failure with anasarca and requiring continuous oxygen administration, was transferred from the department of internal medicine for subacute care. His medical history was remarkable for myocardial infraction, coronary artery bypass graft ten years ago, systolic heart failure (the left ventricular ejection fraction was 20% in the presence of severe mitral regurgitation), arterial hypertension, type 2 diabetes mellitus, dyslipemia, and chronic renal failure. Lately, his condition deteriorated and he could no longer attend the visits in the heart failure clinic where he regularly had received intravenous infusions with furosemide and 'renal dose' dopamine. He had been admitted four times to hospital during the previous six months because of worsening heart failure. The patient had rejected the proposal to receive an ICD devise, though, being himself a physician he was aware of the possible consequences of his refusal. Important findings on recent evaluation included pulmonary congestion on chest x-ray and high levels of B-type natriuretic peptide. The current medications were clopidogrel 75 mg/day, aspirin 75 mg/day, ramipril 2.5 mg/day, furosemide 160 mg/day and insulin levemir. Metolazone 2.5 mg/day and thiamine 100 mg/day were added recently.

On admission to our ward the patient was alert, the BP 95/60 mmHg, respirations 28/min, SaO2 by pulse oxymetry 88% in ambient air. The jugular veins were engorged. Grade 4 pitting edema extended along the lower extremities and up to the mid scapula, and infiltrated massively the scrotum. A few wet rales were audible at the lung bases. The heart rate was regular. A mid-systolic gallop sound and a pansystolic grade 3/6 murmur were perceived at the cardiac apex. The liver was enlarged, elastic and pulsatile. There was evidence of sensory-motor polyneuropathy. The patient needed assistance in all activities of daily living. Laboratory values included hemoglobin 12 g/dL, serum creatinine 1.9 mg/dL, BUN 74 mg/dL, albumin 3.3 g/dL, alkaline phosphatase 436 U/L (x 3 times upper limit of normal), while levels of AST, ALT and bilirubin were normal, and the CRP was 15 mg/L. The glycemia was poorly controlled. The ECG showed sinus tachycardia and tall R waves in lead V1, consistent with true posterior myocardial infarction. A chest x-rays showed cardiomegaly and pulmonary venous congestion.

*The patient's goals of management* were acknowledged: his first wish was to be delivered from the massive edema which hindered his movements, in particular the scrotal edema. He strived for a better quality of life and was against prolongation of a life of suffering. The patient was assertive in his desires and often interfered with the physicians' recommendations. So, he sometimes refused to receive the prescribed dose of insulin in spite of exceedingly high blood glucose levels. He persisted in his refusal to receive an ICD device. Having discussed with his spouse and children, the patient did not reach a decision whether to return home or to enter a hospice.

*The physicians' goals of management* were to explore reversible factors which possibly aggravated the heart failure, to comfort the patient, and to come to a decision whether he had entered the phase of terminal heart failure. Regarding the latter subject, the following clinical features are known to be associated with poor prognosis in a patient with chronic heart failure: old age, male sex, presence of a third heart sound, elevated jugular venous pressure, low systolic BP, reduced ejection fraction, functional class IV according to criteria of the New York Heart Association (NYHA), comorbidities, anemia, renal insufficiency, elevated brain-type natriuretic peptide (all were present in the propositus).

*Prognostication* has important implications for deciding between therapeutic options for the patient and his family. One might expect that physicians have an understanding regarding their patients' prognosis, especially if they know the patient well. This belief is countered by data of a prospective cohort study of terminally ill patients, showing that the physicians' predictions were accurate in only 20% of cases, 63% being optimistic and 17% pessimistic. Moreover, the likelihood of erroneous prediction increased as the duration of the patient-physician relationship increased [1]. Hence, the goal of determining with accuracy which individual patient with heart failure will die within 6 months is unrealistic; patients tend to live for variable lengths of time in a continuous state of poor health, with intermittent exacerbations of heart failure, and the immediate cause of death is often a sudden and unpredictable event. Clinicians may be reluctant to refer individuals with heart failure for palliative and hospice care because the unsure prediction of the time of death [2-4].

*The recent position statement on palliative care in advanced heart failure* by the European Society of Cardiology proposed a staged management [4]. Accordingly, for patients with NYHA class I to III heart failure the goals are to provide effective therapies to prolong survival, symptom control, active monitoring, and supported self-management. Repeated admissions to hospital (as witnessed in our patient) may herald the need for supportive and palliative care (NYHA class III to IV). In this situation, the goal of care shifts to maintaining optimal symptom control. Palliative care consultation should be considered. Multidisciplinary assessment of the patient's needs is recommended. Interventions to promote patient self-management skills and caregiver skills result in fewer hospitalizations and lower costs.

*The terminal phase of heart failure* is recognized when, despite maximal treatment, the patient has persistent edema, fatigue, anorexia, hypotension and renal impairment. The following recommendations are pertinent to the terminal phase of heart failure: symptom control, advanced directives concerning resuscitation and ventilation, and an integrated care pathway for dying. Information on end of life issues should be provided in an ethno-culturally appropriate manner to patients and their families. Important is the education of health care providers on the art of talking about the end of life. The discussion and the patient's preferences should be clearly documented in the medical record. Increased practical and emotional support should be provided for care givers.

An expert opinion on this issue has been imparted by Lewis EF [5]. Accordingly, the first goal is to ascertain, prove or disprove intolerance to medical treatment for heart failure. For this purpose the patients are challenged with various combinations of medications, including staggered dosing regimens and alternatives to angiotensin-converting enzyme inhibitors and β-blockers. Cardiac resynchronization therapy is considered if the patient meets the criteria. As patients develop progressive hypotension and side effects from medicines, the responsible medicines should be discontinued after careful information for patients and families (so we had to proceed in the propositus having low BP, renal failure and inadequate response to furosemide treatment). For patients with refractory heart failure who are not candidates for left ventricular assist device or cardiac transplantation, their goals for living are discussed with patient and proxies. The approach to the patient should be based upon his/her understanding of the disease process and the significance of the progression to stage D heart failure. Strategies to maximize survival, though limited, should be discussed focusing on their quality of life. Palliative care consultants are often involved at this stage. For the patient who is clearly at the end of life, referral to hospice is considered with focus on comfort.

*Hospice*, as defined by the Medicare Hospice Benefit, is a health care delivery system focused on caring for the patient and family after treatment efforts aimed at substantially changing the course of the terminal illness are no longer effective or when the patient decides to stop treatment with curative intent. In 2005, the most recent year with complete reporting, only 18.36% of patients in the USA who were dying of heart failure and were hospice eligible actually received hospice care. Reasons for this might be the difficulty in prognostication and the lack of a consensus on when to stop life prolonging therapies.

*The indication and feasibility of mitral valve reconstruction* for our patient having severe mitral regurgitation were considered. Current guidelines recommend surgery for moderate-to-severe or severe mitral regurgitation in patients with evidence of left ventricular dysfunction. One surgical approach for mitral-valve repair involves approximation of the mitral leaflets with suture to create a double orifice. Selected patients who have been treated with this technique as a stand-alone procedure have had successful results lasting up to 12 years. A catheterization-based method has been developed for approximation of the mitral leaflets with a clip that is delivered through trans-septal access. The device (MitraClip, Abbott Vascular) grasps and approximates the leaflets of the mitral valve. Mitral repair performed with this device in 107 patients showed significant reduction in the severity of mitral regurgitation. Although percutaneous repair was less effective at reducing mitral regurgitation than conventional surgery, the procedure had superior safety and similar improvements in clinical outcomes [6].

Our patient was obviously at very high surgical risk; therefore, the possibility to perform mitral valve repair percutaneously was discussed with cardiologists. Their opinion was that the risks of the procedure would outweigh the benefits: despite the leaflets' being approximated with a clip, the much dilated left ventricle would live the mitral valve largely open during systole by pulling the chordae tendinae.

*Possible causes of bilateral leg edema,* added on heart failure, were excluded: venous hypertension, restrictive cardiomyopathy, pericardial constriction, decreased plasma oncotic pressure, capillary hyperpermeability, and decreased lymphatic drainage. An estimate of excess extracellular volume in heart failure has been suggested as follows: pitting edema at the ankles corresponds to 3 liter extracellular fluid in excess, edema at knee level 10 liters in excess, edema at knee and thigh 20 liters in excess, anasarca 30 liters in excess (likely to be the case in our patient).

*Restriction of dietary sodium intake* may help to reduce but does not eliminate the requirement for diuretics. Patients who gain weight despite excreting more than 78 mEq of sodium per day (or have urine sodium > urine potassium on a random sample) are not compliant with the diet.

*To achieve symptomatic improvement and challenge the diagnosis of refractory heart failure* our patient was treated with various combinations of medications. Furosemide 240 mg/day by continuous drip was added to the patient's regular medications, but without any effect on the body weight. This was ascribed to the synergistic deleterious effects on the renal microcirculation of low cardiac output, low BP (mostly 85-90/60 mmHg), the effect of ACE inhibition (well known), and aspirin (often ignored). Therefore, ramipril and aspirin were temporarily discontinued. However, there was no improvement in diuresis.

*Diuretics* have not shown to decrease mortality, but are required to relieve pulmonary congestion, dyspnea and peripheral edema [8, 9]. No other treatment relieves symptoms and signs of sodium and water overload as rapidly and effectively. The goal is to achieve a gradual diuresis, knowing that diuretics deplete the intravascular space with imminent contraction of the effective intravascular volume. The intravascular space is subsequently refilled slowly from the extravascular space, only one liter of fluid per day moving from the extravascular into the intravascular space. A negative fluid balance should therefore be limited to 1 liter per day. For a typical daily oral fluid intake of 1400 mL, the daily urine output should be 2400 mL to achieve a negative balance of 1000 mL/day and a daily loss in body weight of 1 kg. A negative fluid balance greater than 1 liter per day can impair the renal function.

The rule is to prescribe the minimum dose of diuretic, usually furosemide alone or in combination with another diuretic, needed to maintain an edema-free state. The usual dose of furosemide 40 to 120 mg/day taken orally is often insufficient to achieve adequate diuresis in patients with advanced chronic heart failure. Furthermore, the efficacy of loop diuretics is inversely related to creatinine clearance; as creatinine clearance decreases, the dose of loop diuretic needed to produce natriuresis and diuresis must be increased. The optimal diuretic dose has been controversial. Although furosemide was reported to be safe at doses as high as 4000 mg/day, more recent studies recommend much lower doses because the increased risk of adverse effects at high doses. Diuretic dosing should be flexible, with temporary increases for fluid retention and decreases in case of low fluid intake or fluid loss (e.g. gastroenteritis or postobstructive polyuria), increased electrolyte loss, or when hypovolemia is evident.

Diuretic use can lead to hyponatremia, hypokalemia, and hypomagnesemia, increased risk of digitalis toxicity, hyperuricemia, and hypovolemia. It is usually recommended that serum potassium be maintained 4-5 mEq/L because heart failure patients are prone to arrhythmia. Diuretics may increase the activation of endogenous neurohormonal systems in patients with heart failure, which can lead to disease progression unless patients are receiving treatment with a concomitant neurohormonal antagonist (an ACE inhibitor or beta blocker). On the other hand, the risk of renal dysfunction is enhanced by concomitant use of diuretics with an ACE inhibitor or ARB. Undue use of diuretics can lead to hypotension, decreased exercise tolerance, fatigue, and prerenal azotemia.

In some patients with milder symptoms of heart failure a thiazide diuretic such as hydrochlorothiazide may suffice. In more advanced heart failure or in patients with concomitant renal dysfunction a loop diuretic such as furosemide is usually needed. Loop diuretics cause a rapid onset of an intense but relatively short-lived diuresis compared with the longer lasting but moderate effect of a thiazide diuretic. The timing of administration of the loop diuretic can be adjusted to the patient's social activities. It needs not be taken in the morning. The dose may be postponed or temporarily omitted if the patient plans an activity that might be compromised by the prompt action of the diuretic.

*Diuretic resistance* may occur on long term diuretic treatment. Factors contributing to diuretic resistance are impaired absorption of orally given diuretics due to gut edema (the oral bioavailability of furosemide is 40% to 79%), arterial hypotension, reduced renal blood flow, and increased sodium reabsorption at the distal tubule under long-term treatment with a loop diuretic. The latter problem can be countered by a combination of the loop diuretic with a thiazide-type diuretic, in order to oppose sodium reabsorption in different segments of the nephron. The combination of furosemide with hydrochlorothiazide (25 mg once daily) or metolazone (initial dose 5 mg daily) can achieve better diuresis, but requires more frequent monitoring of electrolytes and renal function. Patients with advanced heart failure should also receive an aldosterone antagonist which increases excretion of sodium but not of potassium. It should be remembered that use of a potassium-sparing diuretic or aldosterone antagonist along with an ACE inhibitor or ARB requires careful surveillance for hyperkalemia; treatment with all three is not recommended. A period of intravenous loop diuretic may be required in patients who become resistant to the action of oral diuretics.

*Continuous furosemide intravenous drip* was though to be more efficient and safer than the equal dose in boluses. This perception is contradicted by data of a recent randomized double blind study of patients with acute decompensated heart failure [8]. In comparing i.v. bolus furosemide every 12 hours vs. continuous infusion of furosemide, there was no significant difference in efficacy and safety with either regimen. The latter study did not address the population of frail elderly patients; hence, conclusions of this study might not be valid for the typical patient in acute geriatric care.

*Furosemide combined with 'low-dose' dopamine treatment* has been recently reconsidered. When excessive diuresis causes hypotension, hypoperfusion and/or relative dehydration in patients with decompensated heart failure, there is a risk that a preexisting renal dysfunction is aggravated and that tubular or glomerular injury results. One measure that might prevent deterioration of glomerular filtration under intensive diuretic treatment is by dopamine i.v. infusion at low doses. In a recent study, the combination of low-dose furosemide and low-dose dopamine (2 μg/kg/minute) was equally effective as high-dose furosemide but associated with improved renal function and potassium homeostasis [11]. In another study, sixty consecutive patients presenting acute heart failure (age 75.7 ± 11.2 years, left ventricular ejection fraction 35.3 ± 12.1%) were randomized, after receiving a 40 mg intravenous furosemide bolus, to either high-dose furosemide (20 mg/hour continuous infusion for 8 hours), or low-dose furosemide combined with 'low-dose' dopamine (furosemide 5 mg/hour plus dopamine 5 μg kg/minute continuous infusion for 8 hours). The combination of low-dose furosemide with low-dose dopamine was equally effective as high-dose furosemide but associated with improved renal function profile and potassium homeostasis [12]. Time will show whether revival of 'renal dose dopamine' is to follow.

Every effort should be made to prevent a rise in serum creatinine by more than 25% of basal value consequent to diuretic therapy; the same applies to other procedures aimed at rapid fluid removal such as paracentesis of tense ascites and ultrafiltration. The following measures may be useful: addition to i.v. furosemide of osmotic agents able to expand the effective blood volume, i.v. infusion of small volumes of hypertonic saline solution, administration of albumin, mannitol and/or plasma expanders. It is encouraging that transient worsening of renal function during hospitalization for heart failure did not affect the outcomes after discharge from the hospital according to a recent study.

*Drugs that should be avoided,* if possible, in heart failure patients are most antiarrhythmics (with the exception of amiodarone and dofetilide), most calcium-channel blockers (with the exception of amlodipine), corticosteroids, NSAIDs, many antipsychotics, antihistamines, and thiazolidinediones (because the risk of fluid retention). Some salt substitutes contain significant amounts of potassium and should be used cautiously. Other dietary constituents (e.g. grapefruit and cranberry juice) and supplements such as St. John's wart can interact with warfarin and digoxin. The ban on metformin treatment in patients with heart failure has been eased, when recent studies showed that metformin therapy improves the outcome of elderly diabetic patients discharged after hospitalization for heart failure [10]. However, administration of metformin remains contraindicated during exacerbations of heart failure.

*Ultrafiltration*, appreciated for its property to accomplish a more rapid fluid and weight loss in heart failure patients, has produces neurohumoral activation, increase in creatinine, and symptomatic hypotension similar to i.v. loop diuretics; thus, the safety and cost-effectiveness of this procedure in the treatment of heart failure remains to be verified.

*Heart failure with comorbid renal insufficiency*, as witnessed in our patient, is difficult to manage because cardiac and renal functions are strictly dependent on circulating volume.

Hypovolemia induced by aggressive diuretic treatment alone or in combination with an intercurrent illness decreases both the cardiac output and the glomerular filtration. The goal is to normalize the patient's volume status while avoiding overdiuresis and the ensuing renal dysfunction. The first question in the management of a patient with comorbid cardiac and renal insufficiency is whether the patient is hypovolemic. Hypovolemia should be reversed by fluid administration before irreversible renal damage ensues. Careful physical examination will usually resolve this question, although assessment of the central venous pressure will occasionally be necessary. The next question is whether hypotension is present. Is this the case, pressor agents should be administered to maintain a systolic BP >80 mmHg and a mean BP >60 mm Hg. Low-normal systolic BP (80 to 90 mmHg) is acceptable as long as renal function is improving. In the absence of hypotension, cold extremities are an indication of vasoconstriction leading to elevated systemic vascular resistance; these patients often respond favorably to vasodilatation. Drugs that may contribute to renal impairment should be discontinued, including low-dose aspirin, NSAIDs, ACE inhibitors and ARBs. Low-dose aspirin treatment (75–325 mg/day) may negatively influence the renal function, a disturbance that can persist up to three weeks after termination of aspirin intake [7]. Low-dose aspirin alone, and more so in combination with a diuretic, was associated with significantly lower creatinine clearance. However, given the long-term benefit of ACE inhibitor and low-dose aspirin on heart and renal failure, the therapy should be continued or reinstituted whenever possible.

*The optimal hemoglobin level* in heart failure patients is unknown. It seems prudent to treat anemia in patients with advanced heart failure according to the protocol applied to treat anemia in patients with chronic renal failure. A review compiled 27 randomized trials of erythropoietin in patients with anemia and chronic kidney disease. When treatment with erythropoietin resulted in higher hemoglobin levels (12 to 15 g/dL) the risk for stroke increased, hypertension worsened, and there was more vascular access thrombosis compared to strategies that resulted in lower hemoglobin levels (9.5 to 11.5 g d/L). The mechanisms for harm remained unclear. The optimal hemoglobin target for patients with chronic renal failure, and probably in chronic heart failure, should be 10 to 12 g/dL. Complete correction of anemia should be avoided.

*Our patient suggested* increasing the dose of furosemide to 600 mg/day, based on favorable results obtained in the past with such a high dose. We started a trial with furosemide 600 mg/day by continuous i.v. infusion supplemented with metolazone 2.5 mg/day and vitamin B1 300 mg/day orally. A negative fluid balance of 1 to 1.5 kg/day was attained on this regimen without a detrimental effect on the BP, BUN, serum sodium and potassium. The serum creatinine decreased to 1.3 mg/dL, but the BUN/creatinine ratio remained >25. The patient lost 22 kg in weight, the edema withdraw from the level of the mid-thorax to the inguinal ligaments, the scrotal edema receded, and there was no longer need for continuous oxygen administration.

*Vitamin B1 (thiamine)* was included in the patient's drug regimen. Vitamin B1 deficiency is found in about one third of hospitalized patients with chronic heart failure, an incidence widely exceeding the often quoted cliché that 'beriberi in the western society is mainly encountered in alcoholics'. The prevalence and the consequences of thiamine deficiency among elderly patients admitted to acute geriatric wards were investigated in a study from Western Europe. Severe thiamine deficiency was infrequently met among hospitalized elderly persons, but the prevalence of moderate thiamine deficiency approached 40%. Institutionalized subjects were at particular risk of developing thiamine deficiency [13].

It is well known that thiamine deficiency may cause heart failure ('cardiac beriberi'). Also it is known that diuretic treatment may cause urinary loss of thiamine leading to thiamine deficiency. Cardiac beriberi is classically thought to represent a high-output state with oliguria and lactic acidosis. However, cardiac beriberi can also present with low cardiac output and fulminant vascular collapse, or cause sudden death [14]. Therefore, the possible role of thiamine deficiency should be considered before concluding that heart failure is refractory to treatment. A therapeutic trial with thiamine is the practical means to rapidly diagnose 'beriberi heart', a condition which is quickly reversed by thiamine administration. Though controversial, routine administration of thiamine 100 mg/day to patients with heart failure is recommended by some authors. This principle was applied to the present patient, who received thiamine supplementation. Vitamin B1 loading dose 300 mg/day orally was administered for 10 days and 100 mg/day were administered subsequently.

*A three weeks course* of treatment in the acute geriatric ward seemed to have provided much relief to the patient: the massive edema diminished, the SaO2 was constantly above 90% on room air, the renal function improved, he was on physiotherapy and started to walk with a two-wheeled walker, he was in good mood and planning to move to a nursing home. On day 23 of hospital stay, in the late afternoon the patient developed shaking chills and the temperature rose to 38.8$^{0}$C. Dry crackles were perceived over the left lower lung field. Blood and urine was sampled for culture and empirical treatment with ertapenem was started. The BP was 86/62 mmHg. A few hour later hypoglycemia was diagnosed and treated. Laboratory tests showed WBC 27,000/mm$^3$, polymorphonuclears 92%, creatinine 1.8 mg/dL, BUN 85 mg/dL, potassium 4.9 mEq/L. The ECG showed sinus tachycardia 98 bpm. Another episode of hypoglycemia associated with drowsiness was recorded and remitted promptly on i.v. hypertonic glucose administration. Subsequently, a 10% solution of glucose supplemented with potassium was infused continuously; glycemia monitoring showed values in the range 145 to 170 mg/dL. Oxygen was delivered by nasal prongs. Eight hours later the patient died.

*Pneumonia* complicated the course of the patient's disease. There is an increased risk of cardiovascular events, primarily acute myocardial infarction during pneumonia [15]. Mitochondrial dysfunction induced by sepsis places cardiomyocytes at risk of adenosine triphosphate depletion. Sepsis may be associated with elevated serum troponin, indicating myocardial injury. Sepsis-related changes in the circulating volume and vessel tone affect the cardiac performance.

*Hypoglycemia* was a late complication. The neuroglycopenic symptoms resolved promptly with glucose administration. Hypoglycemia in diabetic patients is most often caused by insulin or oral hypoglycemic drugs. Further causes of hypoglycemia are critical illnesses (hepatic, cardiac, or renal failure), sepsis, inanition, endocrine deficiencies (cortisol, growth hormone, or both), and medications (ethanol, haloperidol, salicilates, sulfmathoxazole /trimethoprim in a patient with renal failure). In our patient hypoglycemia can be ascribed to the additive effects of sepsis, diminished food intake, cardiac and renal failure, while the action of the earlier administered glargine persisted.

With increasing age, the 'protective window' between onset of hypoglycemic symptoms and their recognition is lost, making the elderly person more vulnerable to hypoglycemia. Older patients also have a different profile of symptoms during hypoglycemia, with fewer autonomic and more prominent neuroglycopenic symptoms. Hypoglycemic symptoms may be absent or may not be perceived as such. Only 22% of residents of a long-term care facility who suffered from an episode of infection-related hypoglycemia exhibited clinical signs indicating hypoglycemia.

Intravenous glucose 50 cc of the 50% solution is the standard therapy for severe hypoglycemia, to be followed by infusion of 10% solution of glucose; food should be provided as soon as the patient is able to take it safely. Glucagon is an effective emergency treatment for hypoglycemia where intravenous treatment with glucose is not available. Glucagon can be injected subcutaneously or intramuscularly. The standard 1 mg dose can cause substantial but transient hyperglycemia.

Hypoglycemia has been shown to cause QT prolongation, increased QT dispersion, atrial and/or ventricular ectopics and sudden bradycardia, all of which can predispose to sudden cardiac death. Every caution should be taken to avoid hypoglycemia in a brittle cardiac patient. In a cohort of 4946 patients admitted to ICUs in Australia, 22.4% had an episode of hypoglycemia, defined as a blood glucose concentration lower than 81 mg/dL (sic). The patients were stratified by the severity of hypoglycemia. The mortality among patients with hypoglycemia was 36.6% versus 19.7% in those without hypoglycemia. Increasing severity of hypoglycemia was independently associated with increasing risk of mortality [16].

The 2011 Clinical Practice Guideline from the American College of Physicians [17] recommends not using intensive insulin therapy to normalize blood glucose in hospitalized patients with or without diabetes mellitus. According to the latter guidelines, a target blood glucose level of 140 to 200 mg/dL (7.8 to 11.1 mmol/L) is recommended if insulin therapy is used in intensive care patients. This principle guided the treatment with insulin in our patient. He usually received insulin glargine 30 units/day and insulin lispro three times/day corresponding to the actual blood sugar levels. However, glycemia was poorly controlled, in the range 158 to 409 mg/dL (median 250 mg). The patient feared hypoglycemia and often skipped doses of insulin.

The caregivers' attachment and empathy to this colleague of ours made it not easy to accept the patient's unpredicted-predictable outcome. Indeed, 'patients with heart failure live in a continuous state of poor health for variable lengths of time, with intermittent exacerbations, and the immediate cause of death is often a sudden and unpredictable event' [3]: this was sepsis in the present case.

## Learning Points

- Repeated exacerbations of heart failure necessitating admissions to hospital indicate that the patient might have entered the stage of terminal heart failure.
- The terminal phase of heart failure is identified when, despite maximal treatment, the patient has persistent edema, fatigue, anorexia, hypotension and renal impairment.
- It is essential to ascertain that aggravating factors are not operating and that modifiable risk factors and defects have been corrected.
- Empirical treatment with thiamine may benefit some patients.
- As patients develop progressive hypotension and side effects from medications, the responsible medicines should be discontinued.
- Anemia should be treated; the optimal hemoglobin target is 10 to 12 g/dL.

- Hypoglycemia should be carefully avoided in the diabetic cardiac patient.
- The goal of care in the terminal phase of heart failure shifts to maintaining optimal symptom control, with focus on quality of life.
- Clarification of resuscitation status, increased practical and emotional support for patient and care givers is recommended in the terminal phase of heart failure.

# References

[1] Collins LG, Parks SM, Winter L. The state of advance care planning: one decade after SUPPORT. *Am. J. Hosp. Palliat Care*. 2006;23:378-384.
[2] Howlett J, Morrin L, Fortin M, Heckman G, Strachan PH , Suskin N, Shamian J, Lewanczuk R, Arthur HM. End-of-life planning in heart failure: It should be the end of the beginning. *Can. J. Cardiol.* 2010; 26:135–141.
[3] Lewis EF. End of life care in advanced heart failure. *Curr. Treat Options Cardiovasc. Med.* 2011;13:79-89.
[4] Jaarsma T, Ryder M, Rutten FH, et al. on behalf of the Advanced Heart Failure Study Group of the HFA of the ESC Palliative care in heart failure: A position statement from the palliative care workshop of the Heart Failure Association of the European Society of Cardiology. *Eur. J. Heart Fail.* 2009;11:433–443.
[5] Lewis EF. End of life care in advanced heart failure. *Curr. Treat Options Cardiovasc. Med.* 2011;13:79-89.
[6] JM, Mauri L. for the EVEREST II Investigators. Percutaneous repair or surgery for mitral regurgitation. *N. Engl. J. Med.* 2011; 364:1395-1406.
[7] Segal R, Lubart E, Leibovitz A, Iaina A, Caspi D. Renal effects of low dose aspirin in elderly patients. *IMAJ* 2006;8:679-682.
[8] Felker MG, Lee KL, Bull DA, Redfield MM, Stevenson LW, Goldsmith SR, LeWinter MM, Deswal A, Rouleau JL, Ofili EO, Anstrom KJ, Hernandez AF, McNulty SE, Velazquez EJ, Kfoury AG, Chen HH, Givertz MM, Semigran MJ, Bart BA, Mascette AM, Braunwald E, O'Connor CM, for the NHLBI Heart Failure Clinical Research Network. Diuretic strategies in patients with acute decompensated heart failure. *N. Engl. J. Med.* 2011; 364:797-805.
[9] De Vecchis R, Ciccarelli A, Pucciarelli A. Unloading therapy by intravenous diuretic in chronic heart failure: a double-edged weapon? *J. Cardiovasc. Med.* (Hagerstown) 2010; 11:571-574.
[10] Masoudi FA, Inzucchi SE, Wang Y, Havranek EP, Foody JM, Krumholz HM. Thiazolidinediones, metformin, and outcomes in older patients with diabetes and heart failure: an observational study. *Circulation* 2005;111:583-590.
[11] Elkayam U, Ng TMH, Hatamizadeh P, Janmohamed M, Mehra A. Renal vasodilatory action of dopamine in patients with heart failure. Magnitude of effect and site of action. *Circulation* 2008;117:200-205.
[12] Giamouzis G, Butler J, Starling RC, Karayannis G, Nastas J, Parisis C, Rovithis D, Economou D, Savvatis K, Kirlidis T, Tsaknakis T, Skoularigis J, Westermann D, Tschöpe C, Triposkiadis F. Impact of dopamine infusion on renal function in

hospitalized heart failure patients: results of the Dopamine in Acute Decompensated Heart Failure (DAD-HF) Trial. *J. Card. Fail.* 2010;16:922-930.

[13] Pepersack T, Garbusinski J, Robberecht J, Beyer I, Willems D, Fuss M. Clinical relevance of thiamine status amongst hospitalized elderly patients. *Gerontology.* 1999;45:96-101.

[14] Shivalkar B, Engelmann I, Carp L, De Raedt H, Daelemans R. Shoshin syndrome: two case reports representing opposite ends of the same disease spectrum. *Acts Cardiol.* 1998;53:195-199.

[15] Feldman T, Foster E, Glower DJ, Kar S, Rinaldi MJ, Fail PS, Smalling RW, Siegel R, Rose GA, Engeron E, Loghin C, Trento A, Skipper ER, Fudge T, Letsou GV, Massaro Perry TW, Pugh MJ, Waterer GW, Nakashima B, Orihuela CJ, Copeland LA, Restrepo MI, Anzueto A, Mortensen EM. Incidence of cardiovascular events after hospital admission for pneumonia. *Am. J. Med.* 2011;124:244-251.

[16] Egi M, Bellomo R, Stachowski E, French CJ, Hart GK, Taori G, Hegarty C, Bailey M. Hypoglycemia and outcome in critically ill patients. *Mayo Clin. Proc.* 2010;85: 217-224.

[17] Qaseem A, Humphrey LL, Chou R, Snow V, Shekelle P, for the Clinical Guidelines Committee of the American College of Physicians. Use of intensive insulin therapy for the management of glycemic control in hospitalized patients: A clinical practice guideline from the American College of Physicians. *Ann. Intern. Med.* 2011;154: 260-26.

# Case 50. Refractory Pulmonary Edema

An 88-year old woman was referred from the department of internal medicine with the diagnoses congestive heart failure, severe aortic stenosis, diabetes mellitus type II, urinary tract infection and aggravated chronic renal failure. Klebsiella pneumoniae grew in the urine culture and was treated with ertapenem. On echocardiography the estimated transaortic gradient was 90 mmHg and the left ventricular ejection fraction was 55%. Other medications were furosemide 80 mg/day, aspirin 100 mg/day, repaglinide 3 mg/day, omeprazole 40 mg/day, bisoprolol 5 mg, donepezil 5mg, ferrous calcium citrate 50 mg/day, and folic acid 5 mg/day. During the preceding months she has been repeatedly hospitalized for dyspnea and hypoxemia; bilateral pulmonary infiltrates were seen on x-rays on each of these admissions and were attributed to heart failure resulting from severe aortic stenosis. However, x-rays findings following intravenous furosemide treatment were essentially unchanged.

Five years before the present admission a solid mass has been revealed in the patient's right kidney as well as a small subpleural nodule. The renal mass was suspected to be a malignant neoplasm and the pulmonary nodule to be a metastasis. The significance of theses findings was discussed with the patient and proxies; eventually it was decided to renounce to surgery and refrain from interferon treatment. During the last year the patient became cachectic and bedridden. Also remarkable in the patient's history were type 2 diabetes mellitus, chronic renal failure (eCCT 45 mL/min/1.73m$^2$ ) and iron deficiency anemia, treated with oral iron preparations and blood transfusions as requested.

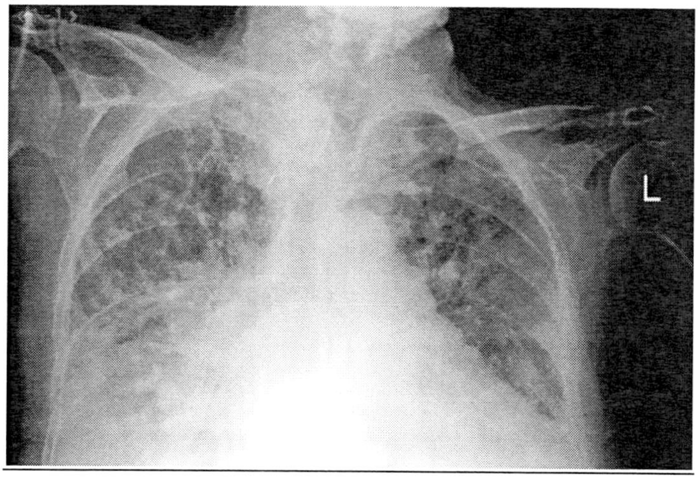


Figure 35. The x-rays shows an enlarged heart, thickened septal lines, disseminated nodules in the lungs, and blunting of the costophrenic angles.

On admission to our ward the SaO2 was 82% on ambient air and increased to 94% with supplemental oxygen, the PaC02 was 40 mmHg. The patient was dependent on continuous oxygen administration. Dry crackles were perceived over the lower lung areas. Chest X-rays (Figure 35) showed an enlarged cardiac silhouette, numerous thickened interlobular septa, and diffusely scattered nodules in both lungs. Intravenous furosemide administered in continuous drip 160 mg/day over four days produced neither clinical nor radiological improvement.

*Numerous thickened interlobular septa*, as seen in this patient, indicate an extensive interstitial abnormality; the underlying disorder may be an inflammatory-fibrosing process, carcinomatous lymphangitis, or an accumulation of fluid, i.e. pulmonary edema [1]. Could natriuretic peptide levels be informative in differentiating between carcinomatous lymphangitis and pulmonary congestion? In reviewing the Medline data base we could not find studies on this issue.

*A nodular pattern* is a feature of both interstitial and airspace disease. The distribution of nodules in the interlobular septa, subpleural and peribronchovascular regions (as observed in the present case) is most commonly seen in sarcoidosis and in carcinomatous lymphangitis. A random distribution of very small well-defined nodules is seen in hematogenous spread of tuberculosis, pulmonary metastases, pneumoconiosis and rarely in pulmonary sarcoidosis. Centrilobular nodules are found in subacute hypersensitivity pneumonitis and respiratory bronchiolitis–interstitial lung disease.

*Lymphangitic carcinomatosis* stands for infiltration of pulmonary lymphatics and the adjacent interstitial tissue by neoplastic cells. Lymphangitic carcinomatosis may be secondary to blood-borne tumor emboli lodging in small pulmonary arteries. Subsequently, cancer cells spread through the vessel walls into the perivascular interstitium and lymphatic vessels, giving rise to bilateral symmetric pulmonary lesions. The radiological reticulonodular shadowing, septal lines and subpleural edema correspond to dilated lymphatics, interstitial edema, tumor cells and secondary desmoplastic response. Pleural effusion is common. CT is more sensitive than plain radiography in the detection of lymphangitic spread and highly suggestive polygonal images can be seen in the subpleural areas [1, 2]. The most common tumors spreading in this manner are carcinomas of the bronchus, breast, stomach and prostate. Alternatively, lymphangitic carcinomatosis may result from the direct extension of a tumor from hilar lymph nodes into the peribronchovascular interstitium; by the latter mechanism lymphangitic carcinomatosis tends to be more localized.

*Renal cell carcinoma* occurs more often in the sixth and seventh decades of life [3]. The three classic diagnostic features of renal cell carcinoma are costovertebral pain, palpable mass and hematuria, but these are seen merely in 10% of cases. Renal carcinoma tends to metastasize widely before giving rise to local symptoms or signs. The most common locations of metastasis are the lungs and bones, followed in frequency by the regional lymph nodes, liver, adrenal, and brain. The presence of a renal tumor in our patient and the subsequent development of a reticulonodular pulmonary infiltrate suggest the possibility of carcinomatous lymphangitis secondary to renal cell carcinoma.

The average 5-year survival rate of patients with renal cell carcinoma is 45% and is 70% in the absence of distant metastases. With renal vein invasion or extension into the perinephric fat the 5-year survival rate is 15% to 20%. Nephrectomy has been the treatment of choice, but partial nephrectomy to preserve renal function is favored with increasing frequency and the outcome is excellent if the mass is completely excised. Medical treatment is generally ineffective. Interferon-alpha provides modest survival benefit [3].

The definite diagnosis in our patient was deferred since relevant diagnostic tests - transbronchial or videoscopic transpleural lung biopsy - entailed unacceptable risks and no prospects of benefit. The probable diagnoses were pulmonary lymphangitic carcinomatosis, renal cell carcinoma, severe aortic stenosis, and possible pulmonary congestion. The prognosis: terminal illness. Palliative care alone was offered to the patient.

### Learning Points

- Persistent shortness of breath and the presence of an interstitial abnormality on chest x-rays demand for a differential diagnosis between pulmonary congestion, interstitial pneumonia, interstitial fibrosis and carcinomatous lymphangitis.
- On CT, pulmonary carcinomatous lymphangitis shows highly suggestive polygonal images in the subpleural areas.
- Pulmonary biopsy, bronchial brushings, or bronchoalveolar lavage fluid usually reveal adenocarcinoma cells.
- Etiological treatment when possible can occasionally improve the patients' survival; if untreated the median survival is 3 months.

## References

[1] Padley S, MacDonal SLS. Pulmonary neoplasms. In: Grainger and Allison's Diagnostic Radiology, 5th ed., 2008.

[2] Hominal S, Falchero L, Perol M, Guérin JC. Carcinomatous lymphangitis. Presse Med. 1999;28:979-984.

[3] Chen DY, Uzzo RG. Evaluation and management of the renal mass Med Clin N Am 2011;95:179–189.

# Case 51. Hyperkalemia Contrary to Expectation

A 62-year-old woman was admitted to our ward on April 28$^{th}$ 2011 for multidisciplinary evaluation. Only two days earlier she had been discharged from the department of internal medicine of a tertiary care hospital with the diagnoses alveolar hypoventilation syndrome, severe pulmonary hypertension, morbid obesity, E. coli urinary tract infection (that remitted on antibiotic treatment), chronic diarrhea, abdominal wall and calf edema, chronic stasis dermatitis, and pulmonary hilar lymphadenopathy. There was hypoxemia and hypercapnia. Transthoracic echocardiography showed severe pulmonary hypertension, tricuspid regurgitation, with normal left ventricular anatomy and function. High resolution CT of the chest showed increased interstitial pulmonary markings, enlarged hilar lymph nodes 1.5 to 3 cm in diameter, and patent pulmonary vessels. The patient did not agree to bronchoscopy and was discharged. Her medications included furosemide 80 mg/day, spironolactone 50/day mg, and citalopram 10 mg/day. She lived in the community alone in poverty.

At the time of admission to our ward the patient was alert, BP 135/72 mmHg, heart rate 92 bpm, respirations 26/min, SaO2 by pulse oxymetry 72% in ambient air, BMI 36. The jugular veins were engorged. There was stasis dermatitis and pitting edema of the calves. The lower abdominal wall was erythematous and exhibited a peau d'orange appearance. A few dry crackles were perceived over the bases of the lungs. The patient needed no assistance in ADL. Neurological examination was unremarkable. The MMSE was 24/30. The patient's behavior was stubborn and bizarre, but she complied to undergo tests and to take the prescribed medications. Laboratory values included hemoglobin 12.4 g/dL, serum creatinine 0.6 mg/dL, BUN 24 mg/dL, albumin 3.8 g/dL, CRP 23 mg/L, $PaCO_2$ 60 mmHg, bicarbonate 24 mEq/L, eCCT by Cockcroft Gault 160 mL/min/1.73m$^2$. No antiendomysial and anti-tissue transaminase antibodies were found in the patient's sera, no occult blood was detected in the stool, and there was no abnormality on urinalysis. She was treated with daily furosemide i.v. 80 mg, oral spironolactone 12.5 mg, citalopram 10 mg, vitamin B1 100 mg, and oxygen 1.5 L/minute through nasal prongs. Soon an additional problem came into focus: the serum potassium levels were progressively increasing, though the patient was not taking potassium supplements, the dose of spironolactone was cut down and the drug was later discontinued (Table 2), and the patient had 4-8 loose stools per day.

*Hyperkalemia* is usually defined as a serum potassium level 5.5 mmol/L or higher, although in some studies 5.0 to 5.4 mmol/L also qualifies for the diagnosis. Hyperkalemia has been reported in 1.1% to 10% of hospitalized patients; in most instances the causes were compound, with reduced renal function, medications, age $\geq$60 years, and hyperglycemia being the most common contributing factors [1]. Hyperkalemia can be asymptomatic, or can manifest as weakness, irritability, paresthesias, decreased deep tendon reflexes, flaccid paralysis, ventricular ectopy, bradycardia, and ileus. In the ECG, mild hyperkalemia is frequently expressed by peaking or tenting of T waves and premature ventricular beats; severe hyperkalemia can show widening of the QRS complex, prolongation of the PR interval, sinus arrest, premature ventricular contractions, ventricular tachycardia, ventricular fibrillation, and cardiac arrest.

*Pseudohyperkalemia* was suspected in the propositus, since hyperkalemia was persistently present in the context of diarrhea, an occurrence which is unexpected and seemingly unreasonable. The finding required validation and explanation. Spurious hyperkalemia or pseudohyperkalemia is an artifactual increase in serum potassium due to the release of potassium from cells during or after venipuncture. There are several potential causes. Forearm contraction, fist clenching or tourniquet use may increase efflux of potassium from local muscle. Thrombocytosis, leukocytosis, or erythrocytosis may cause pseudo-hyperkalemia by release of potassium from the blood's cellular elements. Acute anxiety during venipuncture may provoke respiratory alkalosis and hyperkalemia due to redistribution. Pneumatic tube transport of collected blood can induce the release of potassium from the blood's cellular elements. Cooling of the blood prior to separation of cells from plasma is a recognized cause of pseudohyperkalemia. Hereditary variants of pseudo-hyperkalemia are caused by increased passive permeability of erythrocytes for potassium. The latter can be distinguished from genuine hyperkalemia by in parallel examination of kalium in the serum and in the plasma, and in finding that the kalium concentration in the plasma is normal; for the purpose of this test the blood is sampled in heparinized tubes and allowed to stand at room temperature until the potassium concentration is measured. In the propositus, pseudohyperkalemia and laboratory error were excluded by drawing venous blood without fist clenching and tourniquet, by attesting similarity of serum and plasma kalium levels, the absence of elevated platelet, leukocyte and erythrocyte counts, and by confirmation of the results with another laboratory.

**Table 2. Development and course of hyperkalemia**

| | | | | | | | | | | | | | | |
|---|---|---|---|---|---|---|---|---|---|---|---|---|---|---|
| sK | 4.4 | 4 | 4.3 | 4.3 | 5.06 | 5.6 | 5.3 | 6.5 | 5.8 | 6.4 | 6.2 | 5.1 | 5.3 | 5.1 |
| pK | | | | | | | | | | | | 4.9 | | |
| uK | | | | | | | | | | 38 | | 21 | | 30 |
| pOsm | | | | | | | | | | | | 301 | | 305 |
| uOsm | | | | | | | | | | | | 429 | | 543 |
| TTKG | | | | | | | | | | | | 2.88 | | 3.1 |
| Date | 24 Apr | 25 | 27 | 3 May | 4 | 8 | 9 | 11 | 12 | 15 | 16 | 18 | 19 | 23 |

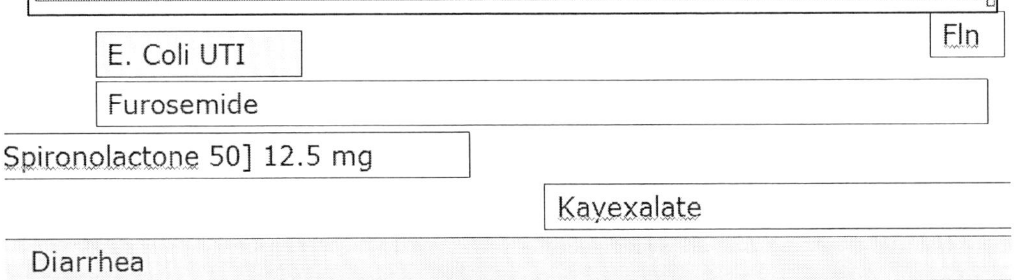


sK (mEq/L) - serum kalium mEq/L; pK (mEq/L) – plasma kalium; uK (mEq/L) urinary kalium; pOsm (mOsm/L) – plasma osmolarity; uOsm (mOsm/L) – urine osmolarity; TTKG - transtubular potassium gradient; Fln – fludrocortisone 0.1 mg/day for 3 days.

*'Paradoxical' hyperkalemia occurring* in the presence of diarrhea (as observed in our patient) has been reported previously. Four patients with renal tubular defect to secrete potassium had hyperkalemia; they had coexisting watery diarrhea. In this particular syndrome it was hyperkalemia which likely stimulated intestinal motility and caused the diarrhea, while potassium loss by diarrhea did not compensate for the renal tubular failure to secrete

potassium [2]. In our patient a similar scenario was unlikely since diarrhea preceded for a long time to the occurrence of hyperkalemia.

The causes of hyperkalemia are classified into the following categories [3]:

*Increased intake of potassium,* even small amounts, may provoke hyperkalemia but only in patients who are unable to excrete potassium in the urine. Several occult sources of potassium must be considered, including salt substitutes, alternative medicines, and alternative diets. Very rarely, marked intake of potassium may provoke severe hyperkalemia in individuals free of predisposing factors. Sustained-release kalium chloride tablets can cause hyperkalemia in suicidal overdoses. None of these causes was relevant to our patient.

*Hyperkalemia can be induced acutely* by *tissue necrosis.* Rhabdomyolysis, red cell transfusion, and tumor lysis may cause hyperkalemia. The tumor lysis syndrome is frequently associated with hyperuricemia, hyperkalemia, hyperphosphatemia, and secondary hypocalcemia that may lead to serious clinical complications, including acute kidney injury and cardiac arrest. Tumor lysis syndrome may occur in response to cytoreductive therapy or spontaneously. In our patient, having lymphadenopathy and diarrhea, the presence of a yet undiagnosed malignancy was a pertinent consideration. However, the rapidly evolving hyperkalemia in the absence of hyperuricemia and hyperphosphatemia makes this a less likely possibility.

*'Solvent drag' hyperkalemia* is secondary to administration of a hypertonic solution: mannitol, hypertonic saline, hypertonic glucose, or contrast dye. This effect is attributed to a drag effect on potassium out of cells as water moves out of cells in response to the osmotic gradient.

*Transcellular shift of potassium* occurs in acidosis, it may be triggered by beta2-blockers, or by insulin deficiency. This was not relevant to the present case.

*Decreased renal excretion of potassium* may occur in severe renal failure, Addison's disease, renin deficiency for example in diabetic nephropathy, as an adverse effect of ACE inhibitors, angiotensin II receptor blockers or NSAIDs, in mineralcorticoid deficiency (hypoaldosteronism) or resistance to mineralcorticosteroids (tubulointerstitial disease, high dose spironolactone, high dose trimethoprim). With such suspicion, the adequacy of the renal response to hyperkalemia should be evaluated by computing the transtubular potassium gradient (TTKG):

TTKG = urinary potassium: serum potassium/urinary osmolarity: serum osmolarity

TTKG less than 7 suggests decreased renal potassium excretion, which usually results from aldosterone deficiency or tubular resistance to aldosterone; measuring the serum aldosterone level should be the following test. However, among patients with underlying renal disease the presence of hyperkalemic renal tubular acidosis is very common and is often due to hypoaldosteronism. In the latter patients a costly and detailed evaluation may not be necessary.

*Elderly subjects* appear to be predisposed to the development of hyperkalemia because the aging-associated disturbances in potassium homeostasis and comorbid disease processes. Hyperkalemia in the elderly is most often precipitated by medications that impair cellular uptake or renal disposal of potassium. Hyperkalemia is best prevented by awareness of hyperkalemia in patients at increased risk, avoidance of therapy with high-risk medications, and monitoring of plasma potassium concentration and renal function at intervals appropriate for the medications prescribed.

In our patient, the urinary excretion of potassium was decreased - 21 mEq/L and later 30 mEq/L vs. normative >40 mEq/L. The TTKG was 2.88 and remained low during challenge by fludrocortisone administration (Table 2). The basal and stimulated cortisol values were normal: basal cortisol 17 mcg/dL and cortisol 1 hour after ACTH stimulation 33 mcg/dL. The differential diagnosis in this situation, theoretically, comprises a drug effect (amiloride, spironolactone, eplerenone, trimethoprim), tubulointerstitial disease, urinary tract obstruction, pseudohypoaldosteronism types I and II, sickle cell disease, systemic lupus erythematosis, and renal transplant. Relevant to our patient were hyperkalemia induced by spironolactone versus hyperkalemia secondary to tubulointerstitial disease.

*Spironolactone* is a nonselective mineralocorticoid-receptor antagonist. It is well absorbed in the gastrointestinal tract. Spironolactone prevents aldosterone from binding to its receptor and thereby decreases potassium excretion by the kidneys. By this mechanism spironolactone can cause hyperkalemia. Spironolactone has a 20 hours half-life attributable to its active metabolites. Spironolactone has a slow onset of action taking several days to develop. Also, the effect diminishes slowly after discontinuation of spironolactone. This is because spironolactone alters gene transcription, and it will take several days for gene products to change - in this case the ENaC and ROMK channels. Coexisting renal abnormalities (hyporeninemic hypoaldosteronism, tubulointerstitial disease, obstructive uropathy, diabetes, or amyloidosis) may converge with spironolactone to lessen potassium excretion and increase the risk for hyperkalemia to occur.

Recommendations for monitoring serum potassium levels during treatment with spironolactone or other aldosterone antagonists include the obtaining of serum potassium levels on days 3–5, 10–14, 35–42, and three monthly thereafter. According to expert opinion, 25 mg daily of spironolactone is associated with acceptable efficacy while minimizing the risk of renal dysfunction and hyperkalemia. If the serum potassium is 5.0–5.4 mEq/L (or 5 to 6 mEq/L according to others) the dose should be decreased; if the level is greater than 6.0 mEq/L the drug should be discontinued. After drug discontinuation the hyperkalemic effect may persist for a few days.

In our patient, discontinuation of spironolactone treatment was carefully ascertained. However, hyperkalemia persisted for longer than two weeks. No longer could hyperkalemia be attributed to this drug.

*Hyperkalemia in our patient shortly followed to urinary tract infection.* This is reminiscent of the syndrome of acquired and usually transient mineralocorticoid resistance belonging to type III pseudohypoaldosteronism. The latter is seen in patients with underlying renal pathologies including infection.

*The urgency of treating hyperkalemia* depends on the cause and the presence or absence of symptoms and signs caused by hyperkalemia. In severe hyperkalemia the diagnostic work-up should be postponed until hyperkalemia is treated [3, 4]. Management of hyperkalemia includes ECG monitoring (with attention to cardiac arrhythmias and to the morphology of T waves and QRS complexes), administration of calcium chloride or gluconate in case of hemodynamic instability, measures to lower serum potassium concentration, and measures to correct the underlying cause of hyperkalemia.

Medications potentially causing or aggravating hyperkalemia should be discontinued, including oral or intravenous potassium intake, ACE inhibitors and ARBs, trimethoprim-sulfamethoxazole, potassium sparing diuretics, and NSAIDs.

When witnessing unstable arrhythmia or hypotension, the treatment aims at immediate antagonism of potassium activity by intravenous administration of calcium chloride or gluconate. Repeated administration of calcium (10 mL of 10% solution) may be required. Because the action of i.v. calcium salts lasts only 20 to 40 minutes, other measures should also be instituted promptly.

Intravenous glucose and insulin (10-20 units given by bolus infusion) induces cellular uptake of potassium. Glucose should be co-administered to prevent hypoglycemia, both to euglycemic and diabetic patients, as long the blood glucose level is below 250 mg/dL. The therapeutic effect of intravenous glucose and insulin combination lasts 4 to 6 hours.

β2-agonists cause movement of extracellular potassium into cells. Treatment with nebulized albuterol (5-20 mg) lowers the serum potassium level for at least 2 hours.

Sodium bicarbonate infusion promotes a shift of potassium into cells. One vial (44 mEq) should be given by slow intravenous push over 5 to 15 minutes. The duration of therapeutic effect is approximately 2 hours. Sodium bicarbonate should be used with caution when hypertonicity, volume overload or alkalosis poses a risk to the patient. Bicarbonate therapy is less efficient than insulin or albuterol.

Exchange resins (Kayexalate) 20 g administered orally, by nasogastric tube (20–50 g Kayexalate plus 100–200 mL of 20% sorbitol) or rectally produces effects after 1 to 2 hours. Kayexalate should be used with caution in patients with poor cardiovascular reserve because the potential to exacerbate volume overload.

Hemodialysis or peritoneal dialysis begins to lower serum kalium within 5 minutes.

*The etiology of the diarrhea in our patient,* which lasted for several months, needed evaluation. Spironolactone can cause diarrhea, an adverse effect which is underreported in the literature. Hyperkalemia per se can cause diarrhea, as recently attested. In our patient the diarrhea came long before institution of spironolactone treatment and long before the onset of hyperkalemia, so the latter two etiologies could be excluded.

Our patient was referred for comprehensive evaluation of diarrhea, hilar lymph-adenopathy, and suspected pseudohypoaldosteronism, but she declined further investigations. She continued taking the kalium exchange resin sodium polystyrene sulfonate (Kayexalate) 30 g x 3 /day. Close follow-up of serum kalium levels was recommended, since hyperkalemia was expected to be transient. It can be anticipated that remission of the renal tubular dysfunction would mitigate renal retention of potassium, and in this phase of the disorder, keeping on with Kayxalate administration might induce hypokalemia.

Since the patient opposed to further diagnostic evaluation a definite diagnosis could not be attained. The limited diagnostic work-up the patient underwent was essential for the short-term management of hyperkalemia. Answers to problems raised in this case might be important for the management of many other patients.

## Learning Points

- Hyperkalemia is defined as a serum potassium level of 5.5 mmol/L or higher.
- The initial step in evaluation of hyperkalemia is to distinguish genuine hyperkalemia from pseudohyperkalemia. Failure to recognize pseudohyperkalemia may result in unnecessary diagnostic testing and potentially detrimental treatment.
- Hyperkalemia can be asymptomatic or can manifest as weakness, paresthesias, decreased deep tendon reflexes, ventricular ectopy, and ileus.
- Severe hyperkalemia can be expressed in the ECG by peaking of T waves, widening of the QRS complex, sinus arrest, and ventricular arrhythmias. The severity of ECG changes does not correlate well with the serum potassium concentration.
- In most hospitalized patients, the pathophysiology of hyperkalemia is multifactorial, with reduced renal function, medications and hyperglycemia being the most common contributing causes.
- Acute hyperkalemia can be induced by the movement of potassium out of the cells (in uncontrolled diabetes mellitus or with increased tissue breakdown), or by the administration of potassium to patients who are unable to excrete potassium in the urine.
- Persistent hyperkalemia usually occurs in patients who ingest normal amounts of potassium but have impaired urinary potassium excretion.
- The urgency of treatment of hyperkalemia depends on the presence of symptoms and signs attributable to hyperkalemia.
- In severe hyperkalemia, the diagnostic work-up should be postponed until hyperkalemia is corrected.
- Management of hyperkalemia includes cardiovascular monitoring, administration of calcium chloride or gluconate to treat hemodynamic instability, measures to lower serum potassium concentration, and treatment of the underlying cause.
- Medications potentially associated with hyperkalemia should be stopped.
- If the cause of hyperkalemia is not evident from the beginning, a stepwise work-up is recommended.
- The patient history, physical examination and ancillary laboratory tests usually hint to the mechanisms involved: increased potassium load, transcellular shift or diminished renal excretion of potassium.
- The next step should be to evaluate the adequacy of the renal response to hyperkalemia. For this purpose the transtubular potassium gradient is computed. Values $>7$ ($>5$ by others) are indicative of an extrarenal cause for hyperkalemia.
- The following step is to establish if low urinary potassium excretion is due to low aldosterone or to resistance to aldosterone effect by measuring serum aldosterone level.
- In patients with underlying renal disease hyperkalemic renal tubular acidosis is a very common finding and is often due to hypoaldosteronism with or without a low renin level. In these patients it is usually not recommended to do costly and detailed evaluation.

## References

[1] Stevens MS, Dunlay RW. Hyperkalemia in hospitalized patients. *Int. Urol. Nephrol.* 2000; 32:177-180.

[2] Taylor JG, Zwillich CW, Kaehny WD, Levi M, Popovtzer MM. Hyperkalemia with concomitant watery diarrhea: an unusual association. *Amer. J. Kidney Dis.* 2003; 42:E9-12.

[3] Rastegar A, Soleimani M, Rastergar A. Hypokalaemia and hyperkalaemia. *Postgrad. Med. J.* 2001; 77:759-764.

[4] Khanna A, White WB. The management of hyperkalemia in patients with cardiovascular disease. *Amer. J. Med.* 2009;122:215-221.

# Case 52. Dizziness, Nausea, Hypomagnesemia

A 69-year-old, community dwelling woman had a six months history of fatigue, pruritus and low-grade fever. On investigation, an adenocarcinoma of the sigmoid colon was diagnosed and resected. The postoperative course was complicated by abdominal wound infection (treated during a 2 months of hospitalization with a gamut of antibiotics), Bell's palsy (that quickly remitted), normocytic anemia (necessitating repeated blood transfusions), and infection with carbapenem resistant Klebsiella Pneumoniae isolated from the operative wound. During the week before her transfer for subacute care the temperature was normal, but the patient continued to complain of ongoing and unexplained nausea and dizziness. Remarkable in her medical history were type 2 diabetes mellitus, morbid obesity (BMI 48), and arterial hypertension. Her medications were ramipril 10 mg/day, hydrochlorothiazide 12.5 mg/day, simvastatin 20 mg/day, aspirin 100 mg/day, metformin 2550 mg/day, omeprazole 20 mg/day and insulin.

At the time of the patient's admission to our ward her temperature was $39.3^0$C. Other vital signs were unremarkable. There were two large wounds in the distal parts of the abdominal wall, clean of secretions, measuring 8 cm and 10 cm in maximal diameter, and reaching the fascia. In the right lower quadrant of the abdomen the skin was slightly infiltrated, exhibiting a peau d'orange appearance. The remainder of the physical examination and chest x-rays provided no hint to the cause of the high fever. Findings on laboratory examinations included hemoglobin 8.2 g/dL, MCV 88 fL, WBC 12,500, neutrophil leukocytes 66% and 19% band forms, plasma albumin 2.8 g/dL, C reactive protein 227 mg/L. Levels of electrolytes, blood glucose, creatinine, transaminases, thyrotropin, serum vitamin B12 and folic acid, and the urinalysis were unremarkable.

After blood and urine cultures were taken, empirical antibiotic treatment was started with gentamicin, vancomycin and metronidazole. The patient received two units of packed cells. Her regular medications were continued. The spiking fever persisted in the following days, so an abdominal CT was performed; there was no intraabdominal collection, but a poorly-defined haziness was noticed in the subcutaneous adipose tissue in an area confined to the right lower abdominal quadrant, corresponding to the finding revealed on palpation. Needle aspiration focused to the center of the indurated area yielded no pus; cultures of the specimen (a few drops of clear fluid) did not grow microbiota. Blood and urine cultures performed on the day of admission were negative. After four days of spiking fever, gentamicin was replaced with Colistin (polymyxin E) whereupon the temperature returned to normal. A few days later there was spontaneous drainage of a large amount of a thick, turbid secretion from the indurated subcutaneous lesion. Cultures from the pus were negative. The subsequently course of infection was uneventful.

Yet, the patient felt sick, suffered from continuous dizziness and nausea, and vomited several times. Lately she complained of paresthesias in the fingers. The cause of dizziness and nausea needed to be evaluated. The possibility of encephalitis was considered in the context of the recent Bell's palsy, but no evidence to this diagnosis was found on examination. Anxiety-induced hyperventilation was neither clinically apparent nor supported by laboratory tests: on October the 9$^{th}$ the PaCO2 was 41 mmHg and bicarbonate 28 mEq/L. Results of orthostatic challenge shoed normal BP reactivity. In considering that dizziness and nausea might be adverse effects to recently added medications the antibiotics were discontinued, however without relief.

*Dizziness is a nonspecific term*, lumping together a variety of unrelated disorders: vertigo, presyncope, disequilibrium and nonspecific dizziness. It has been held that the initial and most important step in the evaluation of dizziness is to fit the patient into one of the four categories mentioned above. However, descriptions of the quality of dizziness are often unclear, inconsistent, and unreliable, casting doubt on the validity of the traditional approach to the patient with dizziness [1].

*Dizziness in the elderly* has a high prevalence, up to 38 percent in a number of studies, and is associated with high risk of falls, disability, institutionalization, and death [2]. Dizziness in elderly patients is often multifactorial: vestibular syndrome, vertigo, cerebrovascular disease, neck disorders, physical deconditioning, depression, medications, and orthostatic hypotension. Treatment should be directed at the most remediable problems [3].

*Useful hints* at the beginning of workup of dizziness have been listed:

- the use of a cane or walker indicates neurological or orthopedic causes;
- use of glasses may suggest an ocular cause;
- facial asymmetry, dysarthria, and hoarseness may suggest a cerebrovascular accident or tumor as the cause of dizziness;
- an otoscopic examination may disclose middle ear effusions, tympanic membrane perforations, cholesteatoma, and neoplasms; pneumatic otoscopy may cause vertigo and nystagmus in patients with perilabyrinthine fistula, Meniere's disease, or superior canal dehiscence;
- the presence of nystagmus suggests vertigo; nystagmus is not always readily visible, although it can be often elicited by provocative maneuvers or electronystagmography;
- tuning fork examination, including the Weber and Rinne test, are essential to evaluate the patient for any hearing loss and to determine if the hearing loss is sensorineural or conductive in nature;
- visual acuity, visual fields, and the fundus may disclose ophthalmic causes of dizziness;

- the possibility of orthostatic hypotension needs to be assessed, whether or not the patient is describing characteristic orthostatic symptoms
- psychogenic dizziness is an important consideration; 60 percent of patients in a series of patients who were referred for evaluation of chronic dizziness had an anxiety disorder [4].

Acute vestibular syndrome versus brainstem/cerebellar stroke is an important differential diagnosis. The presence of nystagmus, gait instability, nausea, vomiting and head-motion intolerance, developing acutely and lasting for a day or longer characterize the acute vestibular syndrome. According to the traditional description, vertigo of peripheral origin is associated with auditory symptoms, vomiting, and/or nystagmus (typically rotational). In most instances the disorder is self-limiting, believed to be of viral nature and is often called vestibular neuritis [5]. The time frame used to define acute vestibular syndromes (one day or longer) excludes most disorders in which dizziness last seconds, minutes or a few hours, such as benign paroxysmal vertigo, transient ischemic attacks, and cardiac arrhythmias.

Vertigo due to lesions of the brainstem or cerebellum is associated with severe imbalance, the patient may be unable to walk or stand, and nearly always there are associated neurologic signs such as diplopia, weakness, numbness, ataxia or nystagmus not suppressed by visual fixation. However, brainstem or cerebellar ischemic stroke can mimic an acute vestibular syndrome, and the diagnosis may be missed on initial presentation. The single best predictor of vestibular neuritis versus stroke is the horizontal head impulse test performed by an expert [5].

Many medications, illicit drugs, recreational drugs, and alcohol may cause dizziness.

Electrolyte abnormalities deserve special attention. The clinical manifestations of hyponatremia include dizziness, headache, nausea, vomiting, as well as seizures, and death. Dizziness, paresthesias, vertigo, irritability, dysarthria, vertigo may be manifestations of hypomagnesemia [6]. Hypokalemia developed during our patient's hospital stay. Administration of the diuretic was discontinued and oral treatment with kalium chloride 1800 mg/day was started, without avail. Parenteral kalium chloride was added, 2000 mg/day in isotonic saline, but the serum kalium continued to decrease. The patient had no apparent cause of hypokalemia, though she vomited once every second or third day. Her stools were formed. There was no evidence of alkalosis and hyperventilation.

The approach to the patient with severe hypokalemia is made easy by using the algorithm proposed by Groeneveld et al. [7]. First, in facing a patient with extremely low serum potassium the patient should be monitored for life-threatening cardiac arrhythmias and weakness of the respiratory muscles, especially if there is a need for increased ventilation. Second, the authenticity of hypokalemia should be confirmed; spurious hypokalemia can occur in patients with leukemia or elevated white cell counts as kalium can be taken up by these metabolically active cells in the test tube. If hypokalemia is genuine, a test for concomitant hypomagnesemia should be ordered since many causes of potassium loss also result in loss of magnesium. The patients are refractory to kalium repletion until their magnesium deficit is corrected. Third, if severe hypokalemia occurred in a matter of hours there might be an important component of kalium shift into cells. Factors which promote the shift of potassium into cells are alkalosis, insulin administration, beta-adrenergic stimulation, stress induced epinephrine release, rapidly growing lymphomas and leukemias, effects of certain drugs (theophylline, albuterol, vitamin B12), hyperthyroid state, and familial hypokalemic periodic paralysis. Fourth, establishing the rate of urinary excretion of kalium distinguishes renal kalium loss from other causes. A random urine potassium-creatinine ratio less than 13 mEq K/g creatinine is consistent with extrarenal mechanisms of kalium loss.

For management of hypokalemia, if mild, oral potassium is preferred. Hypokalemia can be effectively corrected with oral supplements, and large amounts of oral potassium can be given to increase the serum levels rapidly. In case of severe hypokalemia, in patients with arrhythmias and those who are unable to tolerate oral supplements, i.v. potassium replacement should be provided. Intravenous potassium can be given at a rate of 10 to 20 mEq/hour (approx 1g – 1.5 g/hour), but larger doses can be given to patients with severe depletion or respiratory muscle weakness. Doses greater than 20 mEq/hour should be given in a monitored setting through a large-bore peripheral venous catheter or a central line. Burning at the infusion site is the most common side effect of intravenous potassium administration.

Hypomagnesemia 0.7 mg/L and hypokalemia 2.6 mEq/L were found in our patient. Hypomagnesemia is defined by serum magnesium <2.2 mg/L (1.8 mEq/L or 0.74 mmol/L). Clinically important hypomagnesemia is <1 mEq/L (0.5 mmol/L). Magnesium deficiency can be normomagnesemic.

The average daily magnesium intake is 360 mg (15 mmol). Approximately one-third of this is absorbed, principally in the small bowel. Balance is achieved by urinary excretion of approximately 100 mg/day. In the presence of magnesium depletion, the kidney can reduce magnesium excretion to very low levels. Serum magnesium concentration is the main physiologic regulator of urinary magnesium excretion. Hypermagnesemia inhibits loop magnesium and calcium transport, while hypomagnesemia stimulates magnesium reabsorption. There is no hormonal control of renal magnesium reabsorption. The bone is the main reservoir of magnesium, but bone magnesium does not readily exchange with circulating magnesium. The inability to promptly mobilize magnesium stores means that, with negative magnesium balance, the initial losses come primarily from the extracellular fluid; equilibration with bone stores does not begin for several weeks. Thus, serum magnesium concentration falls rapidly with negative magnesium balance. Conversely, there is no protection against hypermagnesemia with loss of renal function. A loop diuretic which inhibits sodium and chloride reabsorption causes decreased magnesium reabsorption, so administration of a thiazide diuretic is occasionally associated with renal magnesium wasting and hypomagnesemia. Gitelman's syndrome, which is due to an abnormality in the gene coding for the thiazide-sensitive cotransporter, is characterized by hypomagnesemia due to urinary magnesium wasting.

Hypomagnesemia occurs in up to 12 percent of hospitalized patients [9]]. The incidence rises to 60 percent in patients in an intensive care setting in which nutrition, diuretics, hypoalbuminemia, and aminoglycosides may play important roles [10]. Hypomagnesemia is frequently occurs on prolonged starvation, protein-calorie malnutrition, in the postoperative state, in patients with abdominal malignancy, on refeeding, in alcoholics, intestinal malabsorption, and prolonged use of laxatives. Excessive renal losses of magnesium may be secondary to increased diuresis (in particular loop and thiazide diuretics, while potassium-sparing diuretics may lower magnesium excretion), interstitial nephropathy, diabetes mellitus, and under the effect of certain drugs (gentamicin, carbenicillin, amphotericin, and digoxin). Hypomagnesemia has been described with the chronic use of omeprazole and other proton pump inhibitors, usually for more than one year. It is not clear why only a small proportion of patients treated with proton pump inhibitors develop hypomagnesemia. Hypomagnesemia is often present in diabetics, but the responsible mechanism is unknown.

Symptoms and signs of hypomagnesemia include twitching, tremor, muscle weakness, arrhythmia, hypokalemia, hypocalcemia, leg cramps, paresthesias, vertigo, seizures, arrhythmia, tetany, dysphagia, esophageal spasm, paralytic ileus, nausea, anorexia, hypertension, depression, delirium, agitation, and confusion. Recognized associated conditions with hypomagnesemia are hypocalcemia, hypokalemia, hyponatremia, hypophosphatemia, diabetic retinopathy, hypertension, increased platelet aggregation, increased sensitivity to digoxin and arrhythmias. The electrocardiogram may show prolonged QT, flattening of T waves, prolonged PR, and a variety of atrial and ventricular arrhythmias. As a result of the associated biochemical abnormalities it is often difficult to ascribe specific clinical manifestations solely to hypomagnesemia.

The diagnosis of hypomagnesemia is established when the serum magnesium is <1.8 mg/dL (1.5 mEq/L, 0.75 mmol/L), but intracellular magnesium depletion can occur with normal serum magnesium and be the cause of several of the symptoms described above. Hypomagnesemia is considered severe when the patient has tetany, hypomagnesemic-hypokalemic ventricular arrhythmias, or serum magnesium < 0.8 mEq/L associated with symptoms (the latter was the case in our patient). The distinction between gastrointestinal and renal losses, if no etiology is apparent, can be made by measuring the 24-hour urinary magnesium excretion or the fractional excretion of magnesium on a random urine specimen.

For treatment of severe hypomagnesemia, 50 mEq of intravenous magnesium are administered slowly over 8 to 24 hours and repeated as necessary to maintain the plasma magnesium concentration >0.8 mEq/L [10]. Alternatively, 1 g (8 mEq) of 10% magnesium sulfate solution is administered intravenously over 15 minutes or magnesium 2 g in 5% dextrose intravenously over 60 minutes. The ECG, BP, respirations, and urine output should be monitored. For nonemergency magnesium repletion a simple regimen is to administer i.v. 8 g of MgSO4 in normal saline over the first 24 hours and then 4 g daily for the next 2 to 6 days. On treatment, serum magnesium rises quickly whereas intracellular stores take longer to replete, so magnesium repletion should continue for at least 1 to 2 days after the serum magnesium level normalizes. Magnesium uptake by the cells is slow and repletion requires sustained administration of magnesium. Patients with concomitant hypokalemia or hypocalcemia should receive potassium and calcium replacement.

In the asymptomatic patient oral replacement should be given, preferably with a sustained-release preparation, in order to prevent abrupt elevations in the plasma magnesium concentration. The underlying disease should be corrected, if possible. When diuretic treatment cannot be discontinued in a patient with hypomagnesemia induced by a thiazide or loop diuretic, addition of a potassium-sparing diuretic may be beneficial (e.g. amiloride). There are two oral preparations of magnesium currently available: Slow Mag™ containing MgCl and Mag-Tab SR™ containing magnesium lactate. These preparations provide 5 to 7 mEq of magnesium per tablet. Six to eight tablets should be taken daily in divided doses for severe magnesium depletion. Two to four tablets may be sufficient for mild, asymptomatic disease. Magnesium citrate is more bioavailable than other forms of oral magnesium.

Patients with eCCT 15-30 mL/min/1.73m$^2$ and symptomatic hypomagnesemia should be treated with 50 mEq of intravenous magnesium given slowly over 8 to 24 hours with a follow-up magnesium level checked prior to subsequent doses. Patients with eCCT 15-30 mL/min/1.73m$^2$ having asymptomatic magnesium depletion should receive half the dose of the selected oral preparation that is recommended for the patient with normal renal function.

Our patient was treated with i.v. 8 g of $MgSO_4$ in normal saline over the first 24 hours and then 4 g daily for the next 4 days, followed by oral magnesium disporal 2 g daily. There was instantaneous remission of symptoms within 24 hours upon correction of hypomagnesemia: dizziness, nausea, vomiting and paresthesias were 'miraculously gone'. The serum magnesium has risen to 1.6 mg/dL and on the following day to 2.4 mg/dL.

Review of the discharge letter from the department of surgery was important in two points: first, hypomagnesemia 1.33 mg/dL was on record by September 18th and second, the patient had not received magnesium replacement. The etiology of magnesium depletion and hypomagnesemia in this case was most likely multifactorial: solid tumor and abdominal surgery, long-term malnutrition (she has lost 16 kg in body weight during the last 2 months), diabetes mellitus, and longstanding thiazide treatment. The possible effect of gentamicin on renal electrolyte excretion might have enhanced urinary magnesium loss.

### Learning Points

- Magnesium deficiency is often underdiagnosed, an omission that may have serious consequences.
- Hypomagnesemia is frequently occurs on prolonged starvation, protein-calorie malnutrition, in the postoperative state, in patients with abdominal malignancy, on refeeding, in alcoholics, patients with intestinal malabsorption, on prolonged use of laxatives or diuretics.
- Malnourished patients should be tested for possible magnesium deficiency.
- Patients with abdominal malignancy should be tested for possible magnesium deficiency.
- The finding of hypokalemia should trigger a test for serum magnesium.
- Hypokalemia resistant to kalium supplementation should be suspected to involve magnesium deficiency, with or without hypomagnesemia.
- Within the gamut of causes of dizziness, the possibility of hypomagnesemia should be kept in mind and routinely tested.
- Magnesium replacement takes time.

## References

[1] Newman-Toker DE, Cannon LM, Stofferahn ME, Rothman RE, Hsieh YH, Zee DS. Imprecision in patient reports of dizziness symptom quality: A cross-sectional study conducted in an acute care setting. *Mayo Clin. Proc.* 2007;82:1329-1340.

[2] Tinetti ME, Williams CS, Gill TM. Dizziness among older adults: a possible geriatric syndrome. *Ann. Intern. Med.* 2000; 132:337- 344.

[3] Sloane PD. Evaluation and management of dizziness in the older patient. *Clin. Geriatr. Med.* 1996; 12:785-801.

[4] Staab JP, Ruckenstein MJ. Expanding the differential diagnosis of chronic dizziness. *Arch. Otolaryngol. Head Neck Surg*. 2007;133:170-176.

[5] Kattah JC, Talkad AV, Wang DZ, Hsieh YH, Newman-Toker DE. HINTS to diagnose stroke in the acute vestibular syndrome: three step bedside oculomotor examination more sensitive than early MRI diffusion-weighted imaging. *Stroke* 2009;40:3504-3510.

[6] Satish R, Gokulnath G. Serum magnesium in recovering acute renal failure. *Indian J. Nephrol*. 2008;18:101-104.

[7] Groeneveld JHM, Sijpkens YWJ, Lin SH, Davids MR, Halperin ML. An approach to the patient with severe hypokalaemia: the potassium quiz. *QJM* 2005; 98; 305-316. 8.

[8] Wong ET, Rude RK, Singer FR, Shaw ST Jr. A high prevalence of hypomagnesemia and hypermagnesemia in hospitalized patients. *Am. J. Clin. Pathol*. 1983; 79:348-352.

[9] Tong GM, Rude RK. Magnesium deficiency in critical illness. *J. Intensive Care Med*. 2005; 20:3-17.

[10] Martin KJ, González EA, Slatopolsky E. Clinical consequences and management of hypomagnesemia. *J. Am. Soc. Nephrol*. 2009; 20:2291-2295.

# Case 53. Hyperphosphatemia after a Single Phosphate Enema

A 91-year-old community dwelling woman was hospitalized in the neurology department with right hemiparesis. Evaluation disclosed uncontrolled hypertension (BP 220/102 mmHg on admission), unstable angina pectoris, right hemiparesis (cerebral CT showed lacunar infarctions and cerebral atrophy), renal failure (serum creatinine 2.2 mg/dL), urinary retention and urinary tract infection, fairly controlled type 2 diabetes mellitus, osteoarthritis, and chronic constipation. The patient's medications were ciprofloxacin 500 mg/day, clonidine 0.225 mg/day, felodipine 5 mg/day, propranolol 120 mg/day, omeprazole 40 mg/day, tramadol 150 mg/day, and lactulose 30 mL/day. She was transferred to our hospital for rehabilitation.

On admission, the patient was alert, BP 143/98 mmHg, heart rate 66 bpm, respiration 22/minute, SaO2 by pulse oxymetry 93% in ambient air. There was right hemiparesis. On digital rectal examination the tonus of the anal sphincter was normal; the rectum was packed with pasty stool. Results on routine laboratory tests were mostly similar to those reported from the neurology department: WBC 10,100/mm3, neutrophils 66%, BUN 38 mg/dL, serum creatinine 1.6/dL, kalium 4.8 mEq/L, calcium 9.3 mg/dL, phosphorus 4.1 mg/dL. Serum levels of AST, ALT, LDH, alkaline phosphatase, albumin 3 g/dL, CK and troponin I, magnesium, bicarbonate, thyrotropin, vitamin B12, and folic acid were within the normal range. There was an enlarged cardiac shadow on chest x-rays. The ECG showed sinus rhythm and first degree atrioventricular block.

Because constipation did not improve on lactulose treatment, a Fleet enema (sodium biphosphate and sodium phosphate) was administered at 6 a.m. On routine blood tests taken later in the morning, serum phosphorus 9.3 mg/dL was found. The serum calcium was 10.1 mg/dL. The patient was free of symptoms; there were neither muscle twitches nor tetany, and the BP and ECG were unchanged with normal QT interval. The high phosphorus finding was confirmed a few hours later. Treatment with intravenous saline and furosemide was started and the patient was rushed to the emergency department for nephrology consultation. Hemodialysis was not required as the patient remained asymptomatic and responded favorably to intravenous saline and furosemide; 12 hours later the serum phosphorus was 5 mg/dL and the calcium 9.2 mg/dL.

In this case, hyperphosphatemia was obviously caused by administration of a phosphate enema: the serum phosphate value was normal before administration of the sodium phosphate enema; there were no other medications or interfering conditions which could explain hyperphosphatemia; quick normalization of phosphate level was attained by enhanced diuresis. Chronic renal failure might have been a predisposing condition to hyperphosphatemia.

*Hyperphosphatemia* is defined as serum phosphate levels above 5 mg/dL. Incorrect laboratory readings (pseudohyperphosphatemia) may occur as a result of interference with the analysis, more commonly in the case of paraproteinemia, while hyperlipidemia and hyperbilirubinemia are rare causes. The main causes of genuine hyperphosphatemia are renal failure (glomerular filtration rate <25), tumor lysis after chemotherapy, administration of phosphate preparations (oral, rectal or parenterally), hypoparathyroidism, pseudohypoparathyroidism, acute respiratory acidosis (by efflux of phosphate from cells), rarely bisphosphonate treatment.

*Hypertonic sodium phosphate enemas* are widely used in both in-patient and out-patient settings. The most common indication is for treatment of constipation, and to a lesser extent in preparation for colonoscopy or surgery. According to the manufacturer (Casen/Fleet), more than 5 00 000 000 U have been sold up to now, illustrating the widespread use of this product. No randomized clinical trials or systematic reviews exist concerning the safety of fleet enema. The reported side effects are minimal, but literature reports refer only to the most severe cases, such as water and electrolyte disturbances. Therefore, publication bias might exist [1]. Indeed, if given to a patient who cannot evacuate the enema promptly, dangerous hyperphosphatemia can develop. Such cases were published as single case reports: a 91 year-old man died after a single phosphate enema [2], coma developed in an adult who was given six phosphate enemas at hourly intervals without evacuation [3], an elderly patient with chronic renal failure developed severe hyperphosphatemia, hypocalcemic tetany and coma after a single sodium phosphate enema [4].

*Symptoms of hyperphosphatemia,* primarily neural hyperexcitability due to the induced hypocalcemia, are paresthesias, muscle cramps, tetany, and seizures. The ECG may show Q-Tc prolongation. Metabolic acidosis occurs frequently. Calcium-phosphate extra skeletal precipitation may occur if the solubility product for phosphate and calcium is greater than 58 mg/dL. Acute renal failure may develop because of direct phosphorus toxicity or because calcium phosphate deposition in the renal interstitium. Adequate hydration does not protect against the effects of hyperphosphatemia. Hyperphosphatemia should be suspected if a patient develops hypotension or neuromuscular irritability after administration of sodium phosphate.

*There are no accepted guidelines* for anticipation and prevention of severe hypophosphatemia after administration of sodium phosphate enema. At increased risk are patients with one or several of the following: age over 65 years, impaired renal function, intestinal obstruction, decreased intestinal motility, increased intestinal permeability, liver cirrhosis, and congestive heart failure. It might be desirable to test serum phosphate levels before choosing the method for colonic preparation and to repeat the measurement before giving the second dose of sodium phosphate in patients at increased risk. Simple tap water or saline solution enemas should be preferred in patients at risk [5].

*Mild hyperphosphatemia* does not require treatment except for the underlying cause. Antacids containing divalent cations including aluminum, calcium, or magnesium are effective intestinal phosphate binders and are the mainstay for preventing hyperphosphatemia of renal failure.

*Severe acute hyperphosphatemia* in patients with normal renal function can be managed with intravenous saline administration plus furosemide, or with glucose and insulin administration to induce an intracellular shift of phosphate. Intravenous calcium administration may be cautiously considered in patients with severe symptoms such as tetany or seizures. However, calcium administration may be complicated by extraskeletal precipitation of calcium phosphate. In the setting of renal failure hemodialysis may be required if hyperphosphatemia has been refractory to standard therapy.

### Learning Points

- Hypertonic phosphate enemas are widely used by medical prescription as well as over the counter. The reported side effects are minimal.
- If given to a patient who cannot evacuate the enema promptly, phosphate enemas can cause dangerous hyperphosphatemia and hypocalcemic tetany.
- At increased risk are patients with older age, renal failure, bowel obstruction, small intestinal disorders, and poor gut motility, to whom alternative treatment has to be considered.

## References

[1] Mendoza J ,Legido J ,Rubio S ,Gisbert JP. Systematic review: the adverse effects of sodium phosphate enema. *Aliment Pharmacol. Ther*. 2007 26:9-20.

[2] Spinrad S, Sztern M, Grosskopf Y, Graff E, Blum I. Treating constipation with phosphate enema: An unnecessary risk. *Isr. J. Med. Sci*. 1989; 25:237-8.

[3] Rohack JJ, Mehta BR, Subramanyam K. Hyperphosphatemia and hypocalcemic coma associated with phosphate enema. *South Med. J*. 1985; 78:1241-2.

[4] Hsu HJ, Wu M-S. Extreme Hyperphosphatemia and Hypocalcemic Coma Associated with Phosphate Enema. *Intern. Med*. 2008;47: 643-646.

[5] Azzam I, Kovalev Y, Storch S, Elias N. Life threatening hyperphosphataemia after administration of sodium phosphate in preparation for colonoscopy. *Postgrad. Med. J*. 2004;80:487-488.

# Case 54. Falls, Cerebrovascular Disease, Orthostatic Hypotension, Warfarin Treatment

This 85-year old community-dwelling man was admitted for a second time to our department. Adenocarcinoma of the sigmoid colon has been recently detected, the rectosigmoid colon was resected with right side colostomy. Two months earlier pulmonary embolism was diagnosed and treated with enoxaparin followed by warfarin. The patient's medical history was remarkable also for arterial hypertension, stable ischemic heart disease, mild renal failure, prostatectomy for benign prostatic hypertrophy, and ischemic stroke, the latter having occurred one year before the present admission. The problems concerning management of cancer-associated venous thromboembolism have been discussed in the context of the patient's first admission, under Case 36. Additional problems came into focus during this second admission.

Over several months he suffered repeated falls, apparently without loss of the consciousness, without convulsive spells or neurological deficit. A fall along with head contusion was the cause for the present admission. Non-contrast cerebral CT performed in the emergency department demonstrated severe cerebral and cerebellar atrophy, periventricular lucency and several infarctions confined to the basal ganglia and to the right hemisphere. The patient's current medications were warfarin 2.5 mg/day, famotidine 20 mg/day, lercanidipine 10 mg/day, and hydrochlorothiazide 12.5 mg/day.

The patient was cachectic. His body temperature was 36.5°C, heart rate 62 beats/minute, supine BP 143/66 mmHg, respiratory rate 24 breaths/minute, oxygen saturation 92% while breathing room air. The surgical wound, stoma and findings on abdominal examination were unremarkable. There was a slightly increased muscle tonus on the left side. The plantar reflex was of the extensor type on the left side. The patellar and Achilles reflexes and results of sensory and proprioceptive tests were normal. There was dysarthria as well as dysphagia for liquids. The balance was steady. The gait exhibited the 'senile gait pattern' and appeared secure while the patient was using a two-wheeled walker. Folstein's Mini-Mental State Examination (MMSE) scored 19/30, clock drawing 1/5. A bedside postural test performed at 10 a.m., 5 minutes supine and 5 minutes standing, disclosed orthostatic hypotension with drop of the systolic BP from 158 to 106 mmHg and diastolic BP from 64 to 57 mmHg, and the heart rate increasing from 69 to 82 beats per minute (Figure 36).

The hemoglobin was 12.2 g/dL, mean corpuscular volume 95 fL, serum creatinine 0.9 mg/dL, PT-INR 2.2. Serum levels of electrolytes, blood glucose, transaminases, thyrotropin, vitamin B12 and folic acid, arterial blood gas analysis and urinalysis were within the normal range. The basic cortisol level was 15 µg/dL; one hour after stimulation with 250 µg i.v. corticotrophin the serum cortisol was 25 µg/dL (normal values).

At this time point the main goals in the management the patient were to uncover and amend, if possible, the causes predisposing the patient to falls, and to revise the choice of anticoagulant treatment in considering the risks entailed with falling.

*There was ample evidence of cerebrovascular disease* which could explain our patient's tendency to fall. CT showed severe cerebellar atrophy, leukoaraiosis and cerebral infarctions; there was no evidence of intracranial bleeding, tumor or hydrocephalus. Other conditions which might mimic symptoms and signs resembling cerebrovascular disorders were excluded, for example brain tumors which occasionally cause sudden-onset symptoms. Seizures, migraine attacks, and faints sometime are difficult to distinguish from transient ischemic attacks. Hypoglycemia, severe hyperglycemia, severe hyponatremia, hypocalcemia, toxic and metabolic conditions occasionally can cause focal brain symptoms [1]; none was revealed in the patient. The presence of fall risk factors, the presence of aggravating conditions, the tempo of onset of falls, and the clinical course may serve as indications, but the diagnosis strongly relies on neuroimaging.

*Risk factors for repeated falls* include older age, history of falls, dementia, slow gait speed, muscle weakness, visual impairment, medical illness, certain classes of medications, medication changes, orthostatic hypotension, and environmental factors. In the patient under discussion, older age, history of falls, dementia, slow gait speed, muscle weakness, and frailty were risk factors which might concur in causing repeated falls. Medications with central nervous system activity, in particular neuroleptics, sedatives, and antidepressants are often implicated, but not so in the present patient who was not taking any of the drugs belonging to those classes. A patient's inadequate judgment of environmental hazards and inadequate judgment of his own motor abilities may be a cause of falls, and was certainly so in our patient as witnessed by nurses and physiotherapist. Orthostatic hypotension might have caused or contributed to falls.

*Orthostatic hypotension (OH),* the definition updated in 2011 by an expert consensus, is diagnosed when a sustained reduction of systolic BP of at least 20 mmHg or diastolic BP of 10 mmHg occur within 3 min of standing or head-up tilt to at least $60^0$ on a tilt table. In patients with supine hypertension, a decrease in systolic BP by 30 mmHg may be a more appropriate criterion for orthostatic hypotension. Patients may feel dizzy, weak or even faint upon standing while orthostatic BP decrement is insufficient to meet the criteria for OH; in the latter case one may still consider OH as a possible diagnosis.

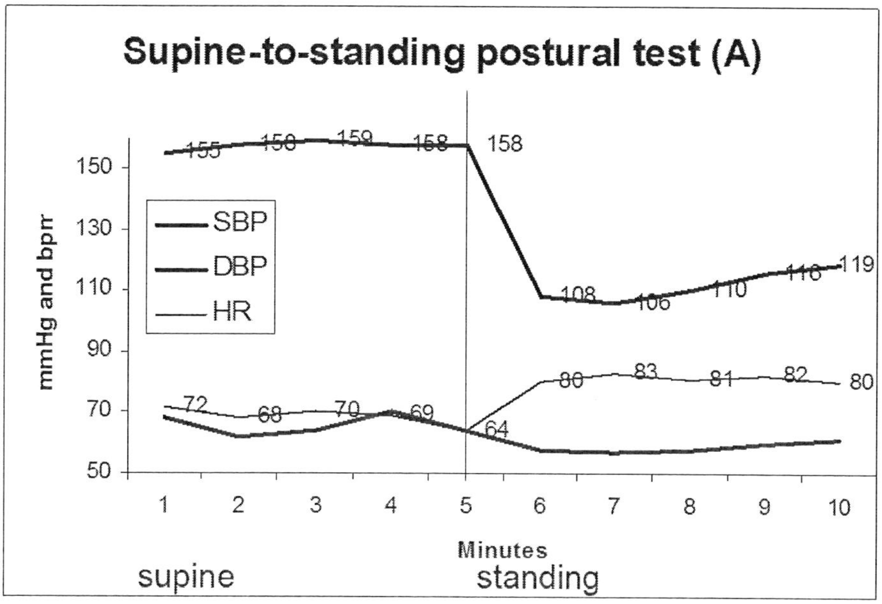


Figure 36. Postural test showing severe orthostatic hypotension.

*The most common causes of OH* are medications (diuretics, nitrates, antihypertensive and tricyclic antidepressant drugs), autonomic neuropathies whether primary (primary autonomic failure, multiple system atrophy and Parkinson's disease) or secondary (diabetic, chronic renal failure, chronic liver disease, alcohol-induced, vitamin B12 deficiency, Guillain-Barré syndrome, paraneoplastic), hypovolemia (dehydration, postobstructive polyuria, bleeding either overt or occult), and blood pooling in large varicous veins [2].

*Aging is associated with an increased risk of OH.* In community dwelling individuals more than 65 years of age, the prevalence of OH is approximately 20%; in those older than 75 years the prevalence is 30%, and in frail elderly individuals living in nursing homes the prevalence of OH may be as high us 50%. Among elderly patients hospitalized for acute conditions the prevalence of OH was 64% in one study [2]. The increased frequency of OH in elderly persons may be explained by age-associated alterations which affect the BP regulation: decreased baroreceptor sensitivity, decreased alfa-1-adrenergic response to sympathetic stimulation, decreased renal sodium conservation, increased vascular stiffness, reduced left ventricular diastolic filling, increased venous system tortuosity. Postprandial hypotension is frequently observed in elderly subjects and may act in concert with OH. Furthermore, for any decrease in BP, elderly persons are more likely to become symptomatic because of the likelihood of coexistent cerebrovascular disease and the rightward shift in cerebral autoregulation (the latter is an adaptative change to arterial hypertension).

*The importance of diagnosing OH* is manifold: OH may underlie symptoms of cerebral hypoperfusion, OH is a marker of frailty, a risk factor for falls, OH is a predictor of ischemic stroke, cardiovascular morbidity, development of chronic kidney disease, and all cause mortality.

*Dizziness and syncope when getting* up, occurring within minutes of standing and obliging the patient to lie down, are typical symptoms of OH. However, the relationship of other symptoms to OH may not be apparent unless one is aware of the wider spectrum of orthostatic disturbances. Thus, weakness, fatigue, visual blurring, vertigo, suboccipital and paracervical pain, chest pain on upright posture, headaches, palpitations, low back pain or dyspnea may occur on standing and disappear when lying flat, being the predominant symptoms of OH in a number of patients [2]. Our patient developed severe OH during the course of the postural test, but no symptoms. So, the warning symptoms that could alert the patient were lacking.

*Three postural tests* are widely applied in practice for the diagnosis of OH: the supine-to-standing test, supine-to-sitting test and the head-up tilt test. Few studies have compared directly the results of different orthostatic tests. A frequently utilized protocol is the short, bedside supine-to-standing postural test [3], which was applied in the work-up of falls in our patient. According to a commonly used protocol, the patient's BP and heart rate are recorded after 5 to 10 minutes of rest in the supine position 5 times, at one minute intervals between measurements. Next, the patient stands up and measurements are taken with the cuffed arm supported at heart level at one minute intervals for 5 minutes. Along the test the patient is asked to report dizziness, faintness or light-headedness, with the examiner recording the transience or persistence of the symptoms. The procedure is aborted for safety reasons if the BP drops precipitously or presyncope ensues. Patients with severe autonomic failure have an immediate drop in BP on standing and OH is easily diagnosed with this simple method. However, when the onset of hypotension on standing is delayed the diagnosis of OH may be missed on the short bedside orthostatic test. The supine-to-sitting postural test has not been standardized. One frequently used protocol involves a single BP measurement after prolonged recumbence followed by BP measurements after 1, 3 and 5 minutes of sitting. Other technical details are similar to the supine-to-standing test.

*Orthostatic BP responses may variate* during the day or from one day to another. OH is most prevalent and severe in the morning when subjects first arise; hence, OH may be underdiagnosed when postural testing is performed in the afternoon. Early morning measurements, especially after a high carbohydrate meal, are useful to identify OH and the possible impact of postprandial hypotension. In one representative study performed in a morning outpatient clinic, 40 elderly persons with orthostatic symptoms of dizziness, falls or syncope were recruited to assess the reproducibility of OH on postural test. All patients had a symptomatic drop in orthostatic systolic BP of more than 20 mmHg documented in the clinic. The BP and heart rate measurements were repeated on two further morning clinic visits: 67.5% of patients had a similar drop in systolic BP on both subsequent visits; in the remainder, the initial response was not reproduced [4]. Hence, detection of OH may require multiple measurements on different days. We use to screen for OH at 10 a.m., the patients having taken their breakfast at 8.30 a.m.; in case of normal result but high clinical suspicion measurements are repeated on another day.

In our patient, the cause of OH was not apparent. There was neither evidence of hypovolemia, glucocorticosteroid deficiency, venous insufficiency, autonomic failure (the adequate increase in heart rate during orthostasis argues against autonomic failure), and he was not taking medications known to cause OH. The difficult to prove possibility of paraneoplastic OH was considered in view of the temporal overlap between the onset of falls and the presence of colonic adenocarcinoma [5].

*Treatment of OH* follows a stepwise approach, described in detail in Case 38 [6, 7]. Medications which might cause OH should be withheld during the hours when the patient uses to be upright; such are antihypertensive medications, nitrates, diuretics, and alpha adrenergic blockers to treat benign prostatic hypertrophy. Among selective alpha adrenergic blockers, alfuzosin causes more often OH than tamsulosin. Heavy meals should be avoided. The patient is encouraged to drink 500 mL of water before the meals. One or two cups of coffee per day are suggested. Increased salt intake is recommended (salt tablets added with meals as necessary). Avoidance of standing up quickly and of standing motionless is advised. The head of the bed should be raised during night-time by 15-30 cm. Anemia needs to be corrected even if mild (our patient was transfused 2 units of blood); recombinant erythropoietin may be of benefit.

Elastic compression, drugs aimed to increase the central blood volume (e.g. fludrocortisone) and drugs which promote venous constriction (e.g. midodrine) are the mainstays of treatment. Short acting pressor agents are prescribed during daytime (and should be avoided during the night), mainly midodrine. Yohimbine, indomethacin, pyridostigmine, octreotide can be added in difficult to treat cases. However, the treatment with short-acting pressor agents is far from satisfactory and the magnitude of response may vary between patients. Mild physical exercise improves orthostatic tolerance by reducing venous pooling and increasing plasma volume. Deconditioning from lack of exercise exacerbates OH. Isotonic exercise in a supine or sitting position is advisable [7].

Our patient was treated with elastic bandages applied to the calves and thighs before rising from bed and taken of before going to bed, and midodrine 5 mg x 2/day. Repeat postural test two days after initiation of the treatment showed a satisfactory BP response

(Figure 37). The test was repeated after other two days and showed, unexpectedly, suboptimal BP response on standing (Figure 38). Therefore the dose of midodrine was increased to 5 mg t.i.d. (to be taken at 7 a.d., 11 a.d., and 3 p.m.). Fall prevention strategies were discussed with the patient and proxies.

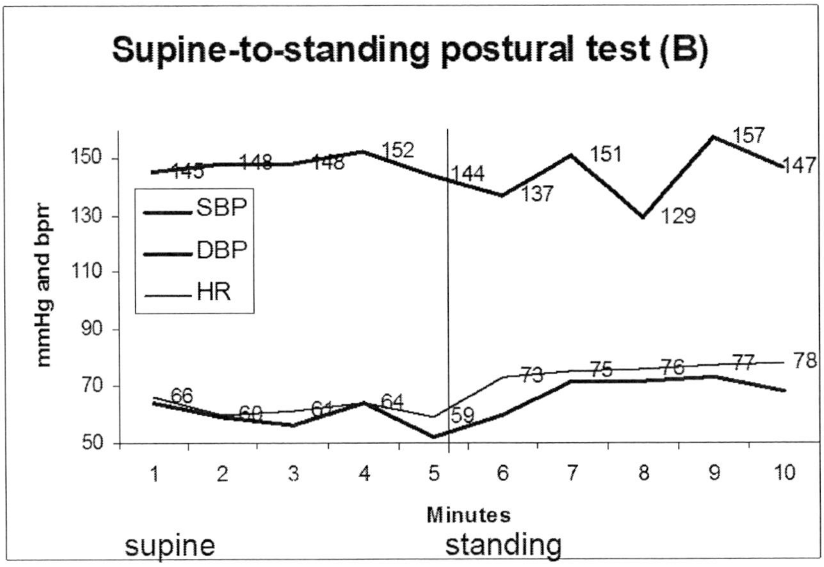


Figure 37. Follow-up examination after two days of treatment, while the patient was on midodrine and wearing elastic bandages. There were large BP oscillations on standing but no OH.

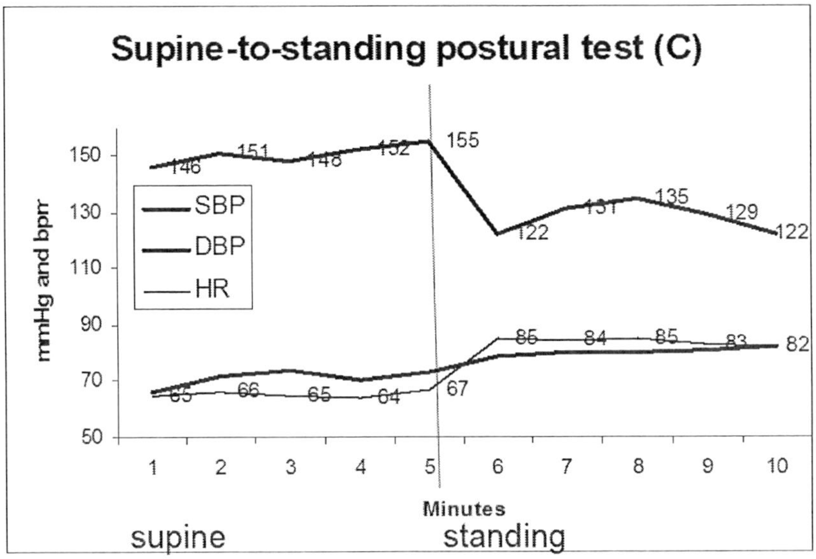


Figure 38. A further test performed two days later, while the patient was on the same treatment regimen, showed again OH, but of lesser magnitude compared to the BP drop before initiation of treatment.

*Fall prevention programs* are widely applied in hospitals, nursing home and community settings. Costs due to injury from an inpatient fall are not covered by Medicare [8]. Regulations have strongly motivated the development of fall prevention programs. Various approaches are used for prevention of falls, but there is inconclusive evidence for effectiveness of most approaches, as shown by two systematic reviews [9, 10]

In hospital patients, a meta-analysis including three trials (131 participants), found a significant reduction in the risk of falling with supervised exercise interventions (RR 0.44), but heterogeneity among studies made it difficult to determine from the pooled analysis which inpatients are likely to benefit from exercise [11]. Analysis of four trials with 6,478 participants found that multifactorial interventions decreased the rate of falls (RaR 0.69, 95% CI 0.49-0.96) [11]. Effective interventions in these trials were balance and strength exercises, environmental modifications, staff education, medication reviews, and a comprehensive geriatric review. Disappointing were the results of another recent study. A comprehensive program, including working with staff members, identifying environmental hazards, behavioral intervention, and using appropriate aids, equipment, and clothing were ineffective in preventing falls [12]. The comprehensive intervention was even harmful for patients with impaired cognitive function: the rate of injurious falls was higher specifically in this group. The authors concluded that cognitive impairment can limit the ability of patients to adhere to the planned safety promoting behaviors [13].

In nursing homes, a meta-analysis of nine trials comprising 3,753 nursing care residents showed no effect of multifactorial interventions on the risk of falls [11]. There is limited evidence from multifactorial intervention trials that education is an effective strategy to reduce falls in the nursing home and rehabilitation settings [12]. In comparing supervised exercise versus usual care in nursing care facilities, a meta-analysis of seven randomized trials of fall prevention interventions (1205 participants) found no decrease in the rate of falls [11].

*The importance of early ambulation* to recovery after hip fracture surgery is well established. Fischer et al. found that early ambulation of geriatric patients admitted for acute illnesses may shorten the length of hospital stay [8]. Yet, a limitation of the latter study is the possibility of reverse causation: patients who increased their step count early during hospitalization may have been less ill.

Experts have debated the tradeoff between early ambulation and the increased risk of fall during acute illness. It is agreed that immobility increases deconditioning and the long-term risk of fall. Early ambulation should therefore be encouraged as a method to prevent falls [8]. Clinical protocols of ambulation should include a recommended schedule and duration or distance of ambulation, patient education regarding safe ambulation techniques, monitoring of the patient's ambulation progress, and guidelines for the role of designated medical staff members in promoting ambulation [8].

Randomized trials of Tai Chi on frail elderly persons did not find statistically significant evidence of benefit. There are no studies evaluating footwear interventions to reduce falls in an institutionalized setting. The effectiveness of hip protectors has been questioned.

*Vitamin D supplementation* is the only intervention with strong recommendation for this patient population in fall prevention guidelines. A systematic review of fall prevention measures in the nursing home [11] included five randomized controlled trials that examined the effect of vitamin D on falls. Among vitamin D users there was a significant reduction in the rate of falls (RaR 0.72), but no reduced risks of complications caused by falls (RR 0.98).

Guidelines for fall prevention from the American Geriatrics Association give a strong recommendation for vitamin D supplementation of at least 800 IU per day for older persons residing in long-term care settings with proven or suspected vitamin D insufficiency [13].

Our patient was taking inadequate and potentially harmful decisions relative to environmental hazards. Therefore, assisted ambulation was recommended, with the patient using a walker along with removal of formal and unformal restraints.

*There is no evidence to support the use of physical restraints to reduce falls.* One study of 263,068 nursing home residents evaluated the effect of full bed rails on all open sides of the bed, half rail one side, trunk restraint, limb restraint, or chairs to prevent rising on falls [14]. A slight increased risk of falls was found among residents who were physically restrained. In reviewing the literature, there is no evidence to support the use of physical restraints to reduce falls in the inpatient or nursing home settings. Moreover, informal restraints such as intravenous catheters, oxygen tubing, urinary catheters, and ECG leads can confine patients to their bed. Although their use may seem indispensable, these devices often lead to complete bed rest and may have deleterious consequences. Limiting informal restraints can improve mobility and delirium. Models of care exist in which patients are treated and symptoms are managed in a restraint-free environment without an increase in the length of stay or cost [15].

Removing restraints may seem to increase the risk of falls, when patients try to get out of bed by themselves or pull on urinary catheters, infusion or oxygen tubing. Practical options are the hiding of unnatural attachments, giving intravenous treatments as boluses instead of a continuous rate, and not overusing oxygen administration. 'Getting out of bed to urinate or just to move around is a natural desire and should be anticipated, encouraged and assisted' [16]. The presence of a family member or sitter may be of assistance in this regard. In general it is recommend not using bedrails or physical restraints for fall protection in long-term care facilities. Only when agitated symptoms present a risk to the patient should chemical restraint with medications be attempted. Uncontrolled pain, retention of urine and feces can cause delirium and should be prevented.

The utility of bed and chair alarms in reducing falls is unclear. Alarm use leads to 'false positive' signals that can be annoying and difficult for the staff to interpret. The effectiveness of bed alarms in preventing falls has not been rigorously evaluated by randomized controlled trials [16].

*The risk of hemorrhagic complications in patients who fall* while receiving antithrombotic therapy may pose difficult dilemmas to the clinician. A 4-year retrospective chart review of consecutive patients who fell during admission to a tertiary-care teaching hospital showed that the fall-related risk of bleeding complications was low. A total of 2635 falls in 1861 patients were reviewed. Six percent of persons taking warfarin suffered a fall-related major hemorrhagic injury. One fall only resulted in a subdural hematoma [17]. Three risk-benefit analyses have been performed and all found that despite risks associated with accurately indicated warfarin treatment its benefits outweigh the risks even in patients who fall [18]. Hence, the risk of falls alone should not automatically disqualify a person from being treated with warfarin. Management of fall risk should be an important part of anticoagulation management and efforts should be made to minimize fall risk.

Furthermore, it is thought that heparin may exercise a direct antitumor effect by the inhibition of extracellular-matrix protease heparanase, the inhibition of angiogenesis and by inhibition of cell–cell interaction by blocking selectins. The direct antitumor effect of heparin might translate into a survival benefit in patients with cancer [19].

We thought that the propensity to fall in our patient was multifactorial. Optimizing treatment of orthostatic hypotension, assisted ambulation, measures to remove environmental hazards, and administration of vitamin D was recommended. Warfarin anticoagulation was aimed for PT-INR 2 to 3. This choice was based on the patient's refusal to receive parenteral treatment (enoxaparin) and unavailability of an effective antidote for dabigatran and rivaroxaban [20].

## Learning Points

- The cause of recurrent falls is often multifactorial; risk factors include older age, a history of falls, dementia, slow gait speed, muscle weakness, visual impairment, medical illness, certain classes of medications, and medication changes.
- Aging is associated with increased risk of OH and OH is a frequent cause of syncope and falls.
- The importance of diagnosing and treating OH is manifold: OH may underlie symptoms of cerebral hypoperfusion, OH is a risk factor for falls, a predictor of ischemic stroke, cardiovascular morbidity, development of chronic kidney disease and all cause mortality.
- Fall prevention programs are widely applied, but there is inconclusive evidence for the effectiveness of most approaches, except for treating OH and administration of vitamin D.
- There is no evidence to support the use of physical restraints to reduce falls; on the contrary, limiting formal and informal restraints can improve mobility and delirium.
- In general bedrails or physical restraints should not be used for fall protection.
- Risk-benefit analyses of warfarin treatment showed that the benefits outweigh its risks even in patients who fall.

# References


[1] Caplan L.R., Hon F.K. Clinical diagnosis of patients with cerebrovascular disease. *Prim. Care* 2004;31:95-109.

[2] Gupta V, Lipsitz LA. Orthostatic hypotension in the elderly: diagnosis and treatment. *Am. J. Med.* 2007;120:841-847.

[3] Naschitz JE. Challenges in acute geriatric care. Nova Sci. Publ, NY, 2010:19-38.

[4] Ward C, Kenny RA. Reproducibility of orthostatic hypotension in symptomatic elderly. *Am. J. Med.* 1996;100:418–422.

[5] Lavi S, Aharon-Pertz J, Haim N, Vlodavsky E, Jacob G. Unusual case of partially reversible severe cardiovascular autonomic failure. *Am. J. Med. Sci.* 2001;326:159-163.

[6] Shibao C, Gamboa A, Diedrich A, Biaggioni I. Management of hypertension in the setting of autonomic failure: a pathophysiological approach. *Hypertension* 2005;45: 469-476.

[7] Figuero JJ, Basford JR, Low PA. Preventing and treating orthostatic hypotension: as easy as A, B, C. *Cleveland Clinic Journal of Medicine* 2010;77:298-306.

[8] Adkins Murphy E. Increasing ambulation of elderly by 12 minutes of slow walking per day reduces length of hospital stay. *Arch. Intern. Med.* 2011;171:269-270.

[9] Oliver D, Connelly JB, Victor CR, Shaw FE, Whitehead A, Genc Y, Vanoli A, Martin FC, Gosney MA. Strategies to prevent falls and fractures in hospitals and care homes and effect of cognitive impairment: systematic review and meta-analyses. *BMJ* 2007; 334:82-92.

[10] Coussement J, De Paepe L, Schwendimann R, Denhaerynck K, Dejaeger E, Milisen K. Interventions for preventing falls in acute- and chronic-care hospitals: a systematic review and meta-analysis. *J. Am. Geriatr. Soc.* 2008; 56:29-36.

[11] Cameron ID, Murray GR, Gillespie LD, Robertson MC, Hill KD, Cumming RG, Kerse N. Interventions for preventing falls in older people in nursing care facilities and hospitals. *Cochrane Database Syst. Rev.* 2010; CD005465.

[12] Haines TP, Hill A-M, Hill KD, McPhail S, Oliver D, Brauer S, Hoffmann T, Beer C. Patient education to prevent falls among older hospital inpatients. A randomized controlled trial. *Arch. Intern. Med.* 2011; 171:517-524.

[13] The American Geriatrics Society Clinical Practice Guideline: Prevention of falls in older person http://www.americangeriatrics.org/health_care_professionals/clinical_practice/clinical_guidelines_recommendations/2010/.

[14] Castle NG, Engberg J. The health consequences of using physical restraints in nursing homes. *Med. Care* 2009; 47:1164-1173.

[15] Hendrich AL, Bender PS, Nyhuis A. Validation of the Hendrich II Fall Risk Model: a large concurrent case/control study of hospitalized patients. *Appl. Nurs Res.* 2003; 16: 9-21.

[16] Hignett S, Masud T. A review of environmental hazards associated with in-patient falls. *Ergonomics* 2006; 49:605-616.

[17] Bond AJ, Molnar FJ, Li M, Mackey M, Man-Son-Hing M. The risk of hemorrhagic complications in hospital inpatients who fall while receiving antithrombotic therapy. *Thrombosis Journal* 2005, 3:1. .

[18] Garwood CL, Corbett TL. Use of anticoagulation in elderly patients with atrial fibrillation who are at risk for falls. *Ann. Pharmacother.* 2008;42:523-532.

[19] Borsig L. Heparin as an inhibitor of cancer progression. *Prog. Mol. Biol. Transl. Sci.* 2010; 93:335-349.

[20] Wartak SA, Bartholomew JR. Dabigatran: will it change clinical practice? *Cleveland Clinic Journal of Medicine* 2011;78: 657-664.

# Case 55. Serendipity

An 84-year-old woman was admitted for subacute care, following to five days of hospitalization in the department of internal medicine. The discharge diagnoses were exacerbation of congestive heart failure, aortic stenosis, severe mitral regurgitation, chronic atrial fibrillation, pulmonary hypertension, pleural effusion, and right renal mass. Laboratory findings were hemoglobin 10.4 g/dL, MCV 84, WBC 5500/mm$^3$, platelets 245,000/mm$^3$, PT-INR 1.45, APTT 51 seconds, serum creatinine 1.5 mg/dL, and BUN 34 mg/dL.

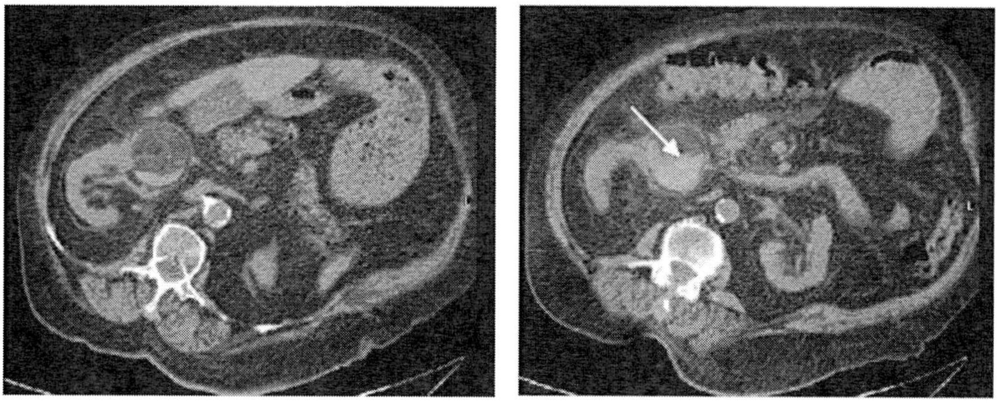

Figure 39 A and B. Non-contrast CT slides at the level of the kidneys. A round mass in the mid-anterior aspect of the right kidney is apparent, 5.2 cm in diameter; the mass is nonhomogenous, having a low attenuation component which is clearly seen in the subcapsular area as a rim, and which is consistent with admixed adipose tissue (A). The fluid-hematocrit level within the right renal mass (arrow) is better seen in a more distal section, the attenuation of the fluid is consistent with blood (B).

A non-contrast CT of the chest, performed as part of the diagnostic work-up, showed loculated left pleurisy, enlarged mediastinal lymph nodes, the largest measuring 19 mm in diameter, and a mass lesion in the right kidney. The renal tumor was 5.2 cm in size, nonhomogenous, having a low attenuation component of 15 Hounsfield units that is consistent with adipose tissue, and a fluid level with attenuation characteristic for blood (Figure 39).

Daily doses of medications at the time of transfer to the Acute Care for Elderly Unit were furosemide 80 mg, dabigatran 300 mg, ramipril 10 mg, metoprolol tartrate 100 mg, simvastatin 20 mg, and omeprasol 20 mg. The patient was hemodynamically stable, the vital signs and ancillary laboratory tests were within reasonable limits (hemoglobin 13 g/dL). Revision of the recent CT triggered a 'red flag' signal, in recognizing the dismal significance of hemorrhage into a renal angiomyolipoma.

Angiomyolipomas are hamartomas composed of adipose tissue, smooth muscle, and thick-walled blood vessels. Angiomyolipomas may be confined to the kidney or may be disseminated, involving the skin, brain, kidneys, and other organs; the disseminated variant is called tuberous sclerosis. Renal angiomyolipomas are typically detected incidentally during a radiologic procedure or during the work-up for suspected renal disease. The appearance on ultrasound depends on the proportions of fat, smooth muscle and vascular elements in the tumor, and on the presence of hemorrhage. Typically, angiomyolipomas appear as circumscribed, highly reflective masses, more echogenic than the renal sinus fat. Because of this high reflectivity, even tiny lesions can be detected with ultrasound. CT usually demonstrates a fatty mass intermixed with areas of increased tissue density. An attenuation value of 15HU is considered diagnostic of fat. Detection by CT even of a small amount of fat within a renal mass establishes the diagnosis of angiomyolipoma, with few exceptions. However, if there is coexistent hemorrhage, the attenuation characteristics change and both ultrasound and CT might miss the diagnosis of angiomyolipoma.

Angiomyolipomas can become large, leading to abdominal or flank pain, bleeding into a lesion, and hematuria. Spontaneous rupture of the kidney may occur - a rare but well-recognized surgical emergency. The resulting hematoma is either subcapsular or extends to the perinephric space. Bleeding into lesions is more frequent with tumors larger than 4 cm (50% risk of bleeding) and most lesions of this size eventually become symptomatic. Patients with ruptured angiomyolipoma present acutely with pain as a result of hemorrhage; up to 20% are in shock at the time of initial presentation. Therefore, it is important to predict the possibility of rupture in caring for patients with an angiomyolipoma. Some patients progress to end-stage renal disease due to replacement and compression of the renal parenchyma. Renin-dependent hypertension can occur due to focal areas of ischemia around lesions.

Anticoagulant therapy increases the risk of angiomyolipoma bleeding. In case of massive retroperitoneal hemorrhage under warfarin treatment, emergency resuscitation and selective interpolar arterial embolization is the treatment of choice. Diagnosis on time is critical; therefore it is imperative to consider the diagnosis early in warfarinized patients and in others at risk of bleeding when presenting with abdominal pain. On dabigatran treatment, as our patient received, the risk of bleeding is similar or higher compared with warfarin. There is no specific antidote for dabigatran, which has a half-life of 12 to 17 hours.

In patients with angiomyolipoma the primary indications for intervention are bleeding, refractory pain and suspicion of malignancy. Prophylactic intervention is indicated for large tumors or in patients in whom access to emergency care may be inadequate. Lesions are often treated with transcatheter arterial embolization, and less often with partial or total nephrectomy. In one study, intervention was required in 20 percent of tumors less than 4 cm in diameter, in 50 percent of tumors 4 to 10 cm, and in all tumors larger than 10 cm. Angioembolization allows rapid patient stabilization in cases of acute hemorrhage. Angioembolization may also be preferred for large masses when partial nephrectomy is not feasible. Surgery should be performed in cases of diagnostic uncertainty or complex vascular anatomy that is not amenable to angioembolization.

Though there was no evidence of actual bleeding, the patient was referred urgently to a tertiary care hospital in considering acute intervention.

## Learning Points

- Renal angiomyolipomas when becoming large may complicate with bleeding into the tumor, with a greater than 50% chance of significant bleeding in lesions larger than 4 cm.
- Anticoagulant therapy increases this risk.
- It is imperative to consider the diagnosis early in patients receiving anticoagulant treatment.
- Selective transcatheter arterial embolization allows rapid patient stabilization in case of acute hemorrhage.
- Prophylactic transcatheter arterial embolization is effective and durable in preventing large angiomyolipomas from bleeding.

# References

[1] Nelson CP, Sanda MG. Contemporary diagnosis and management of renal angiomyolipoma. *J. Urol.* 2002; 168:1315-1325.

[2] Peh WC, Yip KH, Tam PC. Spontaneous renal pseudoaneurysm ruptures presenting as acute intraabdominal hemorrhage. *Br. J. Radiol.* 1997;70:1188-1190.

[3] Wright T, Sooriakumaran P. Renal angiomyolipoma presenting with massive retroperitoneal haemorrhage due to deranged clotting factors: a case report. *Cases J.* 2008;1:213.

[4] Chan CK, Yu S, Yip S, Lee P. The efficacy, safety and durability of selective renal arterial embolization in treating symptomatic and asymptomatic renal angiomyolipoma. *Urology.* 2011;77:642-648.

# Epilogue

In recent years, when gerontologically adjusted medical services became the norm for the highest standard of care, hospitalists had to incorporate principles of geriatric medicine into hospital practice and geriatricians had to assimilate hospitalist skills when providing acute geriatric care. It is the Acute Care for Elderly Unit which is devised to provide trained acute hospital care for elderly patients with geriatric syndromes, disabilities and frailty. Teamwork is here a routine, based on collaboration between hospitalists, geriatricians, nurses, social workers, pharmacist, physical therapist, occupational and speech therapists and dietician, which cooperate to improve the patients' hospital course, to minimize functional decline, and advance discharge planning.

Traditional bedside skills retain their primary importance in acute geriatric care. Yet, clinical skills assume in the high-tech era additional dimensions. Such are the skills to make relevant choices among imaging modalities, laboratory tests, endoscopic procedures, tissue sampling, the ability to consult electronic sources of information, select cost-effective options, discern between different levels of evidence, and integrate the different data and to act in accord with the best evidence. Indeed, physicians should critically evaluate guidelines and the evidence on which they are based, and decide whether the recommendations are relevant in keeping with their patients' preferences and setting. The fifty-five case studies presented in this work provide a real life picture of acute geriatric care: the challenges, successes, mishaps, physicians' attitudes, well integrated routines and topics not covered by textbooks.

At the end of the day physicians wish to be wiser and more competent.

# Index

## A

## B

## C

## D

## E

## F

## I

## J



## K



## L

## N

## O



## P

## Q

## R



## S

## T

## U



## V

## W



## X



## Y



## Z